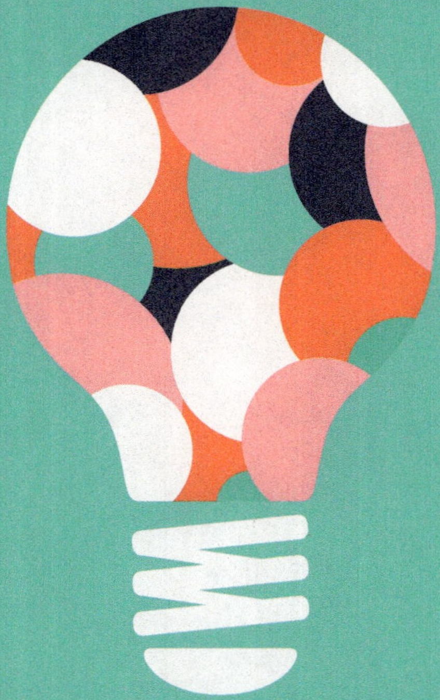

UNDERSTANDING HABITS

The roots of the word 'habit' can be found in the Latin word 'habitus', which translates as 'a state of being' or 'condition'. As with most words, there have been many iterations of the meaning of 'habit', an appropriate series of transformations given the ever-changing nature of human habits throughout history. And yet, whether it's hitting the gym, drinking too much or spending too long in front of the TV, once our individual habits become hardwired into the brain they can be incredibly difficult to change. So why does this happen, how do we alter them, and are we alone in having them? In **Understanding Habits** you'll delve into the science of how habits form, explore why we develop good and bad practices, learn how to break your own worst routines, uncover the ways of the world's most successful organisations and much more.

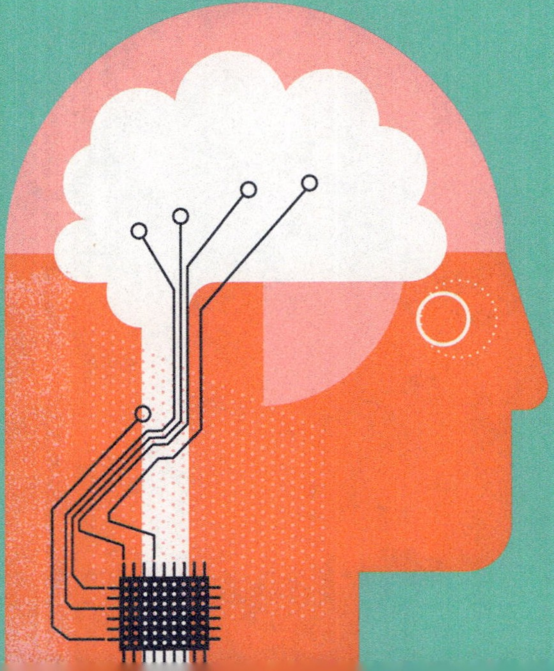

UNDERSTANDING
HABITS

Future PLC Quay House, The Ambury, Bath, BA1 1UA

Editorial
Editor **Charles Ginger**
Designer **Katy Stokes**
Compiled by **Zara Gaspar & Andy Downes**
Senior Art Editor **Andy Downes**
Head of Art & Design **Greg Whitaker**
Editorial Director **Jon White**

Cover images
Getty Images

Photography
All copyrights and trademarks are recognised and respected

Advertising
Media packs are available on request
Commercial Director **Clare Dove**

International
Head of Print Licensing **Rachel Shaw**
licensing@futurenet.com
www.futurecontenthub.com

Circulation
Head of Newstrade **Tim Mathers**

Production
Head of Production **Mark Constance**
Production Project Manager **Matthew Eglinton**
Advertising Production Manager **Joanne Crosby**
Digital Editions Controller **Jason Hudson**
Production Managers **Keely Miller, Nola Cokely, Vivienne Calvert, Fran Twentyman**

Printed by William Gibbons, 26 Planetary Road, Willenhall, West Midlands, WV13 3XT

Distributed by Marketforce, 5 Churchill Place, Canary Wharf, London, E14 5HU
www.marketforce.co.uk Tel: 0203 787 9001

Understanding Habits Fourth Edition (HIB5154)

FUTURE

Connectors.
Creators.
Experience
Makers.

Future plc is a public company quoted on the London Stock Exchange (symbol: FUTR)
www.futureplc.com

Chief Executive **Zillah Byng-Thorne**
Non-Executive Chairman **Richard Huntingford**
Chief Financial and Strategy Officer **Penny Ladkin-Brand**

Tel +44 (0)1225 442 244

Part of the
HOW IT WORKS
bookazine series

Widely Recycled

ipso. For press freedom with responsibility

Contents

"THE KEY TO OUR SURVIVAL AS A SPECIES IS OUR ABILITY TO USE PAST EXPERIENCES TO PREDICT WHAT'S GOING TO HAPPEN NEXT. OUR MOST VALUABLE TOOL IS GOAL-DIRECTED LEARNING – THE FOUNDATION FOR MAKING HABITS"

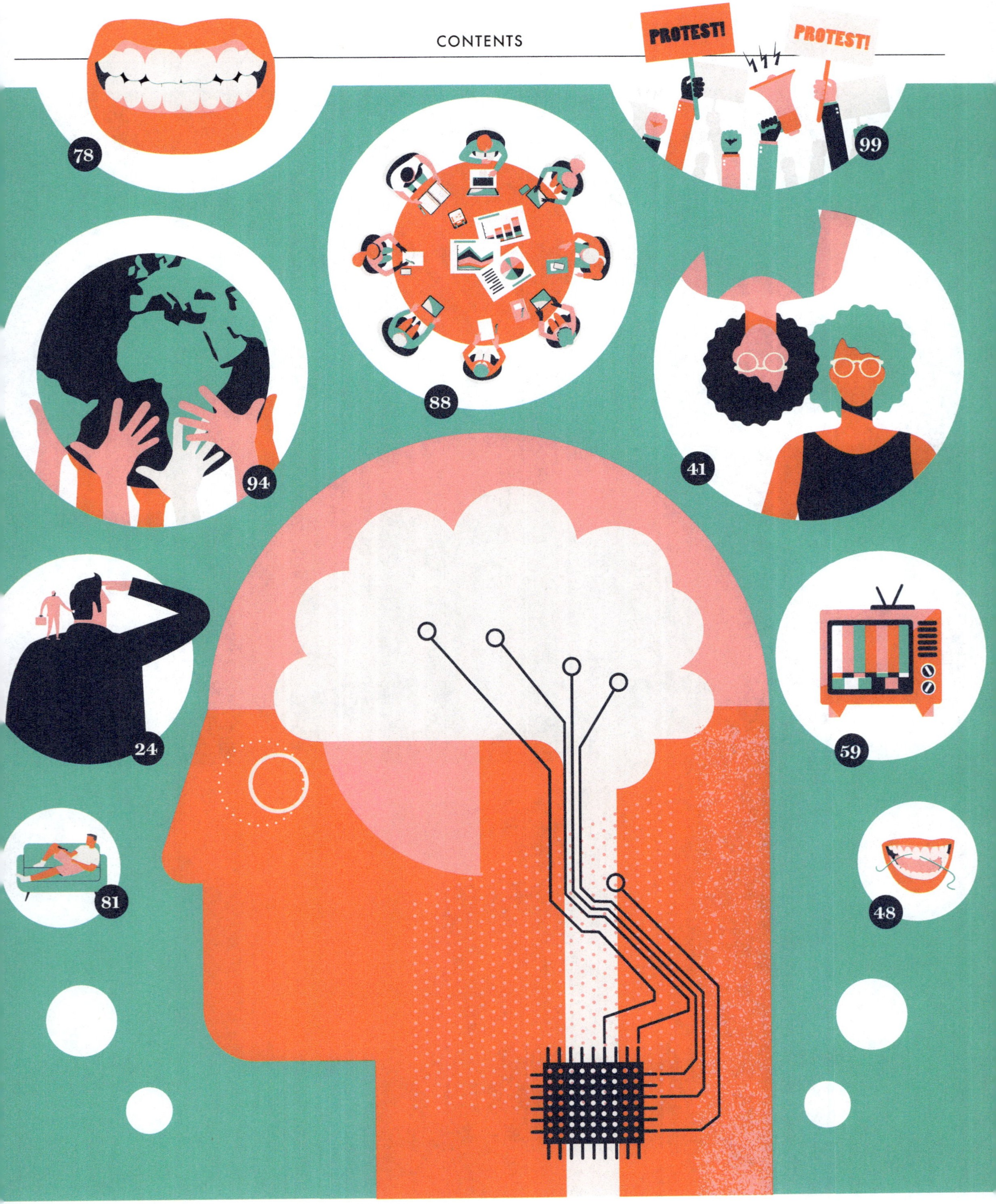

IMAGE SOURCE Getty Images

The power of habit

Be they good or bad, we've all got them, but just how influential are our daily routines?

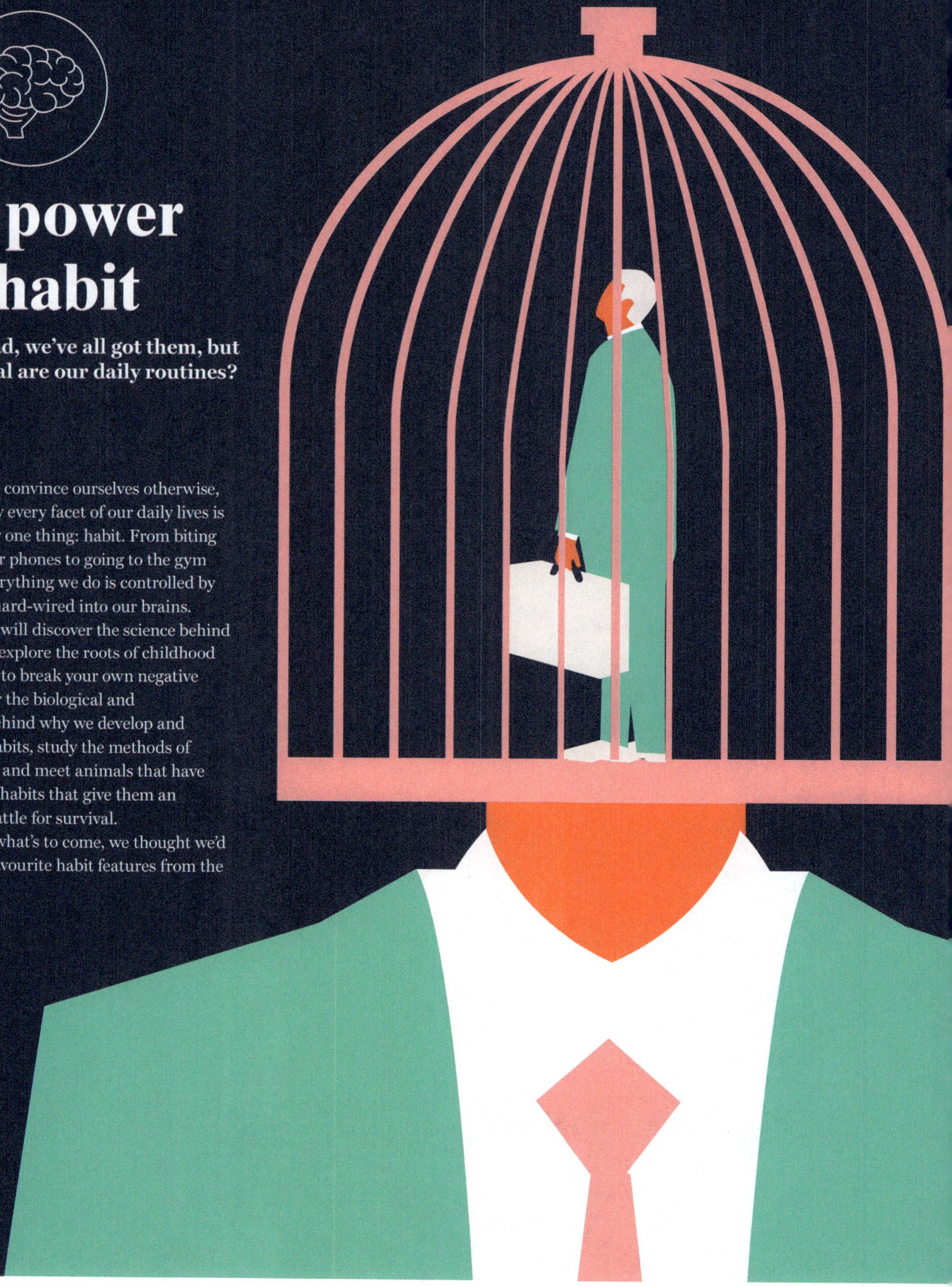

We may try to convince ourselves otherwise, but virtually every facet of our daily lives is governed by one thing: habit. From biting our nails or checking our phones to going to the gym and eating healthily, everything we do is controlled by learned habits that are hard-wired into our brains.

In this bookazine you will discover the science behind the formation of habits, explore the roots of childhood practices and learn how to break your own negative ways. You'll also uncover the biological and psychological reasons behind why we develop and maintain detrimental habits, study the methods of successful organisations and meet animals that have mastered mathematical habits that give them an invaluable edge in the battle for survival.

To give you a taste of what's to come, we thought we'd start with some of our favourite habit features from the Live Science archives.

'Neanderthal' means 'human of the Neander Valley', which is in western Germany.

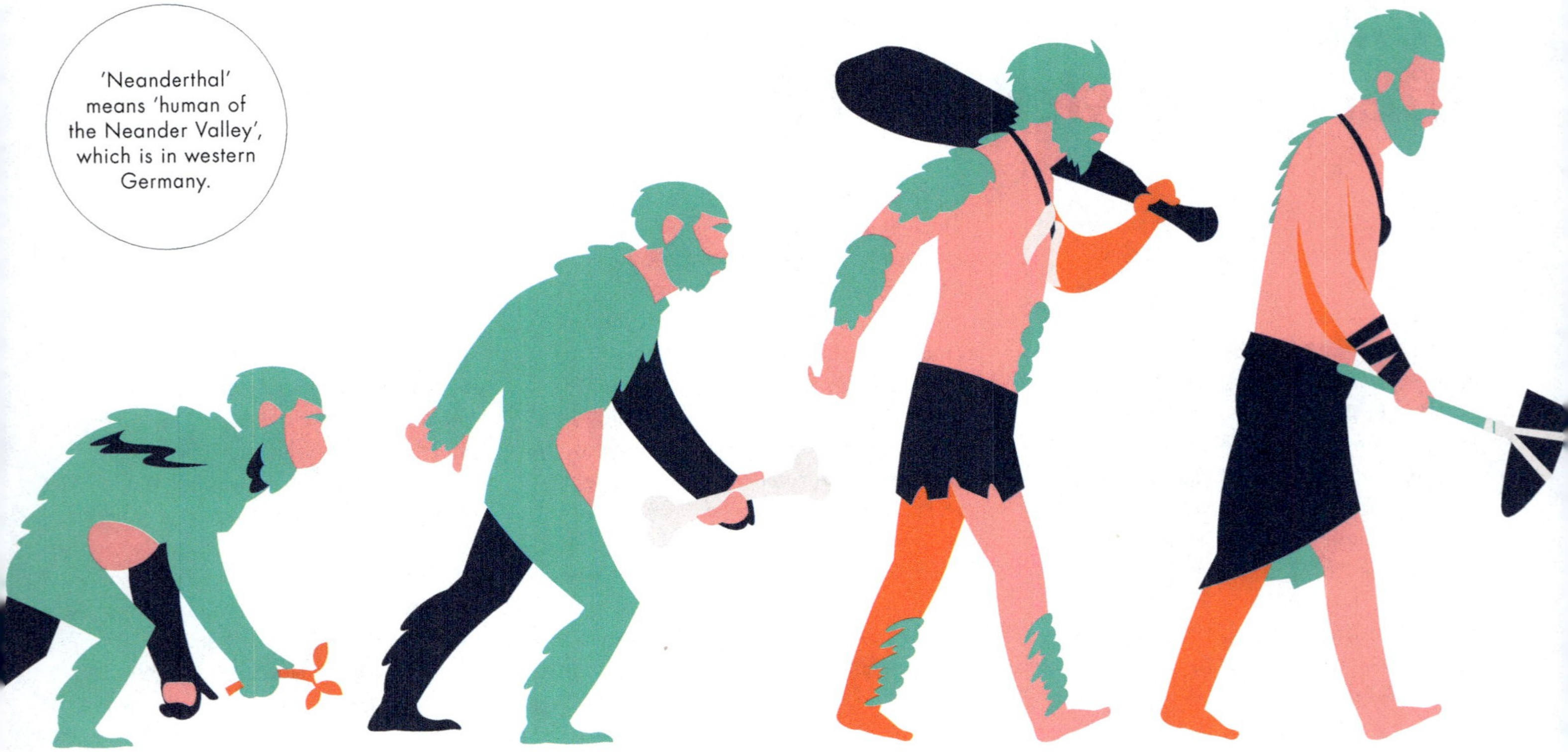

Your hair colour and sleep habits may come from Neanderthals

Neanderthal DNA could influence your skin tone, hair colour, sleep patterns, mood and even smoking behaviour, a new study has found. The finding sheds light on the role Neanderthal genetic variants play in modern human biology in addition to disease, the researchers said.

Neanderthals, the closest extinct relatives of modern humans, died off in Europe about 40,000 years ago. Research over the past decade has revealed that Neanderthals interbred with the ancestors of modern humans who migrated out of Africa. Currently, scientists believed that the genomes of modern human groups that originated outside Africa hold between 1.8 and 2.6 per cent Neanderthal DNA.

Prior work found that Neanderthal gene variants play roles in a wide variety of health-related problems in modern humans, such as depression, heart attacks, nicotine addiction and obesity. However, researchers wanted to see what role Neanderthal DNA might play in nondisease-related traits in modern humans.

The researchers analysed the genetic data of more than 112,000 volunteers in the UK Biobank, a database of health information collected from 500,000 participants over time. This database also noted many other traits, such as diet and behaviour.

"Neanderthal DNA is one source of variation for many traits in modern humans," said study lead author Michael Dannemann, a computational biologist at the Max Planck Institute for Evolutionary Anthropology in Leipzig, Germany.

For instance, DNA from Neanderthals may influence modern humans' hair colour, skin colour and tendency to tan, study senior author Janet Kelso, also a computational biologist at the Max Planck Institute for Evolutionary Anthropology, said in a statement. In addition, modern humans with certain Neanderthal gene variants tend to be smokers, and other Neanderthal gene variants are found more frequently in people who are "night owls".

The researchers also noted that some Neanderthal gene variants were linked with lighter skin tones and hair colour, while others were linked with darker ones. "These findings suggest that Neanderthals might have differed in their hair and skin tones, much as people now do," Dannemann said in a statement.

Kelso noted that many of the traits they saw that were influenced by Neanderthal DNA – including skin and hair colour, mood and sleeping patterns – are linked to the level of sunlight people receive. She noted that Neanderthals had already lived in Eurasia for millennia before modern humans migrated there about 100,000 years ago.

As such, Neanderthals were likely better adapted to the lower and more variable levels of ultraviolet radiation from the Sun compared with the new arrivals from Africa – traits they passed on to the offspring of their liaisons with modern humans.

"This work and future work will help us understand what Neanderthals contributed to variation in modern humans, and perhaps in the future also let us learn more about Neanderthals," Dannemann said.

IMAGE SOURCE Getty Images

Cultural pressures may affect your sleep habits

Our biological clocks may not dictate our bedtimes, but they do influence when we wake up in the morning, a study has found. Cultural pressures and daily responsibilities may override our biological clocks and dictate when we go to sleep, according to the study published in the journal *Science Advances*. However, people's wake-up times are still highly dependent on their biological clocks, as opposed to their morning responsibilities.

The new findings show "Bedtime is more under the control of society, and wake time is more under the control of the [biological] clock," according to Olivia Walch, a graduate student at the University of Michigan and a co-author of the study. The biological clock (circadian rhythm) is the primary driver of human sleep schedules and is affected by environmental cues like sunlight.

In the study, the researchers looked at sleep data from more than 8,000 people in 100 countries who used a smartphone app that helps travellers adjust to new time zones. To use the app, you enter your typical sleep schedule as well as the times when you are normally exposed to light. Using this information, the app suggests custom schedules of light and darkness to help you adjust to a new time zone. In other words, the app suggests that you be exposed to bright light at one point during the day and to darkness at another point.

When the researchers looked at the average amount of time that people in each country slept, they found that people in Singapore and Japan got the least amount of sleep, with an average of about seven hours and 24 minutes per night, whereas people in the Netherlands got the most sleep on average with eight hours and 12 minutes.

Though the difference in average sleep duration between these countries may not seem huge, every half-hour of sleep actually has a big impact on people's cognitive function and long-term health, the researchers said.

The researchers noted that countries that are geographically and culturally close to each other, such as Japan and Singapore, tended to have similar sleep patterns.

They also looked at how sleep times varied among people of different ages and between the sexes. They found that middle-aged men got the least sleep – often less than the recommended seven to eight hours per night.

When the researchers then compared sleep times between the men and women they examined, they found that the women in the study scheduled 30 minutes more sleep than the men per night on average, with the women going to bed earlier and waking up later than the men.

Moreover, the researchers found that people's sleep schedules seemed to become more similar to the habits of their peers as they got older. For example, there were more similarities among the sleep schedules of people older than 55 compared with those younger than 30. One possible explanation for this is that older people tend to have a narrower window of time within which they can fall and stay asleep.

The new findings are a reminder that sleep is more important than many people may realise. Even if someone is getting six hours of sleep per night, which is less than the recommended seven to eight hours, that person is still building up a sleep debt.

Sleep debt is the effect that sleep deficiency can have on the body, which can rapidly lead to physical and mental fatigue, with potentially serious consequences.

"It doesn't take that many days of not getting enough sleep before you're functionally drunk," explained Walch.

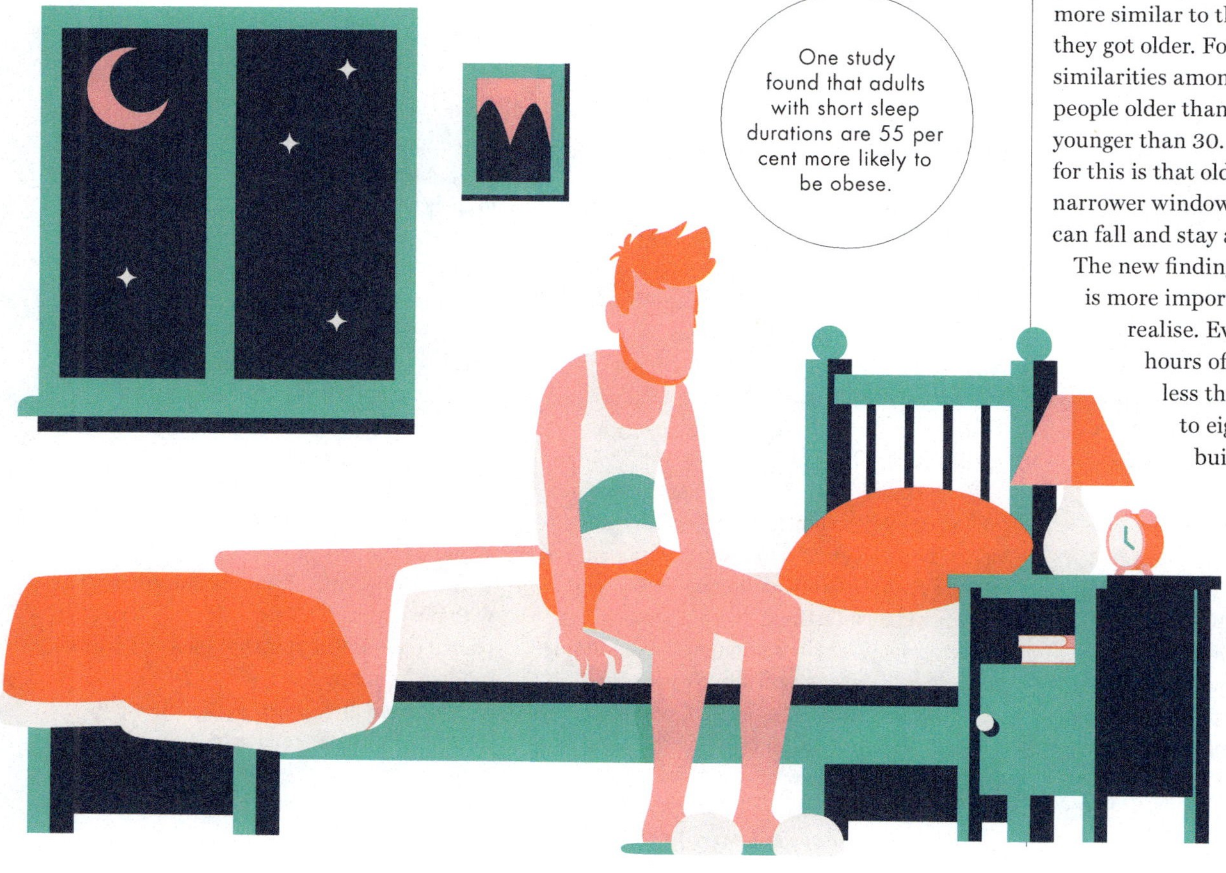

One study found that adults with short sleep durations are 55 per cent more likely to be obese.

What the 'phub'? Your cellphone habits might hurt your relationship

Are you a phubber? That is, do you snub others by constantly looking at your cellphone? If you're guilty of this, you may want to change your ways: a recent survey suggests interrupting real-life to stare at your phone can damage personal relationships.

"Our findings suggest the more a couple's time together is interrupted by one individual attending to their cellphone, the less likely it is that the other individual is satisfied in the relationship," said Meredith David, assistant professor of marketing at Baylor University in Texas and one of the researchers who conducted the survey.

In the survey, the researchers looked at a particular kind of 'phone snubbing' known as 'pphubbing' (yes, with two P's), which occurs when one partner snubs his or her significant other in favour of their phone. It found that pphubbing leads to lower levels of relationship satisfaction.

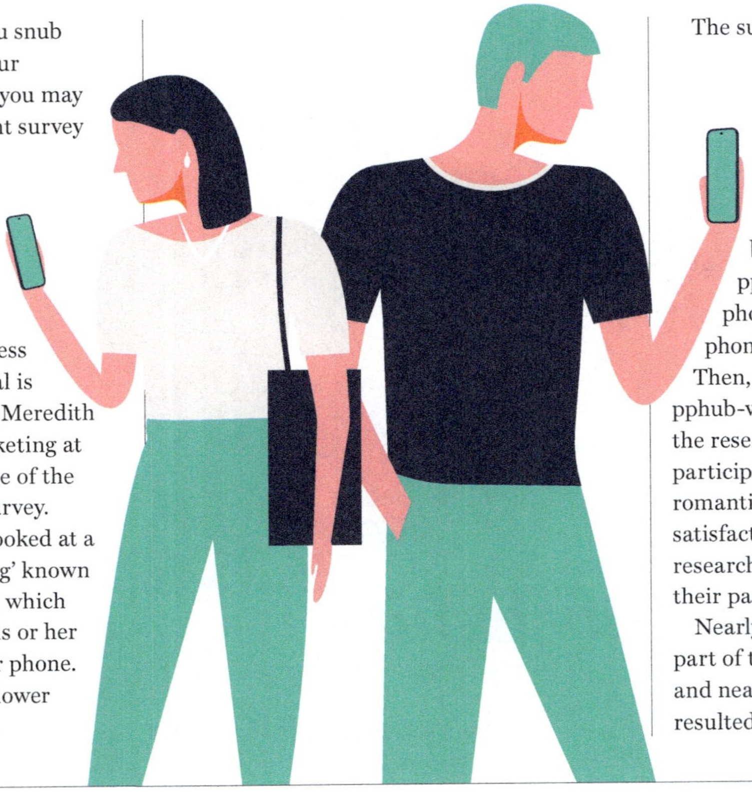

The survey was split into two parts, the first of which was completed by more than 300 people. This first series of questions helped researchers identify which cellphone-related behaviours are perceived as 'pphubbing'. The behaviours most associated with pphubbing included glancing at your phone when talking and checking your phone during lulls in a conversation.

Then, using the behaviours identified as pphub-worthy in the first part of the survey, the researchers asked a separate group of 145 participants, each one of them having a romantic partner, to rate their level of satisfaction with their relationships. The researchers also asked participants whether their partners' cellphone use caused conflict.

Nearly half of those who took the second part of the survey reported being 'phubbed', and nearly a quarter said that this pphubbing resulted in some kind of conflict.

Couples share unhealthy habits

A lot of sharing goes on in a relationship, including unhealthy habits, according to a study. The results suggest people in both married, straight and cohabiting gay and lesbian relationships pick up their partner's tendency to eat unhealthy foods or skip the gym.

Previous studies have found marriage can promote good health habits, such as regular doctor checkups. Indeed, a recent study found married men who have heart attacks seek medical attention faster than unmarried men. However, this latest study suggests the effect of marriage and cohabitation on health isn't always so rosy.

The researchers reported two ways habits can change in a couple: one partner has bad habits and influences the other, or both may 'sync up' their bad habits. In heterosexual partnerships men were nearly always viewed as the 'bad influence' according to the study.

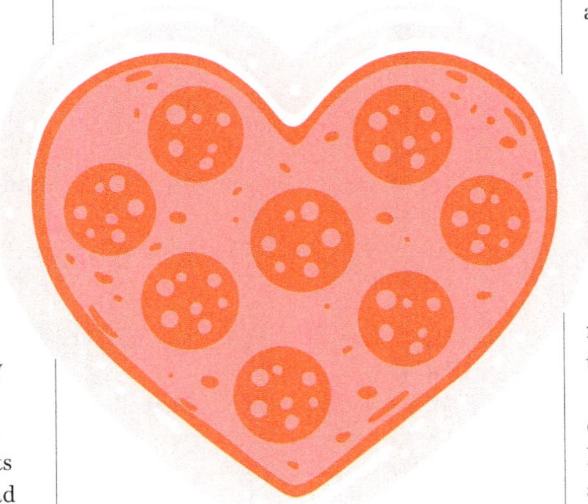

"The finding that one partner is a 'bad influence' suggests that individuals converge in health habits across the course of their relationship, because one individual's unhealthy habits directly promotes the other's," said study researcher Corinne Reczek, an assistant professor of sociology at the University of Cincinnati.

Gay and lesbian couples more often reported a phenomenon the researchers termed 'habit synchronicity'.

"For these individuals, one partner may not engage in what they consider an unhealthy habit on their own, but when their desire for such a habit is matched by their partners, they partake in unhealthy habits," Reczek wrote in her conclusions.

IMAGE SOURCE Getty Images

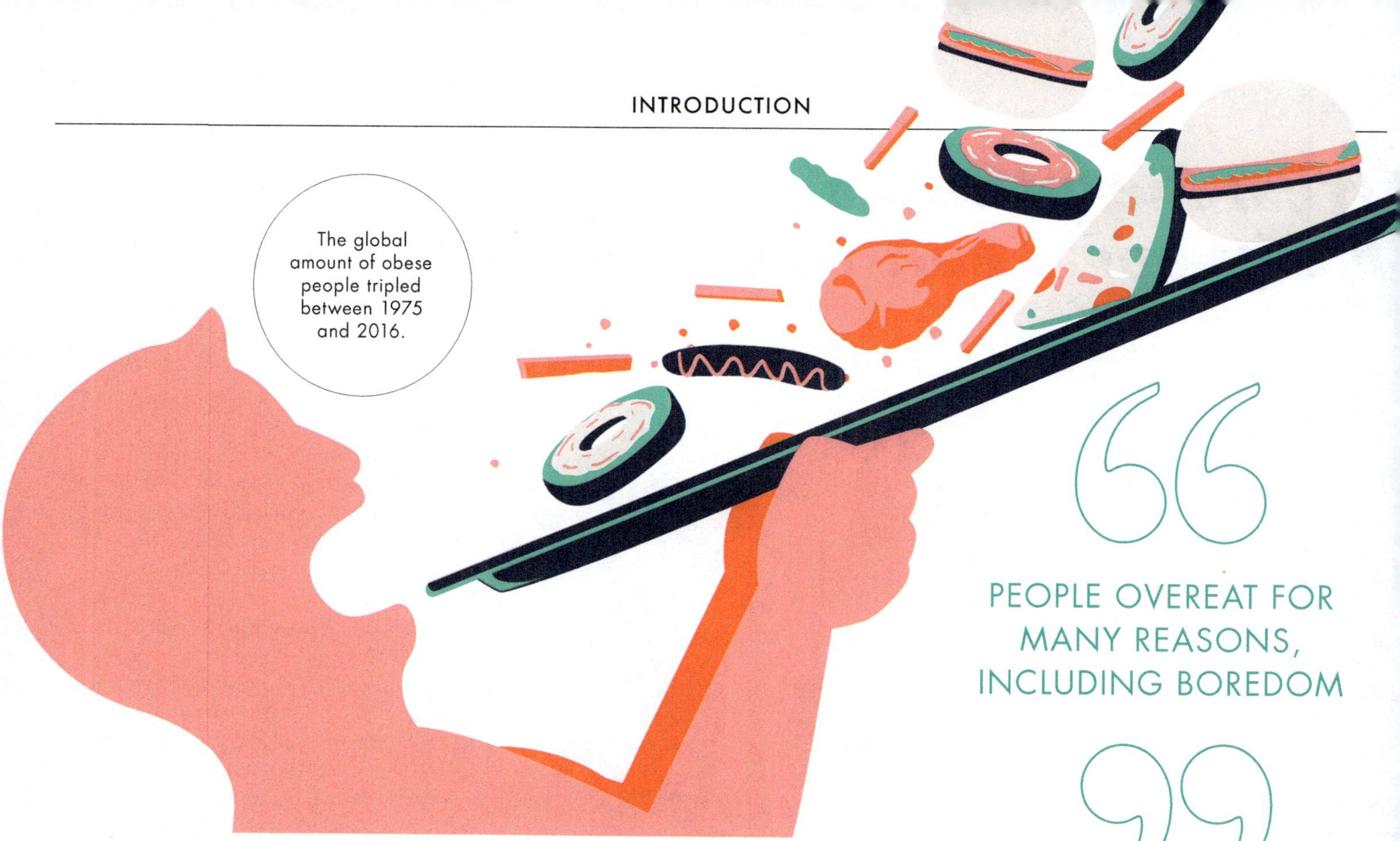

The global amount of obese people tripled between 1975 and 2016.

> PEOPLE OVEREAT FOR MANY REASONS, INCLUDING BOREDOM

Common nervous habits

You know you shouldn't, but you just can't help it. Whether it's nail biting, thumb sucking or overeating, nervous habits plague many individuals, who just can't seem to stop. But why do we engage in these behaviours, and what effect can they have?

Despite the perception of these habits as behaviours set off when we're nervous or stressed, they can occur at any time depending on the individual. People may engage in them when they're bored, relaxed, by themselves or watching TV. People likely continue these habits because they receive some satisfaction from the behaviour.

"Any habit that is perpetuated is rewarded," said Carol Goldberg, a psychologist in New York City. "So in some way it makes them feel more relaxed, or it gives them something else – if it weren't rewarded they wouldn't keep doing it; they're getting something from it." So what are the motivations behind some common habits?

Nail biting: This is by far the most common nervous habit, affecting about a third of young children, 44 per cent of teenagers and 19 to 29 per cent of adults, according to psychologist Penny Donnenfeld. The urge to gnaw may be "an outgrowth of things that were self-soothing in childhood," Donnenfeld said. She added that babies are very mouth oriented, and so the prevalence of the habit in toddlers and young children could be some leftover urge from infancy. The habit can even start from copying someone else, explained Goldberg, who observed children begin biting their nails after watching a popular classmate doing it.

Thumb sucking: Babies are born with the impulse to suck anything in their mouth, a reflex that enables them to breastfeed. While many children will continue to suck their thumbs until they are about two to four years old, most grow out of it on their own.

Overeating: People overeat for many reasons, including anxiety, boredom or frustration. Sometimes people turn to eating as a way to self-medicate, since certain foods can promote feelings of happiness, Donnenfeld explained.

Smoking: More than just a mild habit, smoking can be physically addictive, with frequent users becoming dependent on the drug nicotine. The drug causes changes in the levels of certain brain chemicals, resulting in feelings of calm and pleasure, which smokers can come to crave.

Impact: While the consequences of overeating and smoking are well documented, nail biting and thumb sucking can also carry certain risks. For instance, biting your nails can be unsanitary and spread germs, Goldberg said. "From that point of view, of catching something, having your dirty fingernails in your mouth is not a very good idea at all."

Nail biters may also be judged negatively by their peers. "Socially, it doesn't look very nice," Goldberg said. "If you bite your nails, it doesn't show you off as well to others."

Thumb sucking is not without its risks either. If children don't give it up by the time that their permanent teeth start to develop it can lead to oral problems, including the misalignment of teeth and changes in the roof of the mouth, according to the American Dental Association.

Kick the habit: 8 scientific quit-smoking tips

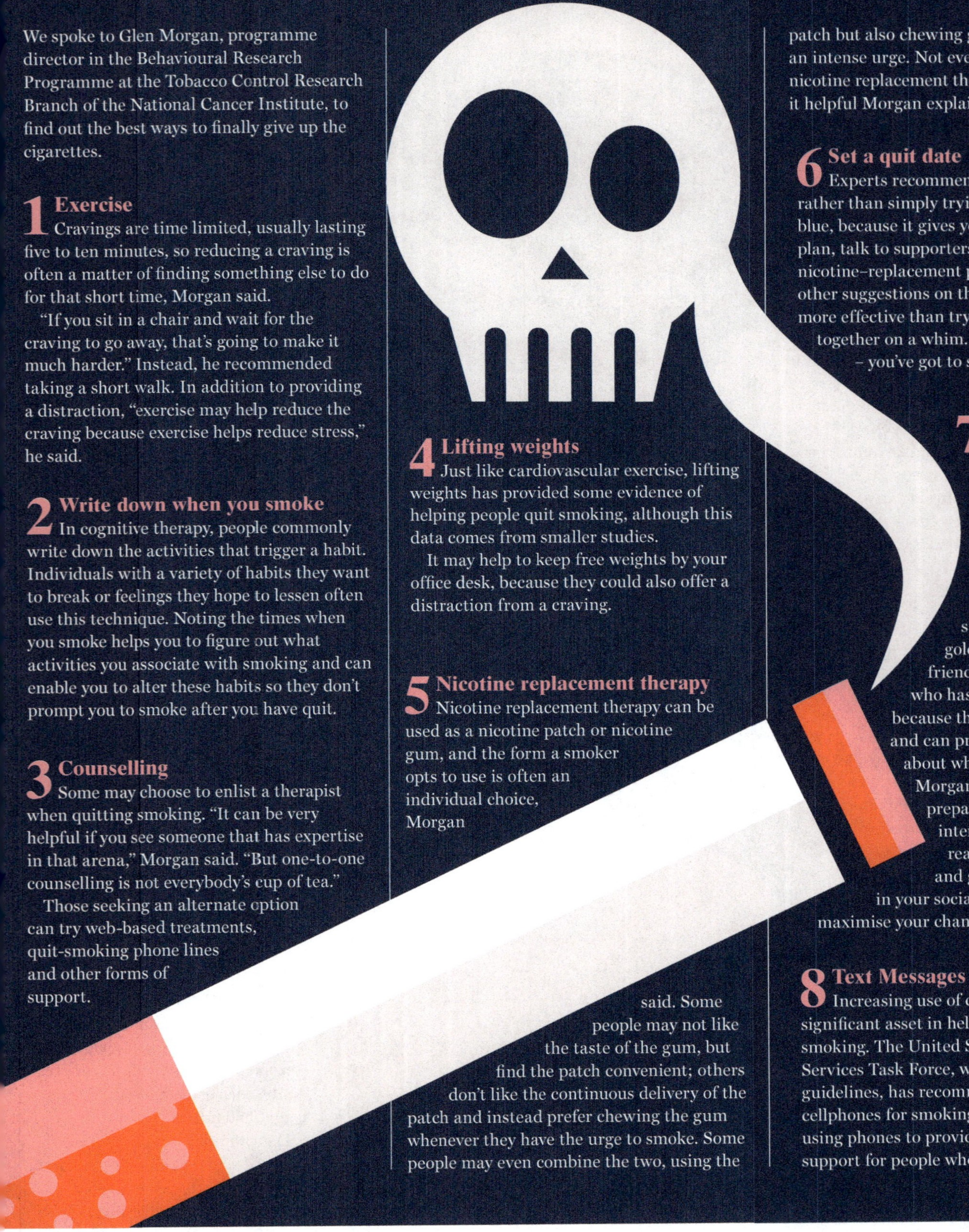

We spoke to Glen Morgan, programme director in the Behavioural Research Programme at the Tobacco Control Research Branch of the National Cancer Institute, to find out the best ways to finally give up the cigarettes.

1 Exercise

Cravings are time limited, usually lasting five to ten minutes, so reducing a craving is often a matter of finding something else to do for that short time, Morgan said.

"If you sit in a chair and wait for the craving to go away, that's going to make it much harder." Instead, he recommended taking a short walk. In addition to providing a distraction, "exercise may help reduce the craving because exercise helps reduce stress," he said.

2 Write down when you smoke

In cognitive therapy, people commonly write down the activities that trigger a habit. Individuals with a variety of habits they want to break or feelings they hope to lessen often use this technique. Noting the times when you smoke helps you to figure out what activities you associate with smoking and can enable you to alter these habits so they don't prompt you to smoke after you have quit.

3 Counselling

Some may choose to enlist a therapist when quitting smoking. "It can be very helpful if you see someone that has expertise in that arena," Morgan said. "But one-to-one counselling is not everybody's cup of tea."

Those seeking an alternate option can try web-based treatments, quit-smoking phone lines and other forms of support.

4 Lifting weights

Just like cardiovascular exercise, lifting weights has provided some evidence of helping people quit smoking, although this data comes from smaller studies.

It may help to keep free weights by your office desk, because they could also offer a distraction from a craving.

5 Nicotine replacement therapy

Nicotine replacement therapy can be used as a nicotine patch or nicotine gum, and the form a smoker opts to use is often an individual choice, Morgan said. Some people may not like the taste of the gum, but find the patch convenient; others don't like the continuous delivery of the patch and instead prefer chewing the gum whenever they have the urge to smoke. Some people may even combine the two, using the patch but also chewing gum when they have an intense urge. Not everyone needs to use nicotine replacement therapy, but many find it helpful Morgan explained.

6 Set a quit date

Experts recommend setting a quit date rather than simply trying to stop out of the blue, because it gives you time to set up a plan, talk to supporters about that plan, get nicotine-replacement products and prepare other suggestions on this list. That's much more effective than trying to pull it all together on a whim. "It's like taking a test – you've got to study."

7 Enlist your social network

Because counselling is not a popular choice for many, you may also want to enlist the aid of friends, family or co-workers for suggestions. "It's golden if you have a friend or significant other who has quit smoking, because they have been there and can provide suggestions about what helped them," Morgan said. "Like preparing for a job interview, you want to get ready, develop strategies and get help from people in your social network in order to maximise your chance of succeeding."

8 Text Messages

Increasing use of cellphones has been a significant asset in helping people quit smoking. The United States Preventive Services Task Force, which issues treatment guidelines, has recommended the use of cellphones for smoking cessation, such as using phones to provide counselling or support for people who are trying to quit.

IMAGE SOURCE Getty Images

Hurricane Sandy dealt a blow to healthy habits

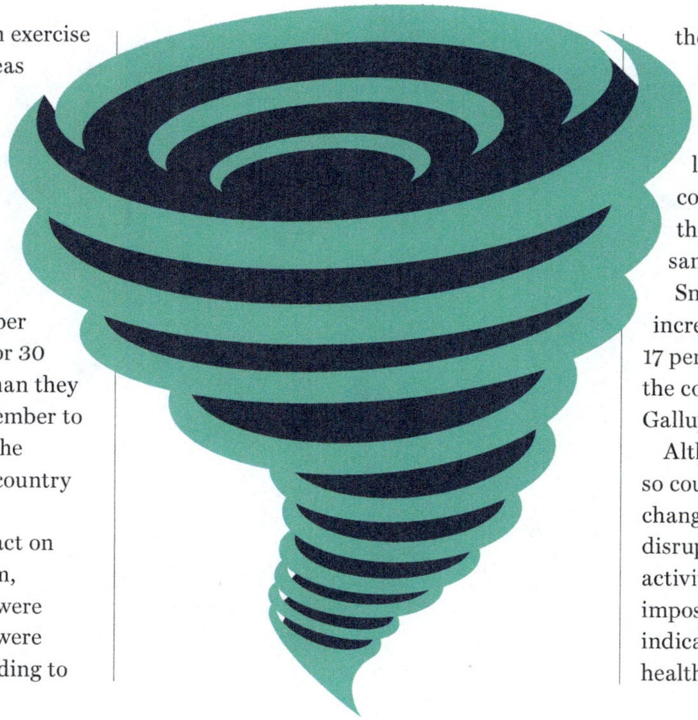

Health officials normally see a dip in exercise during the winter months, but in areas affected by Hurricane Sandy, the drop in physical activity after the storm was twice that of the rest of the country, according to a new poll.

Between 1 November and 15 December 2012, after Hurricane Sandy, residents of New Jersey, New York and Connecticut were 12 to 13 per cent less likely to report exercising for 30 minutes at least three days a week than they were before the storm (from 15 September to 28 October). Over the same period, the decline in exercise in the rest of the country was just six per cent, on average.

Hurricane Sandy also had an impact on healthy eating habits. After the storm, residents in the most affected areas were seven per cent less likely to say they were eating healthily than before it, according to the poll, which was conducted by the Gallup-Healthways Index.

Residents in less-affected areas of the three states were three per cent less likely, and those in the rest of the country were one per cent less likely to say they were eating healthy food over the same period.

Smoking rates after the storm also increased in areas most affected (from 14 to 17 per cent), while smoking rates in the rest of the country did not change in that period, Gallup-Healthways said.

Although the study was correlational and so couldn't say whether Sandy caused the change in healthy habits, natural disasters disrupt normal life and can make everyday activities such as exercise impractical or impossible. The poll numbers provide an indication of just how much disasters affect healthy habits.

Why old habits die hard

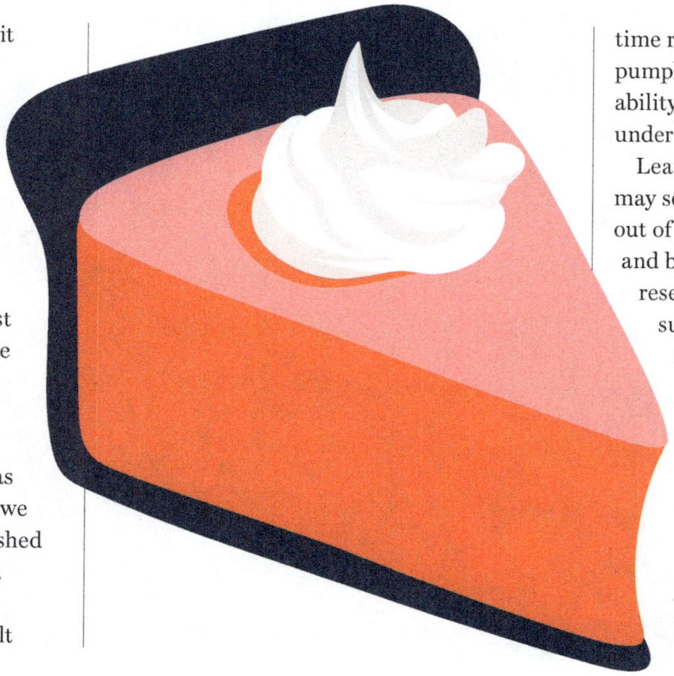

Despite your best efforts, you may find it hard to avoid the eating and drinking habits of the holidays when you return to normal life. The problem, research shows, is your brain's tendency to revert to deep-rooted memories.

"It may not be only the deliciousness of traditional holiday treats that makes them hard to resist but their familiarity," Cindy Lustig, a psychologist at the University of Michigan, said. "The urge to engage in those old behaviours seems to be especially strong in our unconscious memory."

That unconscious memory is known as automatic memory, and it is the reason we tend to revert to older and more established reactions when multitasking or harried.

"Those stressed or tired from holiday shopping may have an especially difficult time resisting their traditional slice of pumpkin pie... stress and fatigue impair our ability to keep those unconscious influences under control," Lustig said.

Learning new behaviours and information may sometimes seem to push old thoughts out of the brain, but it is the early memories and behaviours that stick according to research. In the study Lustig taught subjects to call a coffee cup a 'cup' first, and later to call it a 'mug'. When asked what they named the object, initially the responses were split, but by the second day the individuals referred to the objects more often as a 'cup', as they had initially learned it.

"This procedure let us separate controlled versus automatic processes, and we saw the return of the old memories," Lustig explained.

Healthy habits are most contagious among similar friends

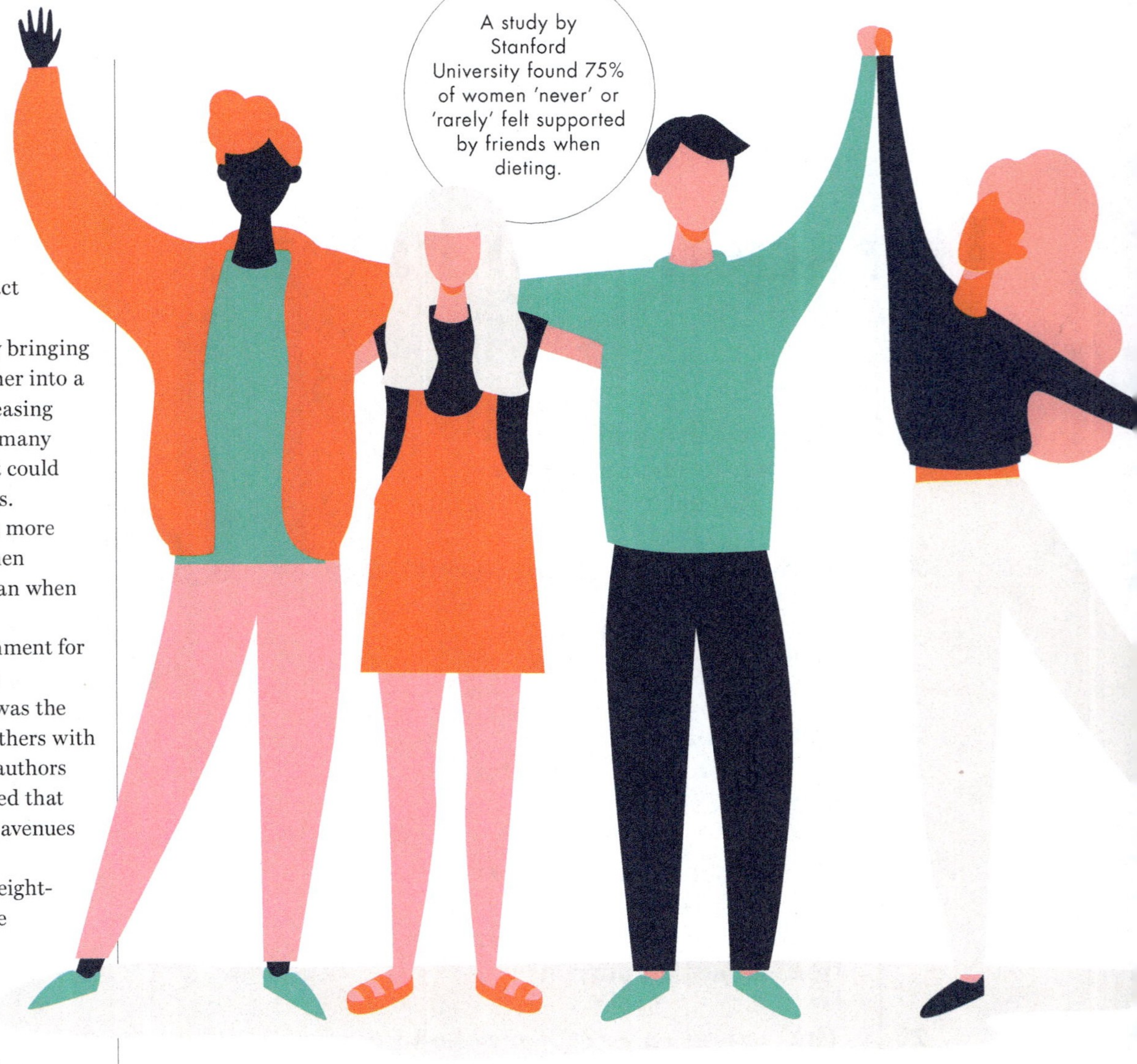

A study by Stanford University found 75% of women 'never' or 'rarely' felt supported by friends when dieting.

Obesity spreads "contagiously" through social networks, claimed a highly publicised 2007 study, and since then, some researchers have been working to use social networks to reverse the obesity epidemic. A study published recently suggests that this may in fact be possible.

Researchers at MIT found that by bringing people who had similar traits together into a social network with the aim of increasing physical fitness they increased how many people picked up a new activity that could bring about healthy lifestyle changes.

Even people who were obese were more likely to pick up the new activity when grouped with other obese people than when grouped with thinner people.

"The most effective social environment for increasing the 'willingness' of obese individuals to adopt the behaviour was the one in which they interacted with others with similar health characteristics," the authors wrote in their conclusions. It is hoped that this study will in time open up new avenues of research in the area.

"You're going to see a lot more [weight-loss] interventions coming down the road that are thoughtfully designed around social networks. And as a result, I think those interventions are going to be more successful," said Ray Browning, a physiologist at Colorado State University who has studied health interventions and social networks but was not involved with the study.

While not well-studied, Browning noted that researchers have observed that some people who sustain weight loss for a long period also change who they spend their time with – for example, a divorce or a move might be involved.

"Some of those individuals completely change their social network, and get out of one and move into another," he said. "The social network they land in has more of these healthful behaviours."

And so, changing your behaviours may be easier if you bring someone new into your group, such as a personal trainer, who can encourage better habits and activities that promote health, Browning said.

"Take the social network you have and bring in that seed individual," he said.

However, while the study showed some success, Browning noted the results may not apply to everyone. There were proportionately fewer obese people in the study than in the general population, and as the sample was obtained from a fitness group those involved were already looking for ways to be healthier.

Additionally, it remains unclear how other new health behaviours might spread through a group, because keeping a log of what you eat is easier than beginning a rigorous exercise programme, which takes a lot of commitment to stick at.

"What we probably have here is a best case in terms of adoption of behaviour. You have a lot of things working in your favour." Still, the study pushes the research in the right direction, Browning said.

"This is a nice, elegant way to start the discussion of how to do interventions with regards to social networks."

IMAGE SOURCE Getty Images

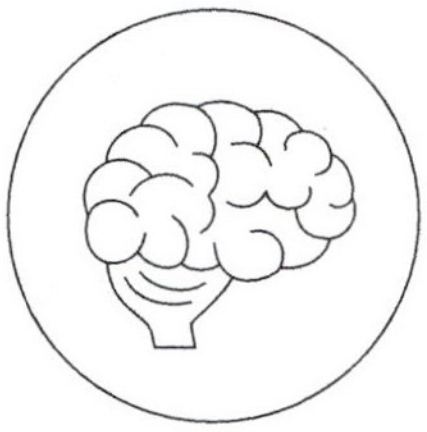

The science of habits

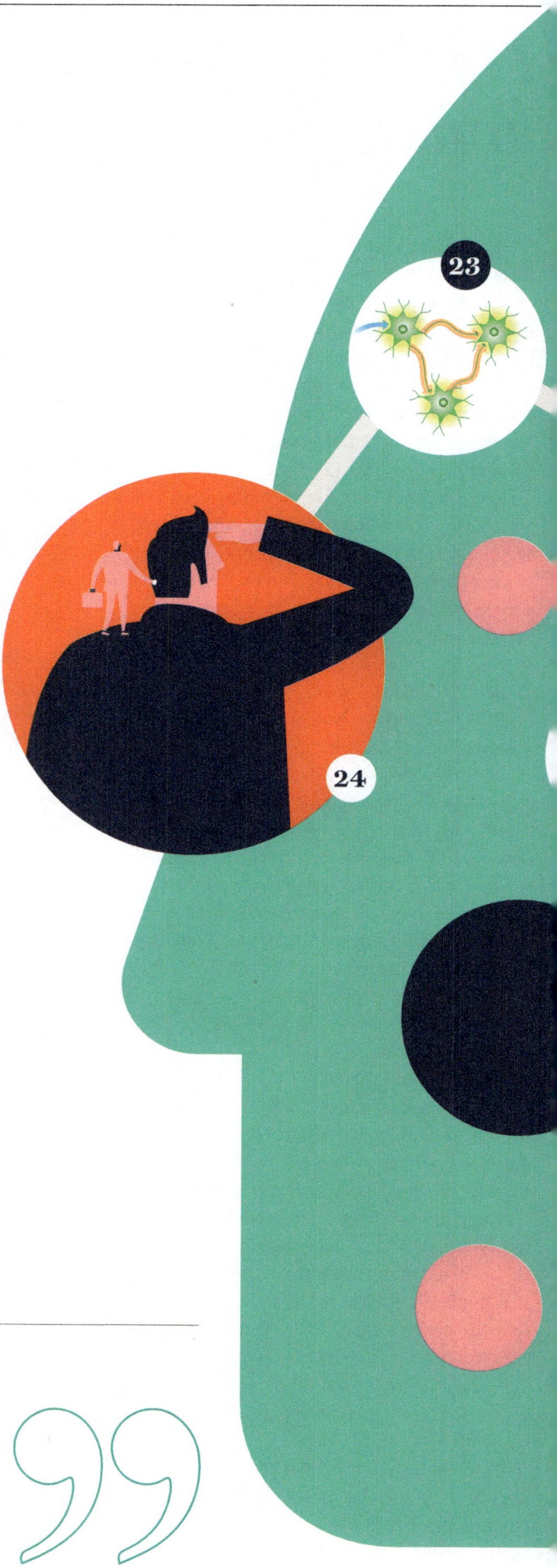

“EVERY HABIT HAS A DIFFERENT COMBINATION OF TRIGGERS AND BEHAVIOURS, BUT THEY ALL START OUT WITH GOAL-DIRECTED LEARNING”

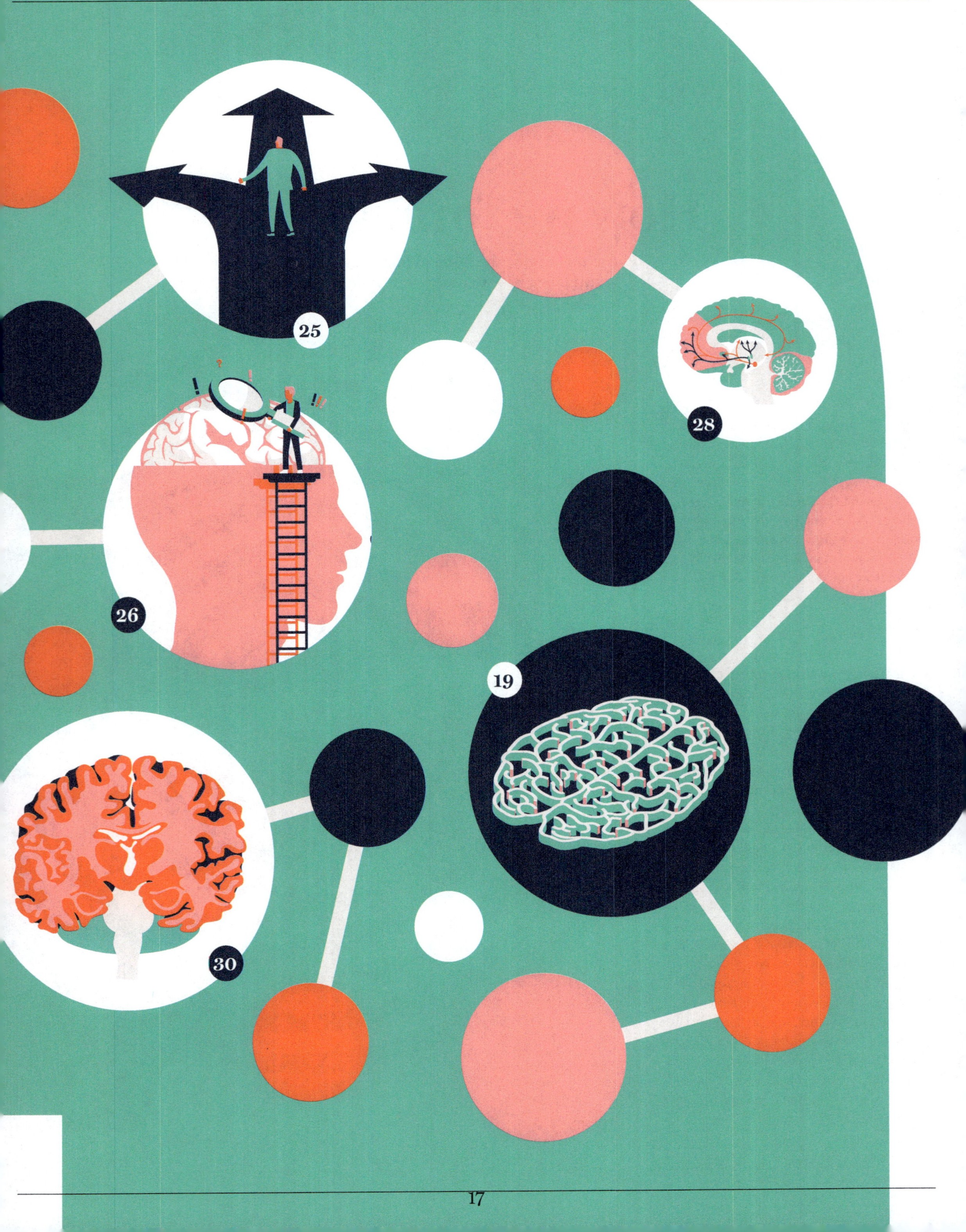
25
28
26
19
30

How we form habits

Take a look under the hood of habit formation and learn how to hack your biology

Humans are creatures of habit. We might have the most powerful brains in the known universe, but we're at our best when we're running on autopilot. The ability to make, break and use habits emerged deep in our evolutionary history, allowing us to perform repeat actions automatically so that we could save processing power for more important tasks.

Learning to make predictions

The key to our survival as a species is our ability to use past experiences to predict what's going to happen next. This allows us to choose the behaviour that best fits each situation. Our most powerful tool for this purpose is goal-directed learning.

When we're working towards a goal, we take in information about the situation, combine it with memories and emotions, weigh it all up, and make a custom decision based on what's likely to happen next. This type of learning uses the full force of the brain's processing power, and it's under conscious control.

Goal-directed learning is hyper-flexible, and it can produce any combination of complex behaviours. But we don't always have the time to make a considered choice, especially if the choice we make is always the same. So, we evolved ways to make repeat decisions without having to think about them.

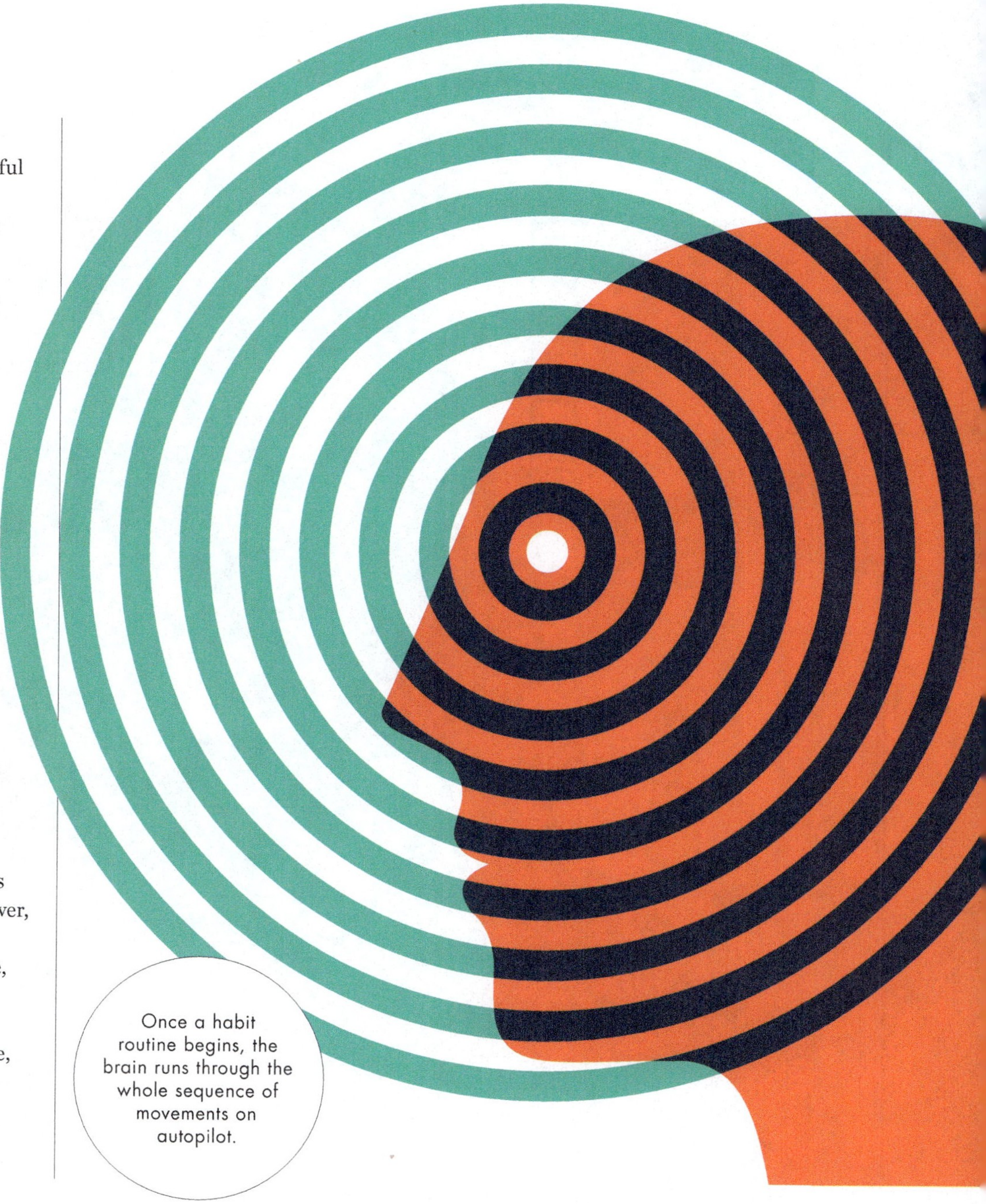

Once a habit routine begins, the brain runs through the whole sequence of movements on autopilot.

The simplest example of this is Pavlovian learning, named after the famous psychologist who experimented on dogs. It's a kind of predictive learning where our brains link up normal reflexes with cues from the environment. For example, we might learn that a ringing bell (the cue) always means that food is coming (the prediction), so we link it with saliva production (the reflex behaviour). This creates a biological shortcut, preparing us for food without the need for conscious thought.

When a trigger and a response are paired together like this, they happen automatically and subconsciously. It's fast and doesn't take much processing, but it's not very powerful. Pavlovian learning always uses built-in behaviours, and there are a limited number to choose from.

Habit learning upgrades this system. It combines the behaviour flexibility of goal-directed learning with the speed of Pavlovian learning.

Habits contain sequences of complex actions, like those created during goal-directed learning, but they remove the need to make them up on the spot. Instead, like in Pavlovian learning, our brains link the behaviours up to a cue or trigger that sets them off automatically. The actions that make up a habit can be sequences of behaviours or sequences of thoughts, and once they start, they run all the way to the end without any effort at all.

Turning a goal into a habit

Every habit has a different combination of triggers and behaviours, but they all start out the same way: with goal-directed learning. Although it takes immense processing power, this type of learning is our most flexible way of predicting the future.

Imagine you're in a maze and you get to a fork in the path. In one direction there is a bar of chocolate, in the other direction there is a dead end.

The first time you run the maze you pick a direction at random, but the second time you use your memory of the last time to make a decision. As you keep rerunning the maze, you start to build up a picture of which direction is most likely to contain the chocolate bar.

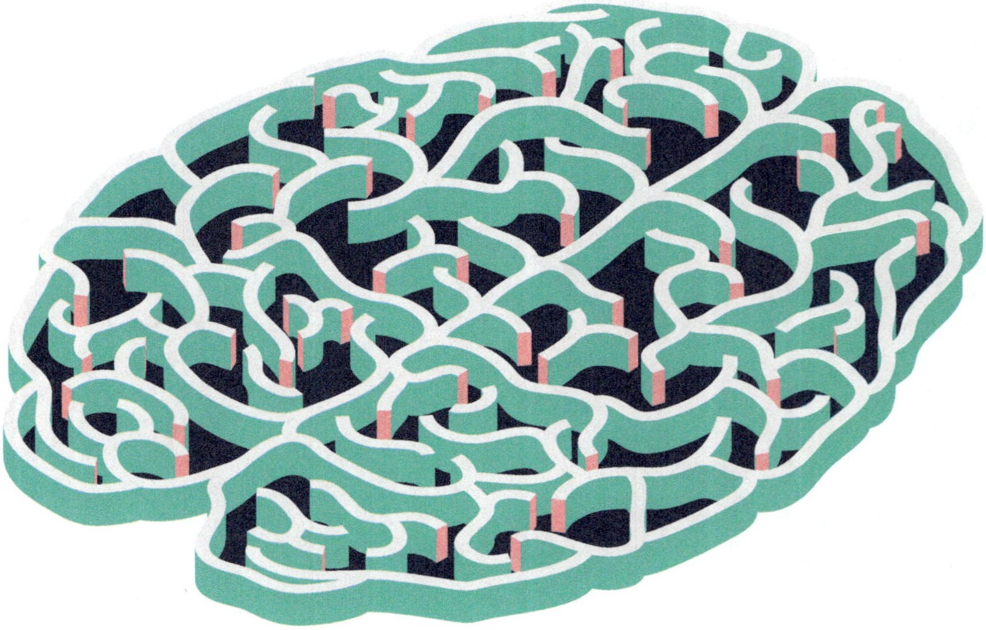

"EVERY HABIT HAS A DIFFERENT COMBINATION OF TRIGGERS AND BEHAVIOURS, BUT THEY ALL START OUT WITH GOAL-DIRECTED LEARNING"

If you're anything like a rat, your maze strategy will start out goal-directed. You might pause when you get to the fork and have a think about which way to turn, but after running the maze a few times you start to notice that the chocolate bar is always on the right. The more you repeat the maze and find the chocolate in the same place, the faster and more automatic your right-hand turn starts to become.

But what if the rules of the game start to change? Now there's a light in the maze. When it's blue the chocolate is on the right, but when it's red the chocolate is on the left.

If the light appears early on in your maze-running experience, you might adjust your strategy and learn to change direction depending on the colour. However, if you've been running the maze for days, chances are you won't even notice. You'll turn automatically, even though there's no reward waiting for you at the end. The decision about which way to turn has become habit. And, once a habit is fixed, it doesn't matter if the reward disappears. You're already running the maze on autopilot.

No reward necessary

The switch from goal-directed learning to habit learning happens in a part of the brain called the striatum, a cluster of brain cells

IMAGE SOURCE Getty Images

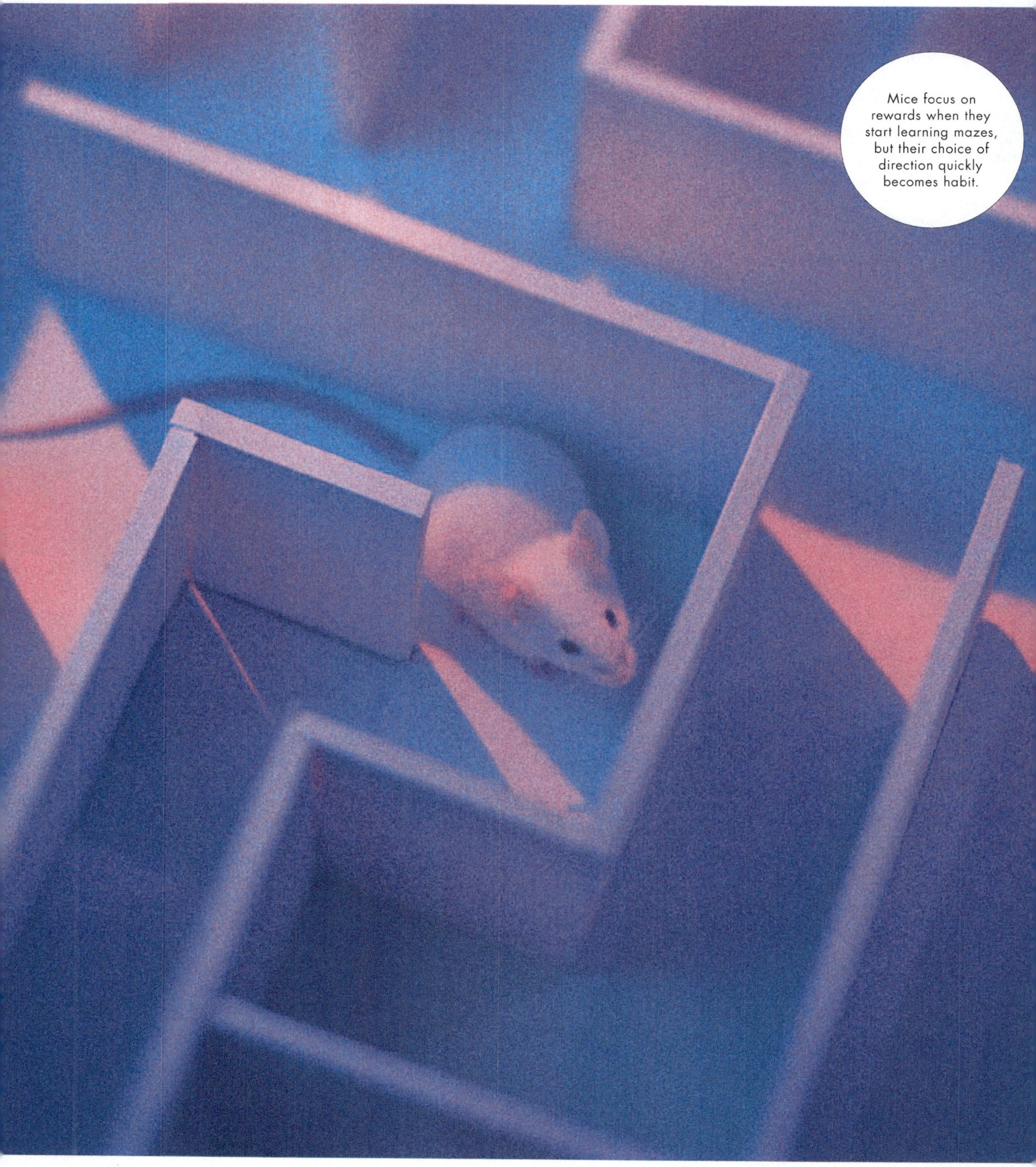

Mice focus on rewards when they start learning mazes, but their choice of direction quickly becomes habit.

responsible for planning, decision-making and evaluating rewards.

When we're working towards a goal, cells in the dorsolateral striatum light up. They talk to cells in the orbitofrontal cortex, the prelimbic cortex and the medial temporal lobe, working together to keep track of goals, weigh up rewards and adjust behaviour.

While these parts of the brain are active we always have the reward in mind, and the brain works hard to weigh up our chances of receiving it. The whole system depends on the brain's reward chemical, dopamine. But habits don't work that way.

If we keep repeating the same set of behaviours in the same situation and always get the same reward, the brain starts to take notice. When we can be relatively confident that the same set of actions will be just as good the 100th time as they were the first, it would be a waste of time to keep weighing up the evidence. So, the brain switches off the circuits involved in reward evaluation and gets right to performing the behaviour.

When we're performing a habit, it's the dorsomedial striatum that switches on. Rather than interacting with the parts of the brain responsible for conscious planning, the cells here talk directly to the basal ganglia and the motor cortex: areas involved in initiating movements. They don't pay attention to the brain's reward circuits at all.

Creating behaviour chunks

To make a sequence of complex behaviours into an automatic habit, the brain performs a technique called chunking. It takes the individual behaviours and sticks them together into blocks that it can play from start to finish without any conscious thought, and part of the process is visible in the cells of the striatum.

When we're first learning to respond to a trigger, the brain cells in the striatum fire all the time, but once we've learnt a behaviour and we're sure it'll always get a reward, this constant activity stops. Instead of a continuous pattern, the cells fire in a burst when the habit behaviour starts, and again when the habit behaviour finishes.

The researchers at MIT who discovered this behaviour think that the two bursts act like a set of start and stop signals to alert the rest of the brain that a habit is in progress. Meanwhile, other cells get to work to keep the rest of the striatum quiet. These cells, known as interneurons, switch other brain cells off, helping to stop them from triggering another habit routine before the first one is finished.

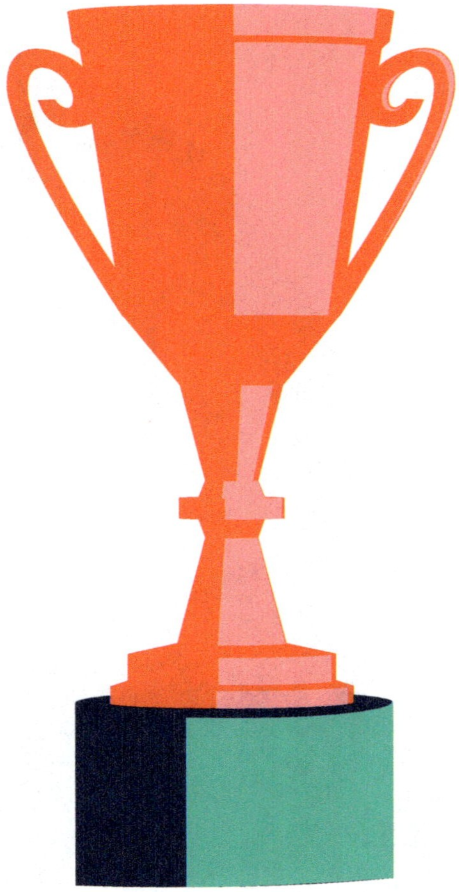

HACK YOUR HABITS

It takes three ingredients to form a habit: a trigger, a reward and lots of repetition

TRIGGER

To hack your own biology and make new habits stick faster, start with a trigger. Your brain needs a cue to set off a habit loop. If you're trying to learn to floss your teeth, put the floss next to your toothbrush for a strong visual sign that it's time to start your new routine.

REWARD

Although established habits are insensitive to rewards, they don't start out that way. You need to give your brain a reason to learn them. Long-term goals, like a clean bill of health at the dentist, are ok, but you might find that you need something more immediate to help get your habit off the ground. Try giving yourself a small reward each time you complete the behaviour to help reinforce the habit.

REPEAT

The trick to turning a goal into a habit is repetition; you need to train your brain to repeat the behaviour without thinking. Until then, there's always a risk that you'll decide the reward isn't worth it, and the habit won't stick. So, repeat the same sequence every day for at least two months. You might even be able to take the reward away once the habit is fixed.

Swapping habits

Anyone who has ever tried setting a New Year's resolution knows that habits can be hard to change. Yet it's not impossible. Although the brain wants to execute habits automatically, we do have the power to interrupt them and change our behaviour. Experiments on rats at MIT have revealed that this ability might depend on a part of the brain called the infralimbic cortex.

Researchers taught rats to turn left in a maze in return for a chocolate milkshake. Then, once the behaviour became a habit, they added a chemical to the milkshake to make the rats feel sick. The rats stopped drinking the milkshake, but they couldn't seem to stop themselves from turning left.

When the researchers interfered with the cells in the infralimbic cortex, the rats were able to change their behaviour. Instead of turning left automatically, they started to think about their decision. Over time, they learnt to turn right instead.

The researchers allowed this new behaviour to continue until it became a habit. Then they tried blocking the cells in the infralimbic cortex again. Unexpectedly, the rats didn't have to re-learn their old behaviour; they started turning left straight away. The old habit was still there inside their brains – all the cells in the infralimbic cortex had to do was switch it back on.

Why make habits if they are so hard to undo?

Habits might seem like a bad idea, but doing everything for a reward would be even worse. Goal-directed learning uses so much processing power that we'd struggle to get through the day if we had to weigh up every little choice. They might be hard to undo, but the fact that we can perform habits without thinking makes it worth the risk.

WORDS Laura Mears

IMAGE SOURCE Getty Images

Memory and retaining information

We take it for granted, but how do we retain and utilise information from our environment?

Memory is the capacity to store and retain information then recall it for use when needed. It is used by most organisms to operate in the most successful manner they possibly can in their unique environment.

There are three main types of memory: sensory, short-term and long-term, although long-term is often split into different types of memory. Sensory memory is a very short-term type of memory that is evoked through the senses. It lasts for a few seconds at most and is not stored.

Short-term memory is a slightly longer-lasting form – around 20 seconds. It's the recording of memories currently being used – i.e. remembering a number to dial in the next 30 seconds. If the information is repeated, however, it causes pathways to form between neurons in the brain and a phrenological loop to be created, causing a memory to be stored as a long-term memory. Unless this repeated firing of the neurons occurs, which is forced by repeating the information, a memory is lost.

When we cannot remember something, it's generally not because we are developing a degenerating brain disease like Alzheimer's – it's far more likely to be that the correct stimuli have not been presented to prompt retrieval of the memory, or that you did not register or retain the original information properly. For example, if you cannot

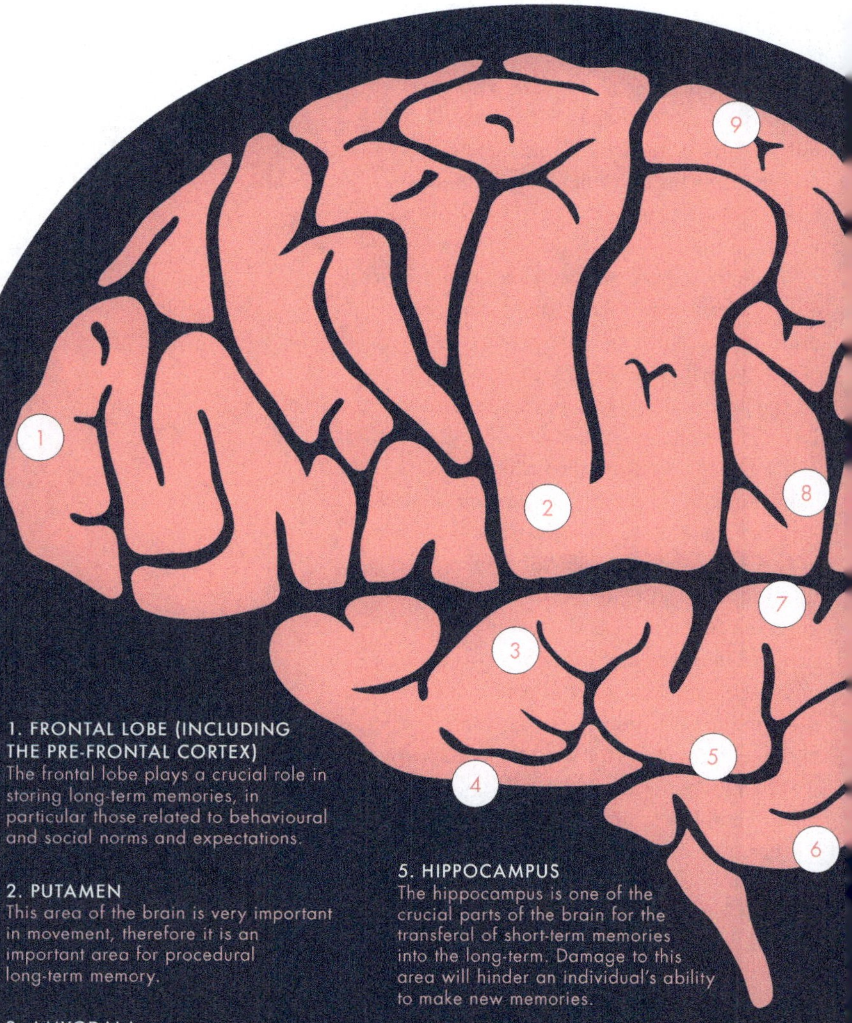

Areas in the brain that are used in memory

1. FRONTAL LOBE (INCLUDING THE PRE-FRONTAL CORTEX)
The frontal lobe plays a crucial role in storing long-term memories, in particular those related to behavioural and social norms and expectations.

2. PUTAMEN
This area of the brain is very important in movement, therefore it is an important area for procedural long-term memory.

3. AMYGDALA
These groups of nuclei play a very important role in the forming of emotional memory, such as reaction to fear.

4. TEMPORAL LOBE
This lobe of the brain primarily stores and processes auditory information and therefore plays a particularly important role in both speech and language. The hippocampus is situated within the temporal lobe.

5. HIPPOCAMPUS
The hippocampus is one of the crucial parts of the brain for the transferal of short-term memories into the long-term. Damage to this area will hinder an individual's ability to make new memories.

6. CEREBELLUM
This is a very important area in motor control and, to some extent, cognitive functions, including language. Damage to this area causes issues with movement, which can influence everything from balance to speaking and walking.

7. CAUDATE NUCLEUS
An important part of a human's memory system, this is linked to feedback processing and response and is thought to regulate activity inside the cerebral cortex.

8. THALAMUS
The thalamus helps to direct the brain's attention to experiences or events by sending signals to the cerebral cortex. It is important for sensation, motor skills and also helps to regulate sleep.

9. PARIETAL LOBE
This large area of the brain plays a crucial role in bringing together sensory information. It is particularly important for the processing of visual information and spatial awareness.

remember where you put your shoes when you took them off, it may be that you were not paying attention when you put them down and consequently have not transferred the memory from short-term to long-term in the first place, rather than having forgotten where they are.

As long as you have registered and retained the event, correct stimuli would cause a refiring of the neurons when creating the original memory, allowing successful retrieval of the information required.

Dependent on its type, a memory is stored in different areas of the brain. This helps people to store related information more easily, as it can be linked to previously stored related material.

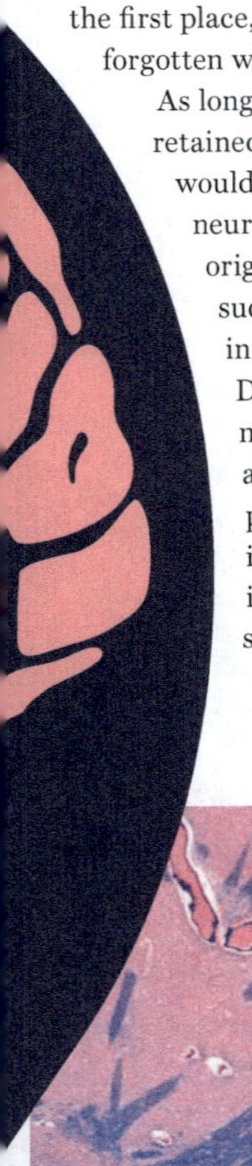

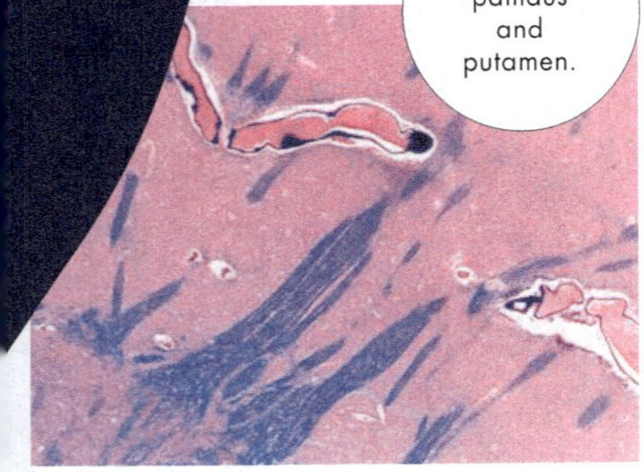

Globus pallidus and putamen.

TYPES OF MEMORY

The complex ways we remember...

SENSORY MEMORY

Sensory memory is evoked through the senses and is the initial perception of something. This is a fleeting memory and will not be transferred into short- or long-term memory unless we focus on remembering the event.

SHORT-TERM

This type of memory is stored temporarily for up to 20 seconds. It can, however, be confused with working memory, a separate type of memory that allows an individual to retain information only for long enough to, say, complete a sum. Unless information is repeated several times to establish a pathway between neurons it will decay and be lost.

LONG-TERM – PROCEDURAL (IMPLICIT)

This kind of long-term memory is how we remember to do things such as ride a bike. It is where we store our 'body' memories – our motor skills.

LONG-TERM – PROCEDURAL (IMPLICIT)

This kind of long-term memory is how we remember to do things such as ride a bike. It is where we store our 'body' memories – our motor skills.

LONG-TERM – DECLARATIVE (EXPLICIT)

This type of memory is how we store facts for retrieval and consists of things such as names and dates.

LONG-TERM – EPISODIC

This is where we store event-related memories and link them together. For example, if you went to a dinner party you wouldn't remember every moment, but you would recall a collection of events, smells and sounds that link together when you think of the overall event.

HOW DO WE STORE MEMORIES?

Memories are formed in our brains through electronic pulses passing between neurons. As neurons fire more than once, the pathway and link between the neurons strengthens; if the first neuron is triggered in the future, it is more likely that the others will too. Memories are stored in different areas of the brain, depending on what they are and what they are used for.

INPUT

The stimulus for a memory can be related or unrelated. For example, if you see a letterbox, you may remember you had a letter to post, therefore stimulating a memory through a related input. However, some people use unrelated stimuli, like a piece of string tied to their finger that they have formed an unrelated link to something else with.

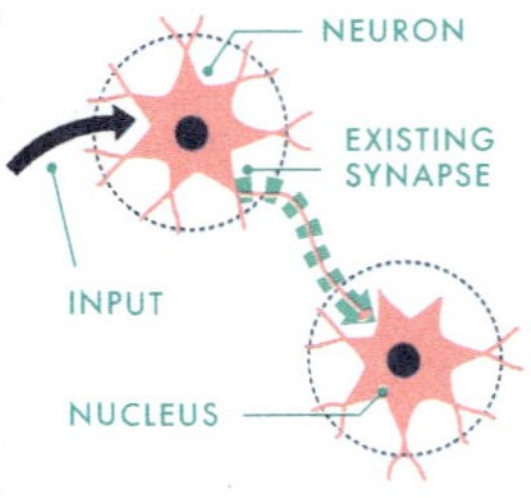

CIRCUIT FORMATION

As a memory is being formed, certain neurons will link together in a circuit to store this memory. It will link related memories, and repetition of this circuit firing will strengthen the memory. This is called a phrenological loop.

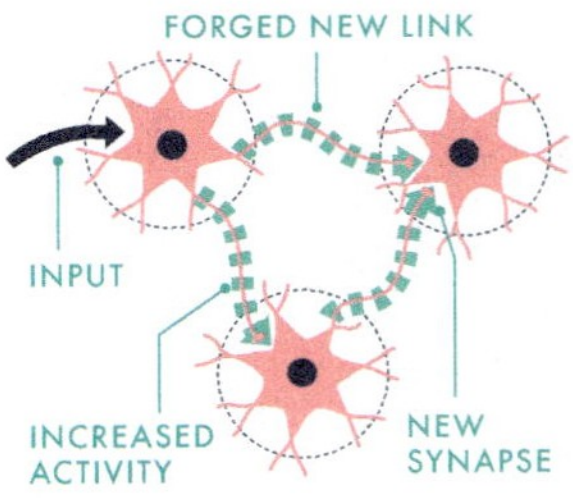

INCREASING ACTIVITY

Repeated firing of the neurons involved in the first memory formation will strengthen the memory, as the neuron pathway becomes stronger.

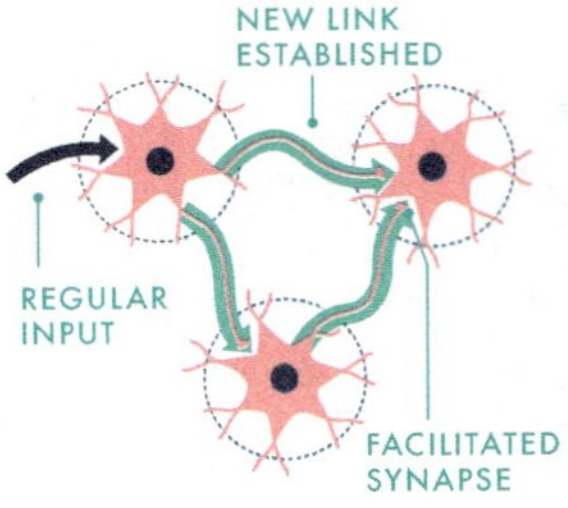

HOW WE FORM AND STORE LONG-TERM MEMORIES

The time it takes for a memory to really stick

ATTENTION 0.2 SECS
If something grabs our attention we're far more likely to remember it. Neurons fire as we continue to focus, ensuring a memory moves from short-term to long-term. The thalamus plays a big role in directing attention.

→

EMOTION 0.25 SECS
Events or things that cause an emotional response are more likely to be remembered because they activate raised levels of activity in the amygdala, and this arousal means more information is taken in and processed.

→

SENSATION 0.2–0.5 SECS
Sensory memory is based on receiving information from our senses – i.e. sight, smell, touch. The lingering feeling you have after someone touches your arm is the sensory memory fading, and this first information from the senses is the starting point for any memory.

↓

WORKING MEMORY 0.5 SECS–10 MINS
Working memory is when information is briefly stored in order to be used in the immediate future. It lasts for a few seconds or so, but if repetition occurs, refreshing the time limit in which it can survive, it will be retained and can move into short- or long-term.

←

HIPPOCAMPAL PROCESSING 10 MINS–2 YRS
If we need to retain a piece of information, or it particularly strikes us, it will travel from the short-term memory, based in the pre-frontal cortex, to the hippocampus, where it is processed and can move into the long-term memory.

←

CONSOLIDATION 2 YRS +
If you use a piece of information repeatedly, the links between the neurons remain strong. These are likely to stay in place for a long time. Repetition and reuse enables the pathways to remain in place and the memory to stay in the brain.

IMAGE SOURCE Getty Images

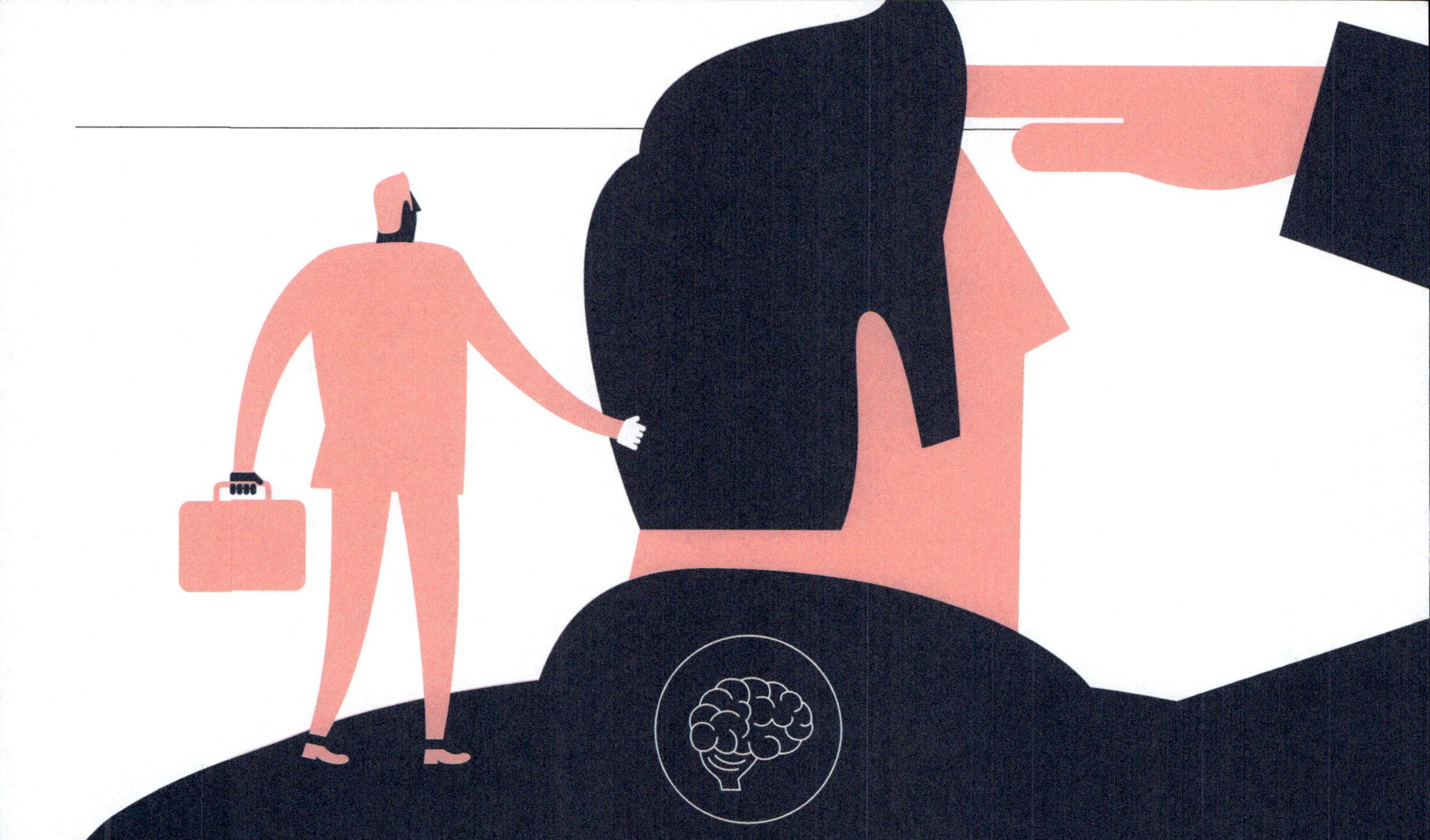

Anticipatory timing

The process that allows your brain to predict the future

The brain is a powerful learning machine; it has the ability to learn from previous experiences in order to 'predict' future events. This is known as anticipatory timing and it is what enables humans to successfully navigate the world that we live in and also plays a key role in helping us to concentrate. But how does the brain do this?

Researchers think two different regions are responsible for its ability to 'predict' the future. These regions are known as the basal ganglia, a group of structures that are found deep within the cerebral hemisphere, and the cerebellum, which is located at the back of the brain. Both structures are associated with cognition and movement.

The basal ganglia is associated with tasks that involve rhythm – such as singing along to your favourite song – while the cerebellum is connected to past memories – for example, being able to predict when a traffic light will change from red to green. The researchers also found that if one of these areas becomes damaged, the other region has the ability to compensate, and this is important in understanding neurodegenerative disorders such as Parkinson's disease. This research challenges previous theories that suggested a single brain system was responsible for all our timing needs.

Most notably, the ability to predict the future is essential for professional athletes – it takes longer to execute a swing than the time a batter has to view the ball travelling towards them.

Furthermore, researchers in another study found that the brain could predict events twice as fast as they actually occurred in real-time. This ability to predict the future could be the reason for the immense success – and stubborn survival – of our species, as we are able to predict the possible consequences of an action.

WORDS Baljeet Panesar

BUILT FOR SPORT

Not only are athletes' bodies finely tuned machines, but their minds are too

In the professional sporting world, the speed and precision with which athletes make decisions can be the difference between success and failure. But it's not just their bodies that are built for sport – it's their brains too. Studies suggest that some areas of athletes' brains are larger than those of their less-able counterparts.

Researchers at the Chinese Academy of Sciences compared the brains of professional divers with those who did not participate in professional training. The researchers found that three regions – the left superior temporal sulcus, the right orbitofrontal cortex and the right parahippocampal gyrus – of the professional divers' brains were significantly thicker than the non-athlete group.

Another study revealed that professional cricket players were more able to accurately predict the trajectory of the ball significantly earlier and with greater accuracy than the non-professional players – a skill that is vital for success in a match and one that has also been demonstrated in other ball sports, including basketball, football, tennis and hockey.

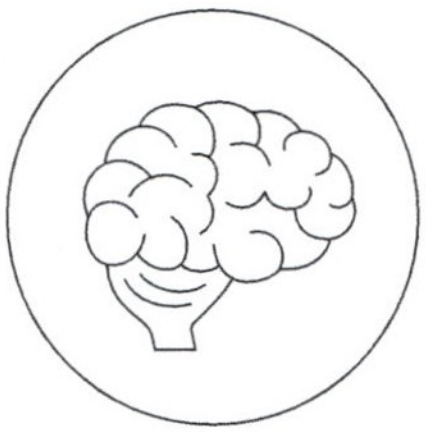

The science of making decisions

To do, or not to do?

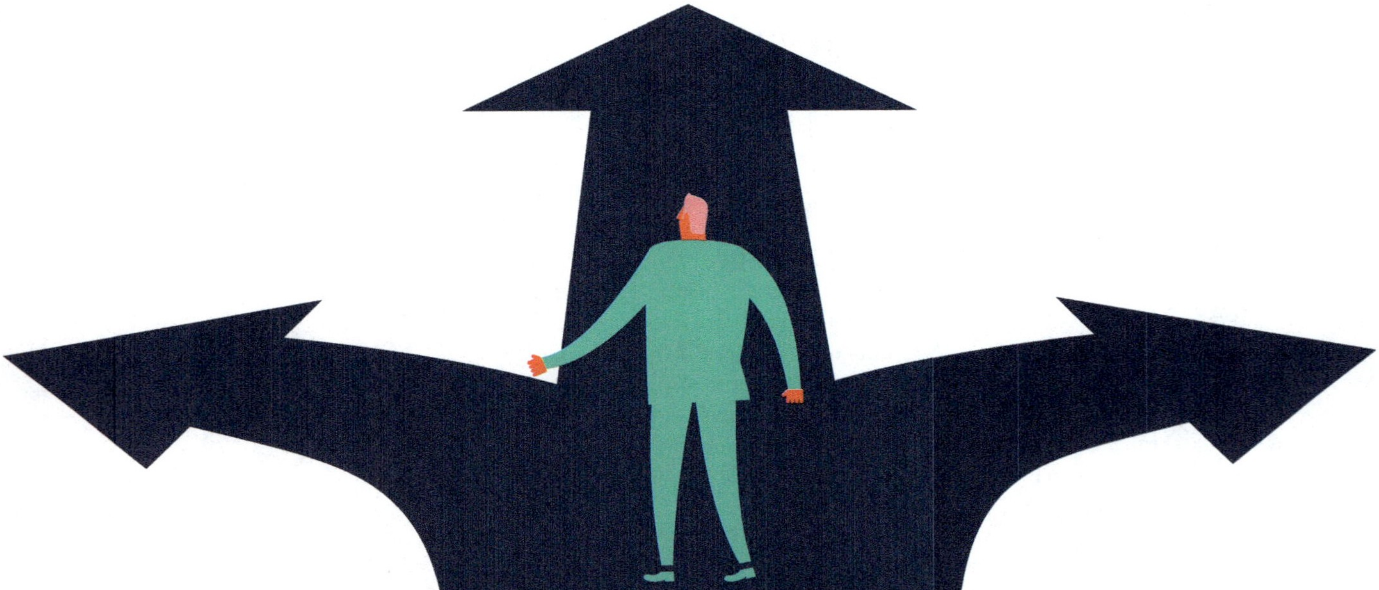

We make hundreds of decisions every day; some are trivial, like deciding what to eat for breakfast, others are more complicated – and have consequences – such as deciding whether or not to apply for that job. Making a decision is one of the most essential human behaviours, but just how does the brain make a decision?

Decision-making is a complex process, and although it has been studied for years, it is a process that we only partially understand. What we do know is that there's not one single decision-making region of the brain but rather various brain regions – including the anterior cingulate cortex, orbitofrontal cortex (a region in the prefrontal cortex) and ventromedial prefrontal cortex – that work together to make a decision. Scientists think that the ability to stop or modify a decision is controlled by two individual locations within the prefrontal cortex and the frontal eye field that requires ultrafast communication between the two areas. It's also thought that emotions may play a role in decision-making.

It has long been suspected that injuries or damage to the anterior cingulate cortex or ventromedial prefrontal cortex can affect a person's ability to make decisions. In 1848, American railway worker Phineas Gage suffered a severe brain injury when a metre-long iron rod was impaled through his skull. Although Gage survived, he experienced major changes in his behaviour and personality, and since then it has been thought the orbitofrontal cortex plays a key role in decision-making.

In a 2004 study, researchers found that different areas of the brain are active depending on whether participants were told to do something or were able to exercise autonomy. Another study found the brain is less able to make important decisions later on in the day as a means of conserving energy.

WORDS Baljeet Panesar

IS FREE WILL JUST AN ILLUSION?

How the brain makes its mind up before you even realise

We believe that we must first have a thought to which we then respond. But in the 1980s the American scientist Benjamin Libet performed an experiment that suggested that the brain shows electrical activity before a conscious decision is made. The results of this experiment proved controversial, and the method was further developed by Professor John-Dylan Haynes from the Max Planck Institute for Human Cognitive and Brain Science in Leipzig, Germany.

Haynes' research team asked 14 volunteers to complete a decision-making task. The task was to press one of two buttons with either their right or left hand, but they had to remember when they made their decision. The researchers found that it was possible to predict the volunteers' decisions by monitoring brain activity in the frontopolar cortex up to seven seconds before – possibly ten seconds before due to the delay in imaging – they reported their decision. Other studies since have also produced similar results, all of which raise some very interesting questions about the concept of free will and whether we truly are in control of our decisions.

IMAGE SOURCE Getty Images

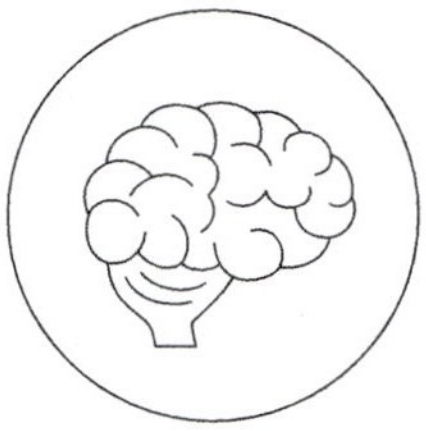

The curious cases of Henry and Eugene

Meet the two patients who revolutionised our understanding of memory and habits

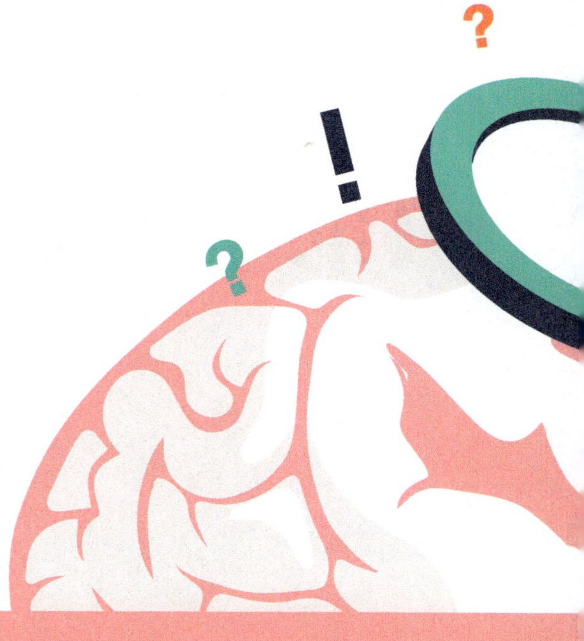

Neuroscience research relies on patients with existing brain damage to provide an insight into the workings of the brain. This reliance is largely because ethical guidelines understandably prevent scientists from manipulating live human brains in order to carry out experiments. However, guidelines haven't always been so strict, and lobotomies – removing chunks of the front of patients' brains to 'treat' mental health conditions – were rife until as recently as the mid-20th century. A similar procedure termed a lobectomy also exists, which is the removal of a lobe of a diseased organ. These used to be performed on the brain but are now usually restricted to the lungs. A misguided brain lobectomy removed the medial temporal lobe of a patient known as H.M., who was later revealed to be a young man by the name of Henry Molaison.

Brain damage can also occur naturally through viral infections such as encephalitis, where a virus spreads from the body into the brain, causing inflammation and the destruction of brain cells. This happened to patient E.P. (Eugene Pauly) and resulted in the loss of his medial temporal lobe. The medial temporal lobe is a collection of brain structures located in the centre of the brain. It includes the hippocampus, entorhinal and perirhinal cortices, amygdala and subicular complex, which work together to process new information and combine it into memories.

Henry Molaison

Henry was diagnosed with a form of epilepsy occurring in the temporal lobe after being hit by a bike at the age of seven. His condition was managed by a cocktail of anti-epileptic medications that allowed him to live a normal life at his home in Connecticut, US. However, his epilepsy gradually worsened throughout adolescence until, at the age of 27, his seizures were so disruptive that he was forced to give up his work on an assembly line. It was then, in September 1953, that Henry sought the drastic medical intervention that was to change his life forever.

Without the complex tools we have today, such as MRI scanners, which allow doctors to peer inside the body, Henry's surgeon, Dr Scoville, removed a 54.5mm-long area on the left side of his brain and a 44mm-long portion on the right: his medial temporal lobe.

Without his medial temporal lobe, Henry's epilepsy was partially alleviated, but the operation was not wholly successful, as he still required anti-epileptic medication. He was also left with severe amnesia, a form of memory loss that can present in different ways. For Henry, this meant he was unable to form new memories after the operation (retrograde amnesia) and had forgotten memories he had formed in the couple of years immediately before his

> "HENRY WOULD FORGET HE'D EATEN HIS BACON ROLL IN THE MORNING AND REPEAT THE TASK, RESULTING IN HIM EATING UP TO FOUR FOR BREAKFAST"

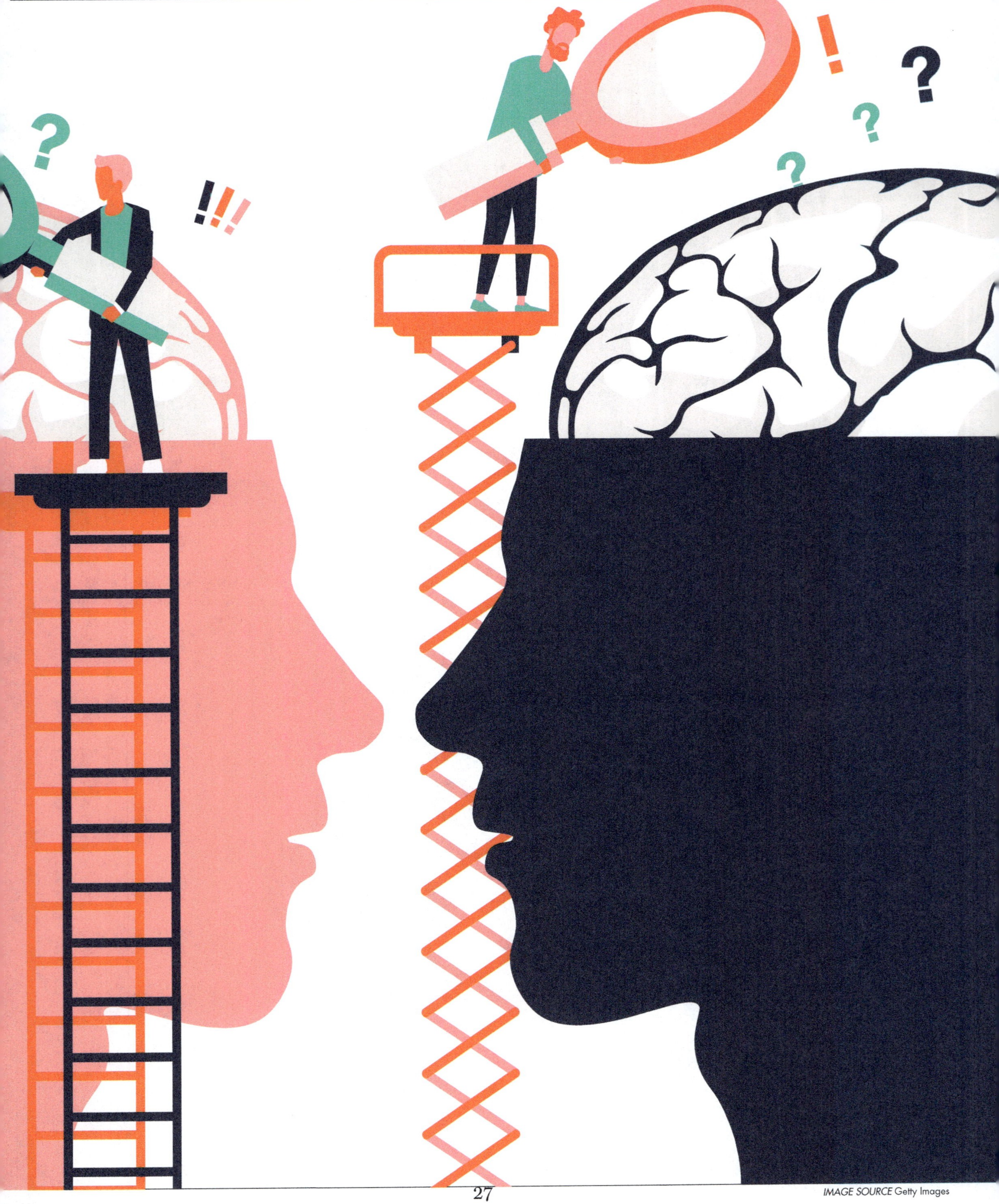

IMAGE SOURCE Getty Images

operation (partial anterograde amnesia). Over his life, there was an increase in the number of years prior to the operation that he could no longer remember.

Eugene Pauly

Eugene was born in 1922 and grew up in California, US, eventually leaving home to become a radio operator for an oil company at sea. Upon his return he worked as an aerospace technician. By 1992 he was enjoying a peaceful retirement with his wife when he suddenly contracted viral encephalitis – a virus spreading to his brain. The virus destroyed his medial temporal lobe and caused damage to areas in the wider temporal lobe by severing connections between brain cells. His resulting amnesia mirrored that of Henry Molaison, but the damage extending outwards through the temporal lobe also cost him his sense of smell, impaired his semantic knowledge and caused anterograde amnesia stretching back up to 50 years.

The word 'semantic' is defined as relating to meaning in language or logic, so semantic knowledge is an understanding of language and how it works, and semantic memory is remembering language, such as the names of objects. The logic aspect was tested by asking Eugene to identify and explain ambiguous sentences. Eugene performed worse on these tasks than 'control' participants (who had no brain damage), whereas Henry did not have any problems. This extra impairment for Eugene was due to the damage inflicted on his lateral temporal lobe, which Henry did not experience. Yet despite this slight difference in the areas damaged, the two displayed many similarities.

Similarities

Although the damage to their brains had been caused by very different circumstances, both men were left without medial temporal lobes. Therefore, neither Eugene nor Henry could form new memories, meaning they forgot events almost instantly. Forgotten events included every new occurrence, from meeting someone new to eating breakfast. In fact, Henry encountered health problems because he would forget he'd eaten his bacon roll in the morning and repeat the task, resulting in him eating up to four of them for breakfast a day.

THE BASAL GANGLIA

The brain area Eugene and Henry used to learn new skills is formed of these parts:

DORSAL STRIATUM
Made of the caudate nucleus and putamen, this is important for planning, carrying out and automating motor behaviour dependent on energy required and potential reward. This processing contributes to its role in forming habits and addiction.

VENTRAL STRIATUM
Containing the nucleus accumbens and olfactory tubercle, it evaluates risks/gains of behaviours.

GLOBUS PALLIDUS
This helps regulate movement, motivation, reward, aversion and control of actions and goals.

VENTRAL PALLIDUM
This receives strong signals from the brain's emotional circuits to govern reward and motivation behaviour and produce motor outputs.

SUBSTANTIA NIGRA
This is important for regulating movement, and it receives information from the striatum directly and via the globus pallidus. It is the site of damage in Parkinson's disease.

SUBTHALAMIC NUCLEUS
This region of the brain is involved in making difficult decisions, plus some motor functions. It combines cognitive (thinking), emotional information and motor processes into an output.

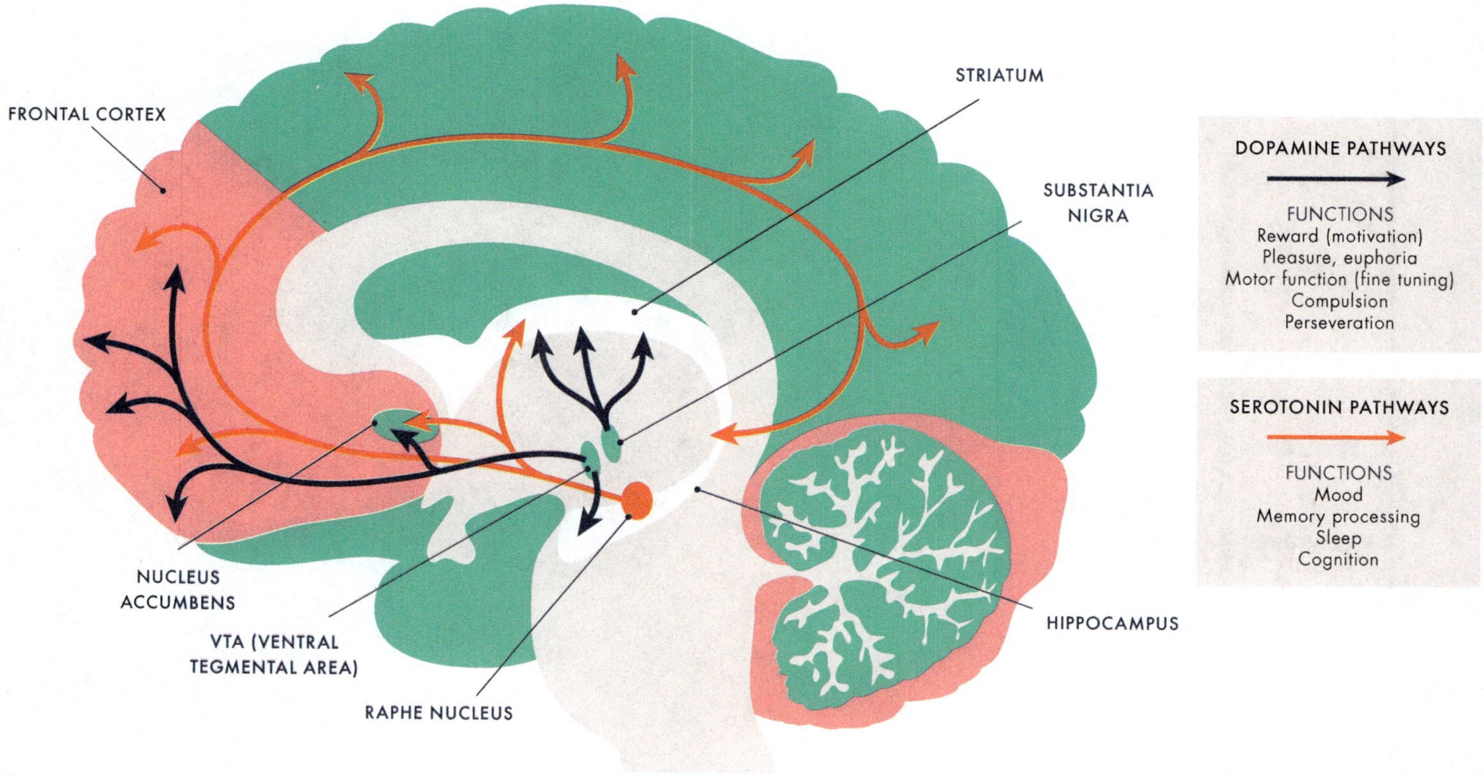

Eugene would also sometimes have multiple breakfasts as it was part of his learnt morning routine, which he would forget he had already done.

The men's amnesia meant they were both confined to the present tense, frozen in a snapshot in time and permanently identifying themselves as being younger than they actually were. They would forget people as soon as they had been introduced and repeat statements they had just uttered as if it were the first time they were saying them. However, both men had normal intellectual and cognitive function aside from their memory issues. Although both remained anonymous for most of their lives, they were very willing to participate in research. The research, which provided a rare insight into how memory works, was initiated with Henry by PhD student Brenda Milner. Following this, more patients with medial temporal lobe damage, like Eugene, were thoroughly analysed by neuroscientist Larry Squire. This intensive research revealed some very specific learning tasks that rely on areas other than the medial temporal lobe.

An alternative form of memory

This potential for learning demonstrates humans have distinct types of memory – declarative and nondeclarative. Researchers have since further classified these into more descriptive subtypes, but Henry and Eugene were pivotal in revealing these two initial distinctions. Declarative memory is the conscious ability to recall facts and events and is processed by the medial temporal lobe. Nondeclarative memory is unconscious and describes things such as motor skills, conditioning and habits. Due to their medial temporal lobe damage, it is declarative memory that Henry and Eugene lacked, but thorough and careful testing revealed their capacity for nondeclarative learning in spite of their injuries.

One such experiment was a memory task where two picture cards were presented to the participants (people with medial temporal lobe damage – also termed amnesiacs – and 'control' participants) in pairs. One card in the pair had 'correct' written on the back. The task was for the subjects to select the 'correct' card of the pair.

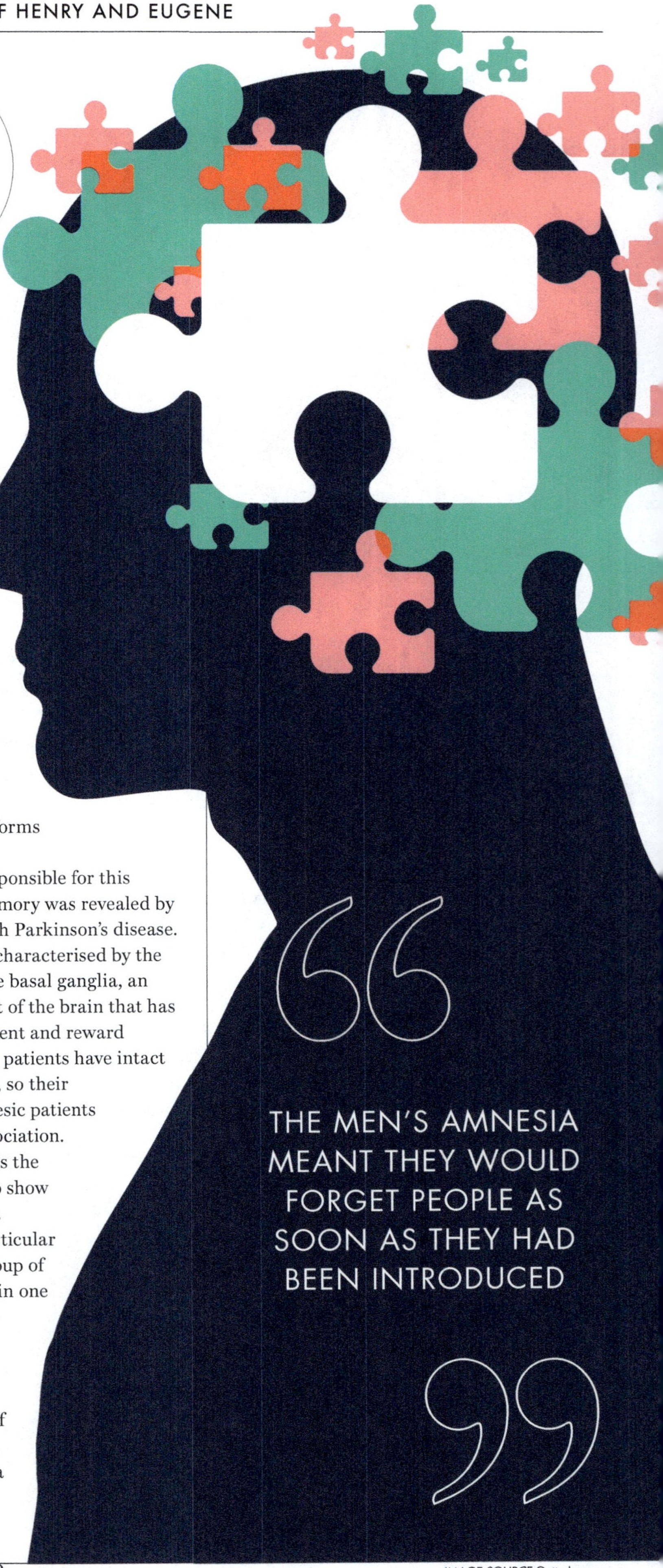

A piece of Henry and Eugene's brains was missing, due to very different circumstances.

The cards were always presented in the same pairs and the same card was always 'correct', so a pattern could be identified and memorised. The amnesic patients were able to memorise this task, albeit more slowly than the controls. This suggested that they were learning the task using a part of the brain other than the medial temporal lobe, which had previously been attributed to all forms of memory.

The brain region responsible for this alternative form of memory was revealed by a group of patients with Parkinson's disease. Parkinson's disease is characterised by the death of neurons in the basal ganglia, an evolutionarily 'old' part of the brain that has roles including movement and reward behaviour. Parkinson's patients have intact medial temporal lobes, so their comparison with amnesic patients presents a double dissociation. A double dissociation is the most conclusive way to show a particular brain area is responsible for a particular task. It compares a group of patients with damage in one area and an otherwise healthy brain with another group with damage to a different area but healthy rest of the brain. In this case, amnesic patients had a healthy basal ganglia

> "THE MEN'S AMNESIA MEANT THEY WOULD FORGET PEOPLE AS SOON AS THEY HAD BEEN INTRODUCED"

IMAGE SOURCE Getty Images

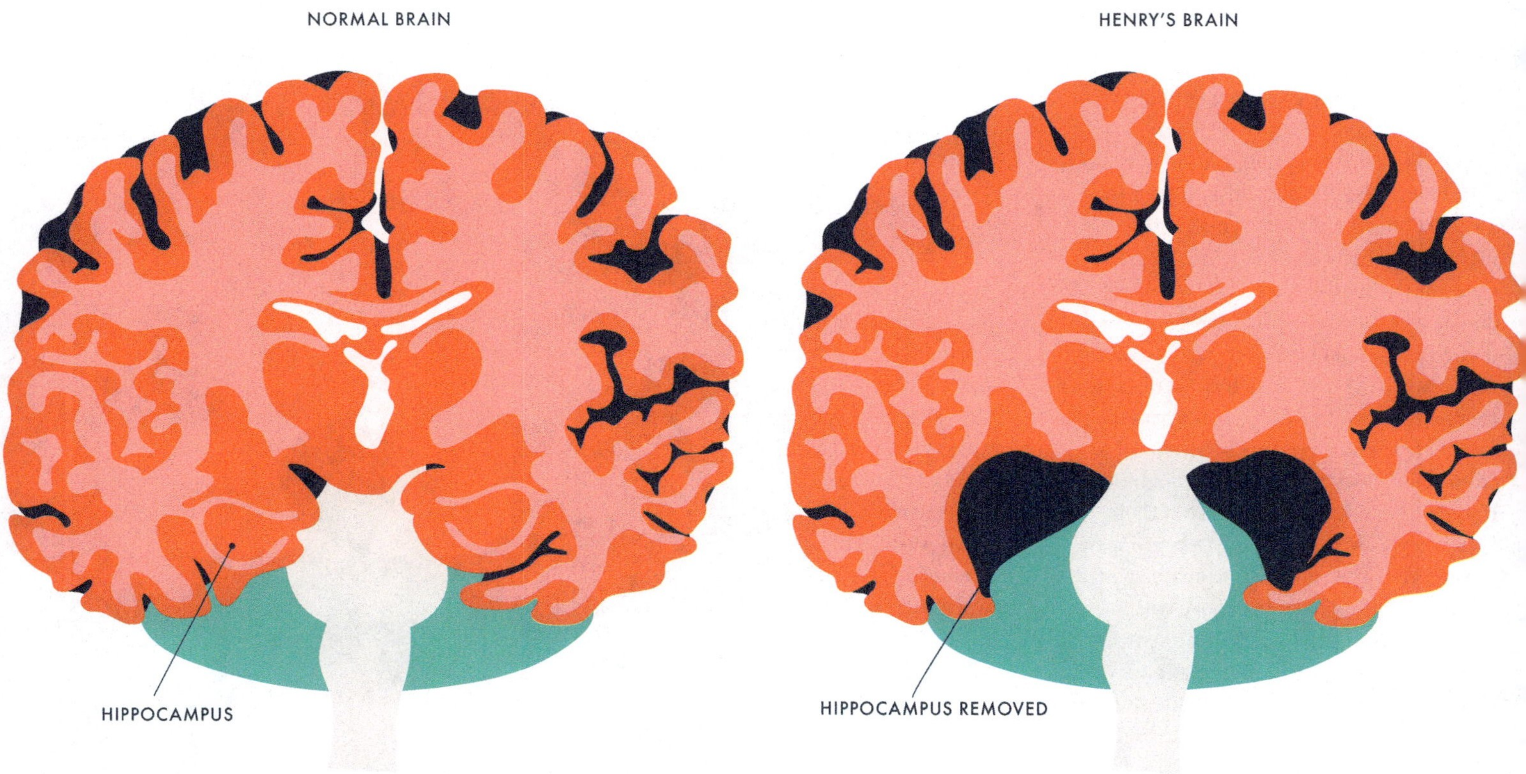

but damaged medial temporal lobe, while Parkinson's patients had a healthy medial temporal lobe but damaged basal ganglia. The Parkinson's patients were able to perform tasks that tested their declarative memory but not tasks like the card-pairing task, which tested their nondeclarative memory. Conversely, amnesic patients performed well in the nondeclarative tasks but not the declarative tasks. Therefore, scientists concluded that the medial temporal lobe is in charge of declarative memory, while the basal ganglia is responsible for nondeclarative memory.

Habitual learning

The nondeclarative memory of the basal ganglia is underpinned by a gradual process called habitual learning. This has now been shown in rats to occur in the neostriatum within the basal ganglia and is guided by the reward system. The reward system relies on chemical signals from the neurotransmitter dopamine. A habit is formed when an individual receives a reward for a certain behaviour that triggers a release of dopamine in the basal ganglia, motivating them to do it again. In animal models, this reward is usually a piece of food, but it can be anything, such as the human participants seeing the word 'correct' and being congratulated by the experimenter when they turn over the right picture card.

> EUGENE WAS ABLE TO GO TO HIS KITCHEN TO GET FOOD, AS THE FOOD WAS THE REWARD, BUT WAS NOT ABLE TO RECOUNT WHERE THE KITCHEN WAS WHEN ASKED

These subtle rewards are how the amnesic patients Henry and Eugene developed habits in their daily lives following their brain injuries. The rewards become the goal and create the motivation to perform the goal-driven behaviour over and over until it becomes a learnt, subconscious habit. For example, Eugene was able to go to his kitchen to get food when he was hungry, as the food was the reward, but he was not able to recount where the kitchen was when asked, as this yielded no reward. Similarly, he learnt a specific route near his home where he would go for a daily walk and find his way home again, despite not being able to consciously identify which house was his.

The key to habitual learning is the cues remaining identical. If a tree or roadworks blocked his path, Eugene would be utterly lost and unable to navigate home because the habit had been disrupted. Similarly, if the picture cards were presented in different pairs or all together, the amnesic patients were unable to identify the 'correct' cards. Sudden changes totally threw them.

Another example are the behavioural changes Eugene showed over the 14 years he was studied. When experimenters first visited him he was hostile and reluctant to be tested, requiring persuasion from his wife. However, after several years of the same researchers visiting him, he greeted them warmly and instinctively went to the table he was usually tested at, even without his wife's presence. Interestingly, he still denied ever having met them or taking part in these tests before. This change in behaviour illustrates habitual learning by Eugene subconsciously and gradually over several years as a result of regular occurrences in a specific environmental context. Therefore, habitual learning is a very specific form of learning that is intrinsically dependent on ritual and repetition.

Repetition also comprised another form of memory Henry and Eugene were able to exhibit: working – or immediate – memory. Through repeating a string of numbers, they could retain the sequence in their minds for up to 20 seconds. However, if their attention was drawn elsewhere they would instantly forget they had even been tasked with remembering numbers. This demonstrated that this working memory was being stored temporarily in an area other than the medial temporal lobe. Research into attention and working memory has pointed to the involvement of several regions, from the prefrontal cortex to areas deep within the brain.

All of these different forms of memory that Henry and Eugene retained show just how complex and nuanced a process memory is. They provided an invaluable insight into the brain's ability to find novel ways to function when the ordinary route is blocked. This incredible ability was cemented by the fact that Henry lived a relatively functional life for 55 years without a medial temporal lobe. Both men's incredible brains are now stored at the Brain Observatory in San Diego, US, and continue to contribute to neuroscientific knowledge to this day.

WORDS Josie Clarkson

THE MEDIAL TEMPORAL LOBE

Eugene and Henry's medial temporal lobes were both destroyed. This part of the brain is responsible for learning and temporary storage of memory and is comprised of the following:

HIPPOCAMPUS

Derived from the Greek for 'seahorse', the hippocampus is responsible for learning and making new spatial (mental maps) and declarative (facts and events) memories. It also links to the emotional centres contributing past experiences to current emotional events.

PARAHIPPOCAMPAL CORTEX

This area is responsible for episodic memory (personal experience) and visuospatial processing (navigating through a scene). These combine into contextual associations, i.e. using context and previous experiences to make sense of surroundings.

AMYGDALA

This combines information to produce emotional responses. It uses emotion to deduce the attractiveness or aversiveness of something.

ENTORHINAL CORTEX

This section consolidates memory with regards to sensory information by two-way communication with the hippocampus.

PERIRHINAL CORTEX

The function of this region is sensory perception that enables an individual to recognise and memorise objects. It transmits sensory information to and from the hippocampus via the entorhinal cortex.

SUBICULAR COMPLEX

With its name taken from the Latin for 'support', the subicular complex receives and processes input from other brain areas, e.g. it amplifies signals from the hippocampus. The front of the subiculum mainly processes memory, movement and spatial information, while the back can soften the body's stress response.

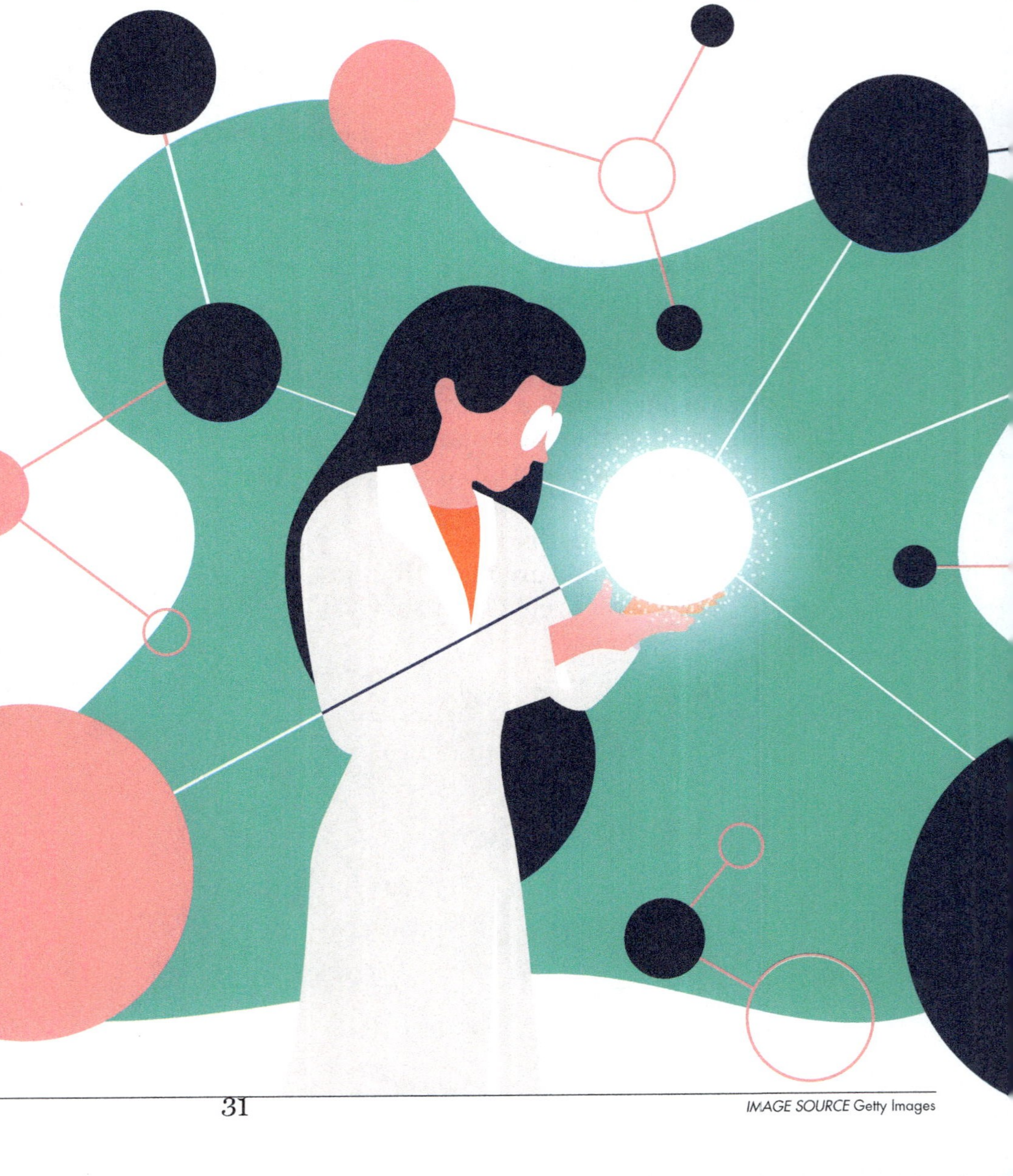

IMAGE SOURCE Getty Images

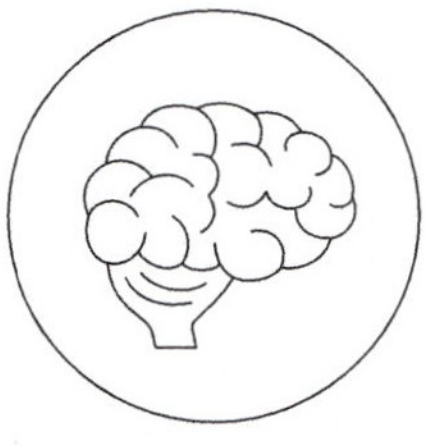

Learning good habits

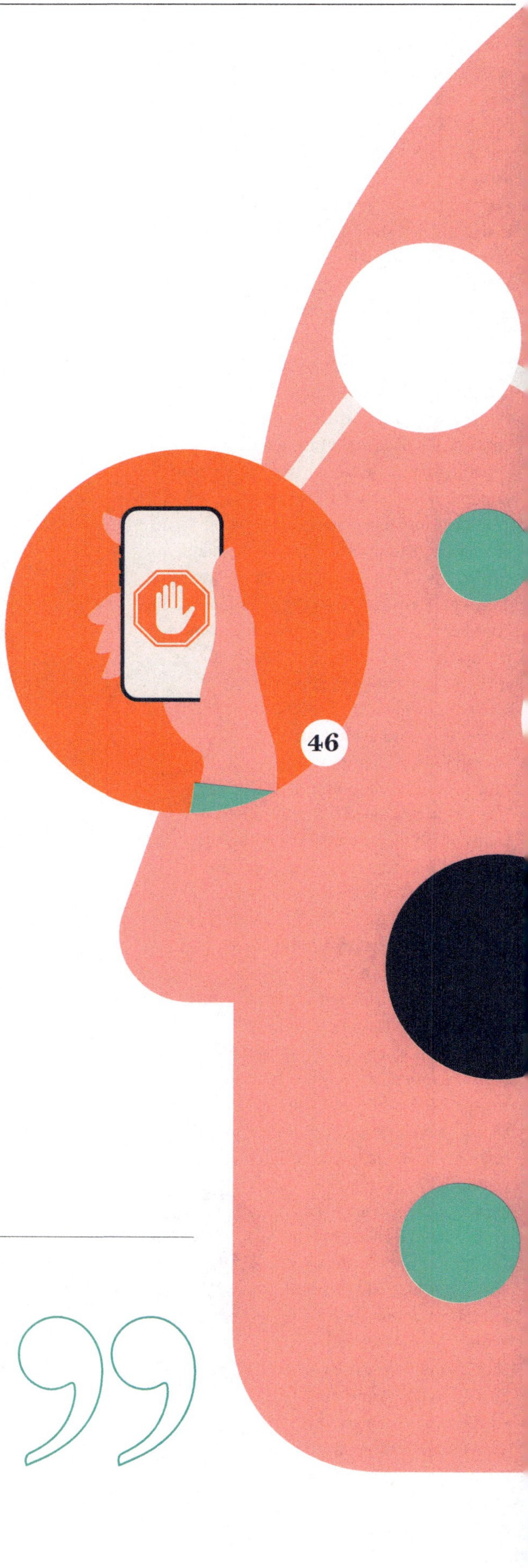

EVEN OUR POLITICAL BELIEFS CAN BE PARTIALLY HERITABLE... VOTING TURNOUT MAY ACTUALLY BE DUE TO ANCIENT GENETIC CONTROLS OF BEHAVIOUR

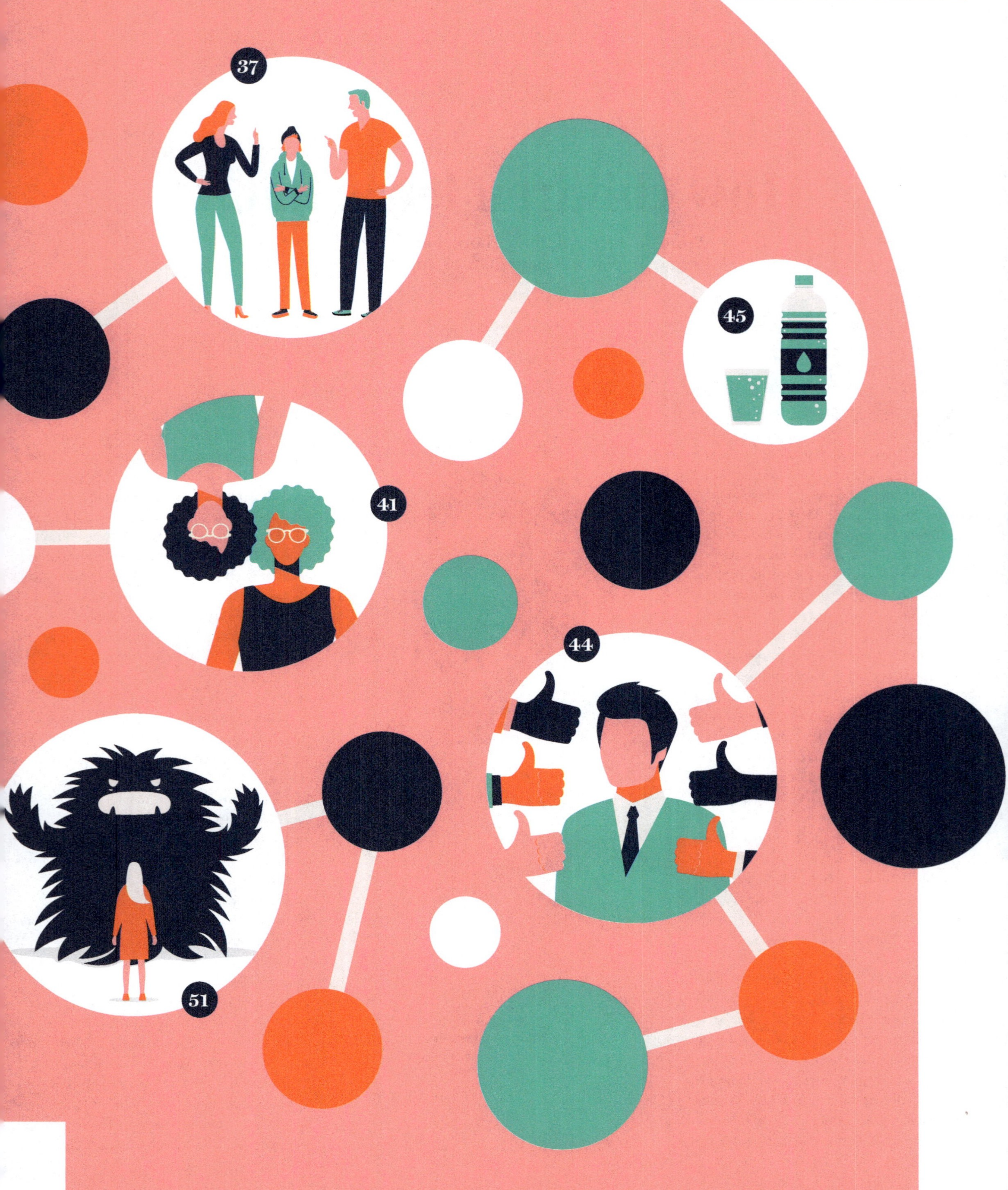
37
45
41
44
51

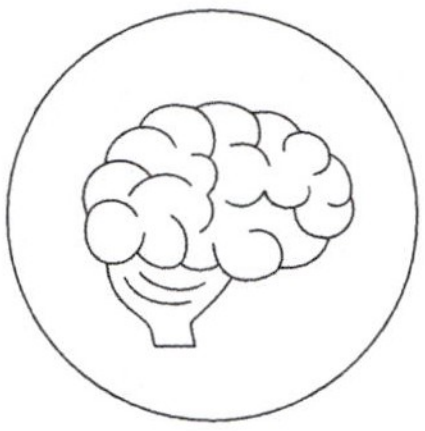

How children learn habits

From the moment they're born, babies begin to store information that will contribute to their habits later in life

Neuroscientists believe that many of the cognitive functions needed for thought and learning are already present and working when a baby is born, or develop in their first years. From birth, children have the ability to recognise patterns and regular occurrences – recognising these patterns, organising things into categories in the mind and applying the information to new situations is known as inductive learning. Inductive learning allows children to use the things they see and hear to make sense of situations and take on unfamiliar challenges.

As babies grow, learn and observe, they begin to understand how the world around them works and how they should act in particular situations. With each new piece of information, connections form between the neurons – nerve cells – in their brains to try and make sense of it all. An infant's brain grows rapidly, increasing in size fourfold in the first five years of life. Connections are strengthened and thoughts are organised more logically when inductive learning happens through experience rather than instruction from someone else.

Very young children have little control over their emotions and impulses; while the foundations and the information begin to accumulate early on, it takes several years for children to make conscious decisions about the way they react to – and learn from – events. Experts have identified three key components needed for self-control: working memory, inhibition and attentional flexibility.

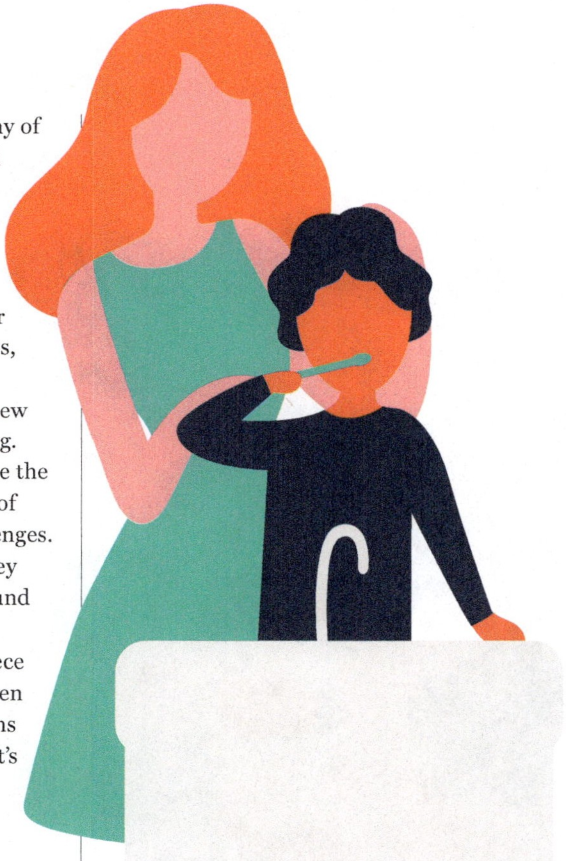

A child who knows their behaviour is being monitored is more likely to stick with a good habit.

Working memory is the ability to temporarily hold information in the mind while it's being processed or used. Inhibition is the ability to suppress natural responses, overriding an instinct or desire and choosing a different reaction. Attentional flexibility is the capacity to switch focus between objects, tasks or thoughts. Together, these components give young children the self-control and cognitive functions they need to learn, plan and make choices. They are constantly developing, but inhibition and attentional flexibility usually improve rapidly between the ages of three and four. Motivating factors like improving skills, impressing peers and receiving praise can all impact how much a child regulates their instincts. Bad habits like nail biting, hair twirling and body rocking often occur when a child is feeling stressed, bored, nervous or overwhelmed; these behaviours can help children soothe themselves, or they may occur because a child's brain is so busy processing other things that their self-control is weakened.

Like many young animals, babies and children learn a great deal through imitation. Trial and error can lead to important discoveries and stronger neural connections, but following the example of someone more experienced is less risky. Despite being safer, imitation is no easier; it takes a great deal of thought to copy the movements and behaviour of another person. Scientists have found evidence of a 'mirror neuron system' that stimulates the same nerve cells when a person is observing an action as when they're trying it themselves. It's through imitation that

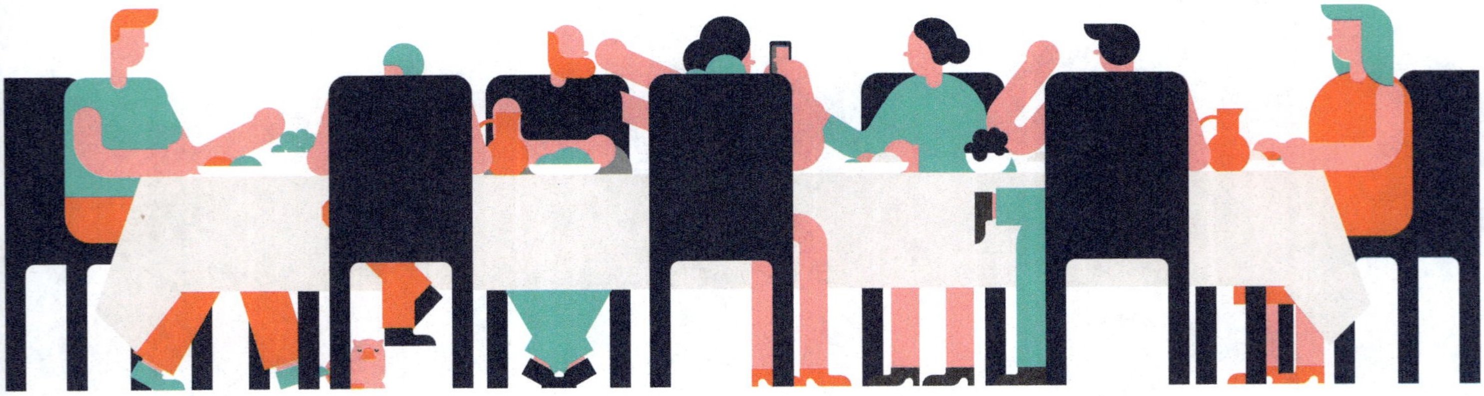

children learn important communication skills like facial expressions and speech, which is why children have accents similar to those with whom they spend the most time.

As children develop more sophisticated cognition, they're able to carry out tasks more efficiently. Activities like walking initially take a great deal of effort and concentration but gradually become easier and more automatic. With so much to process and think about, automating certain actions, reactions and behaviours saves brain power. In this way habits begin to form as children process more information subconsciously. A child's reactions and habits depend on many factors including their personality, confidence, level of interest and previous knowledge.

As the people they usually spend the most time around, parents and other caregivers have an enormous influence on the development of children. Parental style (how authoritative, responsive, indulgent and emotional caregivers are with their children) and parenting practices (specific actions and behaviours caregivers use to teach and interact with their children) determine how children see the world, themselves and their relationships with others. Whether consciously or not, parents and other caregivers reinforce certain habits in children and dissuade them from others. Responding to positive behaviours with praise and rewards forms stronger connections in the brain and makes the child more likely to repeat them, but bad habits can also be reinforced if they result in the child getting attention.

TAKING ROOT

Certain habits and attitudes become 'fixed' when children are as young as nine

A 2014 study of household chores by Brown University revealed that certain routines and habits are ingrained by the age of nine. The survey of almost 50,000 families in America found that habits relating to the home were unlikely to change after this age, with children completing the same chores with the same attitude right up until the end of high school.

Dr. Robert Pressman, Director of Research for the New England Center for Pediatric Psychology and lead researcher on the study, says that parents hoping their children will gradually take on more responsibility by themselves are likely to be disappointed. Caregivers should introduce the chores they want their children to be involved with as early as they're able to attempt them safely. Crucially, they must resist the urge to correct or take over if a child does a job 'wrong'; by attempting and failing, children find solutions for themselves rather than learning that it's easy to get out of helping.

As well as subconsciously learning from adults through mimicking, children choose to follow adults when they want to behave like grown-ups. A child receiving pocket money, for example, might save it in a piggy bank because it pleases their parents and seems like a grown-up thing to do, even if they haven't fully grasped the idea of savings yet and really want to spend it immediately. This requires self-control and the delay of gratification, which involve complex thought and can only be utilised when a child has a solid grasp of 'the future' as a concept. Once the child has saved up enough for a particular object or experience, the payoff of saving becomes clear and the resulting reward and sense of accomplishment reinforce good money habits.

Incentives can play a big part in the formation of good habits; children are more likely to add a behaviour to their unconscious repertoire if they get something out of it. Children – especially young children – operate largely in the present moment and can find it hard to understand that some things don't provide a benefit until sometime later, or that certain behaviours must be repeated over a long time for the impacts to show. A small reward given immediately after the action creates a positive association and encourages a child to keep up this new habit. A 2016 study of healthy eating observed 8,000 children and found that a small incentive given for eating fruit or vegetables (in this case a voucher for 25 cents) doubled the number of children eating at least one of their five a day. The effects of

IMAGE SOURCE Getty Images

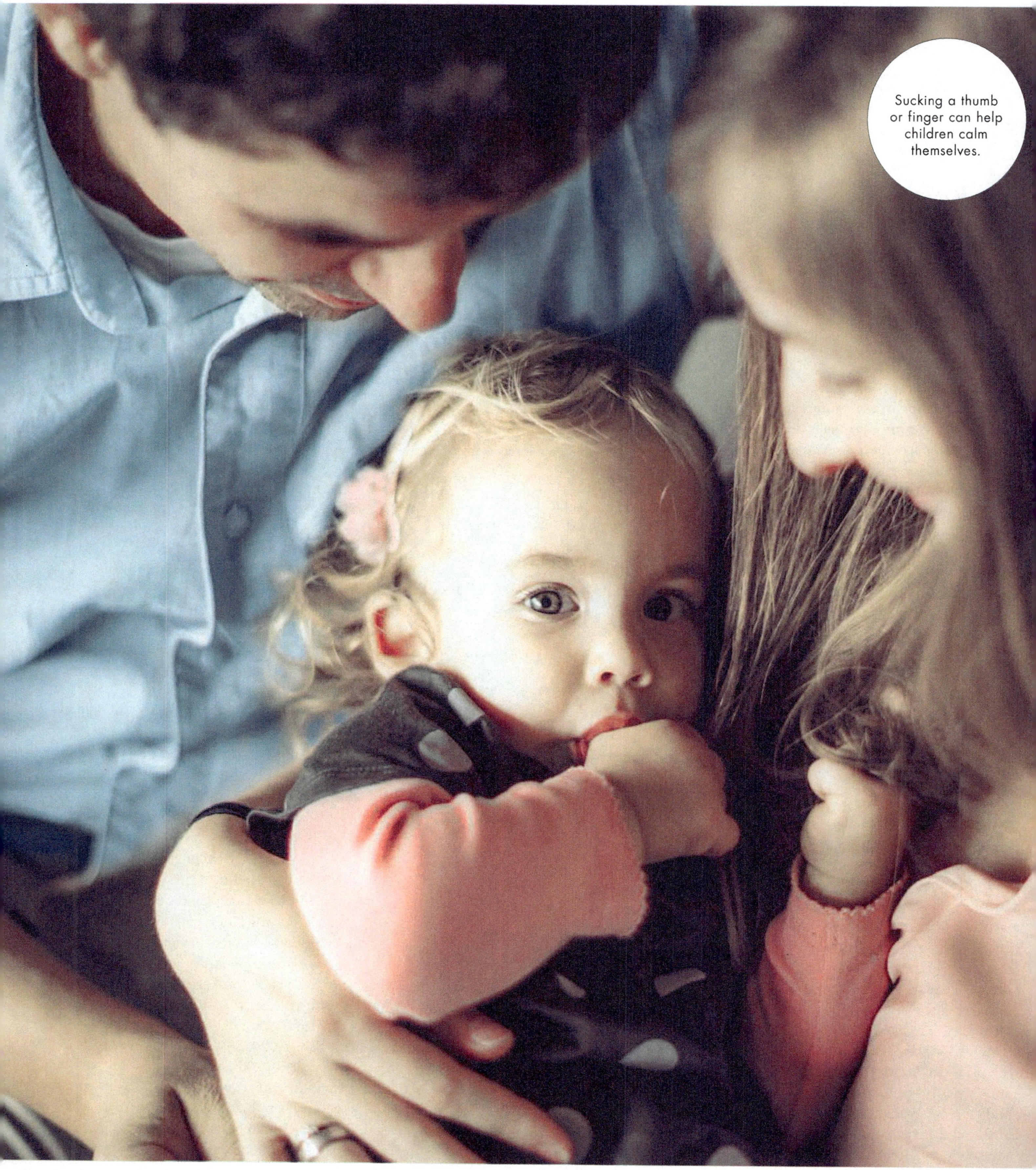

Sucking a thumb or finger can help children calm themselves.

the incentives continued months after the study ended and the children had stopped being rewarded for healthy eating. The use of rewards or incentives for promoting good habits in children is still debated among scientists, but several other studies of school children have produced similar results to the 2016 paper, indicating that small rewards can help establish good habits.

Young children are constantly learning about themselves, their life and the people around them. 'Classic' habit formation involves repeating a behaviour until it becomes second nature, but some scientists suggest that there are other factors that drive or influence habit formation. New information can make a child more likely to pick up a good habit; in the case of the healthy eating study, some children may have started eating a more balanced diet because they were given fruits and vegetables they hadn't tried before and didn't know they liked. As children get older and begin to understand that their behaviour has consequences later down the line, habits like drinking water and brushing their teeth make more sense and so are easier to maintain.

THUMB SUCKING

It's one of the most common childhood habits, but why?

Babies have natural suckling instincts that help them to latch onto their mothers during breastfeeding, and they will automatically suck on any object placed in their mouths. As breastfeeding offers nourishment and closeness with their mother, babies associate suckling with comfort and safety and begin to suck on their fingers or thumbs to soothe themselves. As the habit develops, a favourite finger or thumb usually emerges. The suckling reflex fades at around four months, but the behaviour can continue long after weaning.

Many children drop the thumb sucking habit by the age of four as they find new ways to calm themselves. If a child continues the habit past the age of six, emerging adult teeth can be pushed forward. Experts recommend praising children when they resist the temptation to suck their thumb rather than telling them off when they do, as the distress caused by being scolded could increase the desire to self-soothe. They also suggest looking for the cause of the behaviour and finding an alternative solution – engaging the child in an activity if they suck their thumb out of boredom, providing comfort if thumb sucking results from nervousness, and teaching children alternative calming methods, such as deep breathing.

Just as incentives can help to reinforce good habits, monitoring a child's attempts to implement a new behaviour or routine can improve the likelihood that it will be maintained. While nagging may make a child reluctant to do something, gentle reminders, feedback and the knowledge that an adult is noting whether or not a behaviour is carried out can help children to internalise and develop habits. A study of handwashing found that incentives, monitoring and a combination of the two all increased the likelihood that a child would consistently remember to wash their hands.

Research has shown that infancy is a crucial time for the formation of food preferences and eating habits, as children are still 'plastic' during this period and can be encouraged to develop healthy eating behaviours. Infants are predisposed to prefer sweet and energy-rich foods and reject bitter tastes, and when left unchecked this natural predisposition can lead to unhealthy eating habits. Most children are happy to try a wide variety of new foods up until the age of 18 to 24 months. Exposure to lots of different tastes and textures

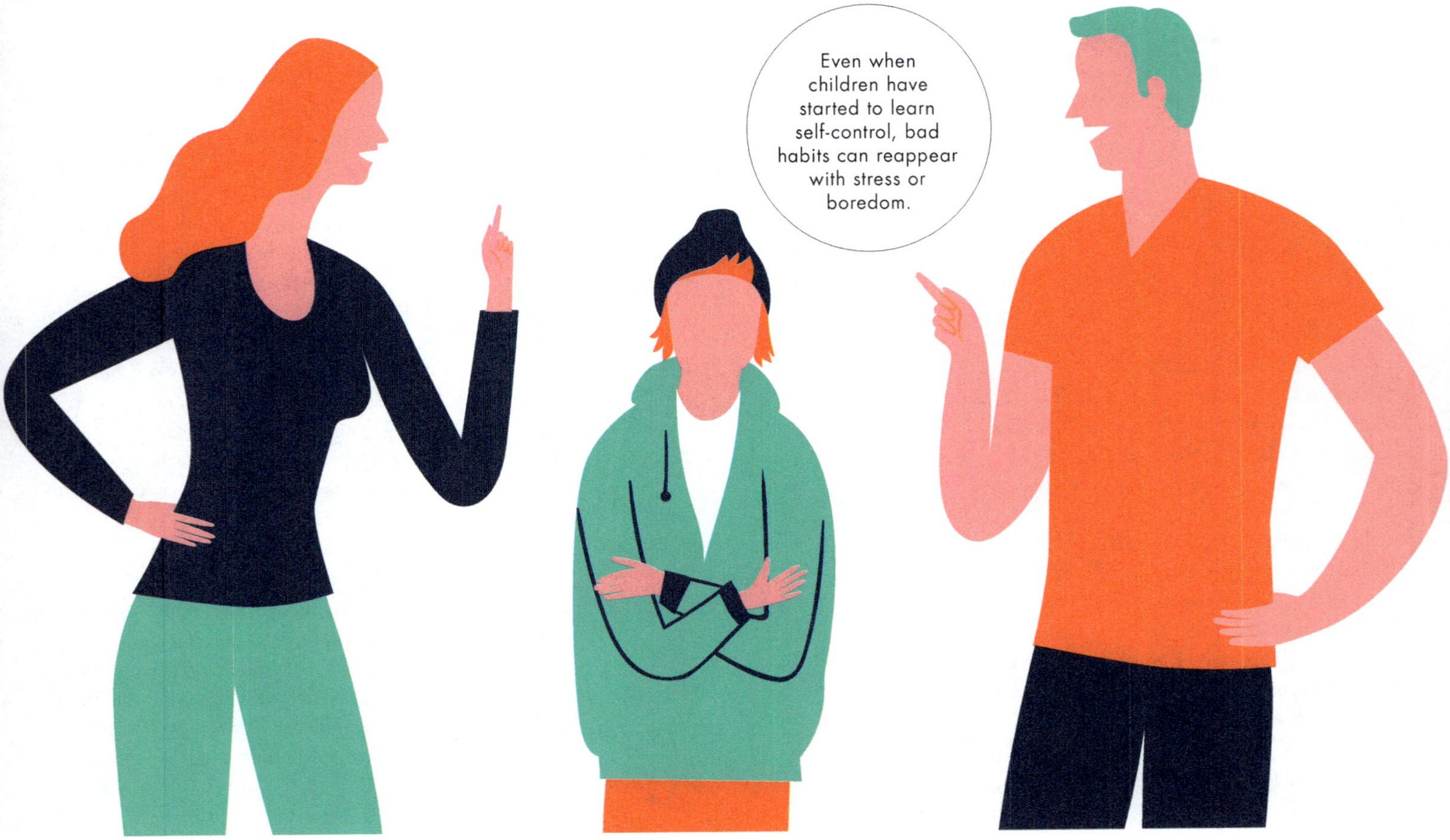

Even when children have started to learn self-control, bad habits can reappear with stress or boredom.

IMAGE SOURCE Getty Images

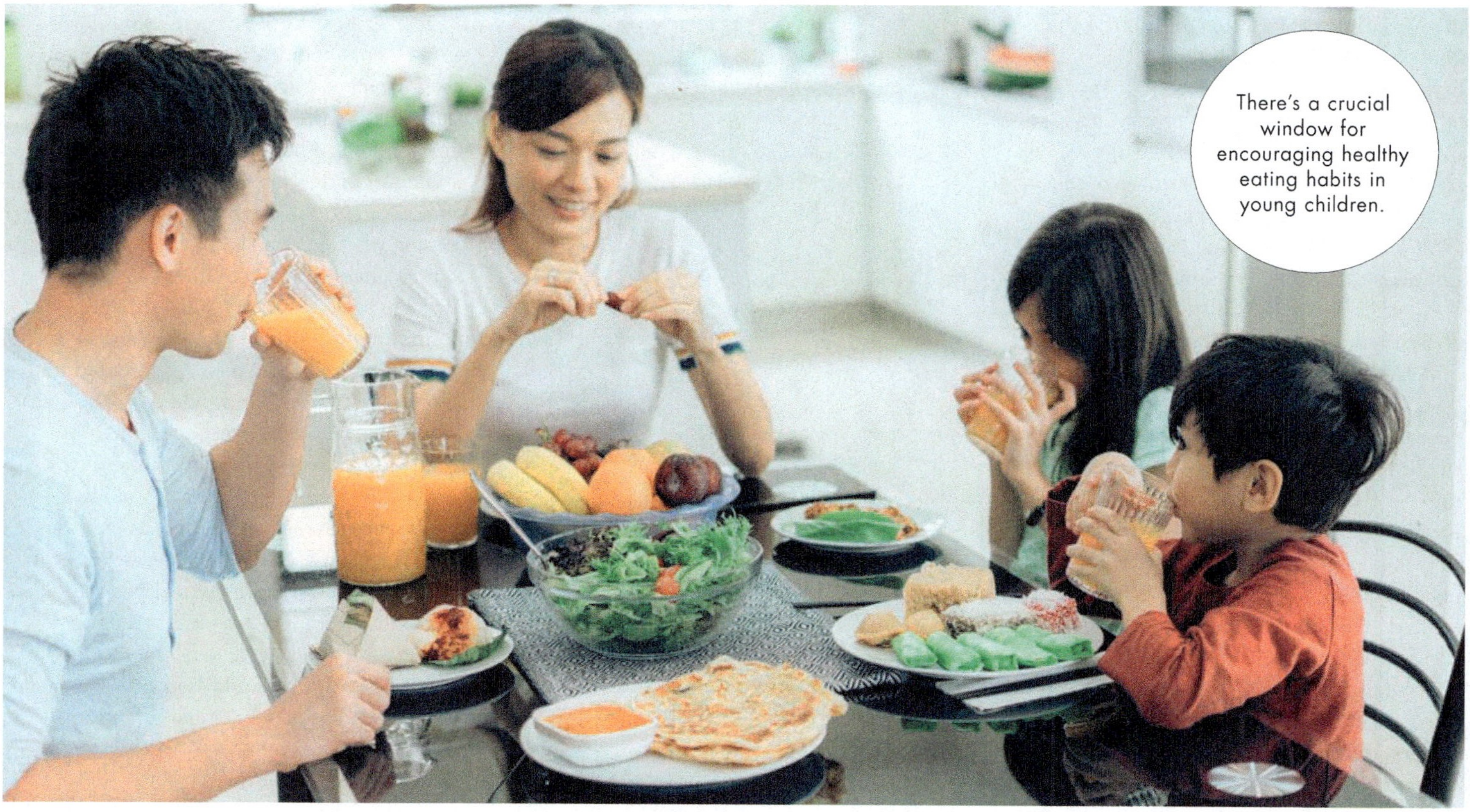

There's a crucial window for encouraging healthy eating habits in young children.

immediately after weaning seems to further increase this natural willingness to try novel food. After this point, they often enter a period of refusing food and eating only a small selection of foods. Scientists believe that at this age children are beginning to process the concept of food and to understand that foods they haven't tried before could either be tasty or horrid, safe or dangerous. This 'fussy' stage peaks around the age of three, after which children become more willing to try new foods again. As eating a meal is usually a social event for a child, the eating habits of others shape their own habits and preferences. Children observe how and what their friends, family members and role models eat and often follow the examples they see. Scientists call this social facilitation.

Social context is hugely influential for children as they consider where they fit in and try to navigate complex interactions and relationships. Bad habits such as swearing and smoking are more likely to be picked up if they're considered 'cool' in a young person's social circle or the social circle they want to be part of, while certain behaviours will be actively avoided if they're considered unfashionable by others. Family members, friends, schoolmates, celebrities and influencers can all drive changes in behaviour or reinforce existing habits.

> IN 2019 AMERICAN PARENTS DESCRIBED THE 'PEPPA EFFECT' – THE APPEARANCE OF A BRITISH ACCENT IN CHILDREN WHO WATCH THE CARTOON *PEPPA PIG*

The media is playing an increasingly large role in children's development. From a very young age children are exposed to TVs, tablets, computers and advertising. Repeated exposure to certain media can create new behaviours and habits; in 2019 American parents began describing the 'Peppa Effect' – the appearance of a British accent in children who frequently watched the English cartoon *Peppa Pig*.

Children are seven to nine years old by the time they begin to understand the purpose and nature of adverts. Until this age, they don't question the messages they see in adverts and other media. This trust in the media and the fact that certain adverts are designed specifically to appeal to children mean that what children see impacts their choices and habits. A child might, for example, develop a preference for a particular breakfast cereal because of the character on their advertising, or begin to show an interest in a new type of toy because of their targeted marketing.

WORDS Victoria Williams

IMAGE SOURCE Getty Images

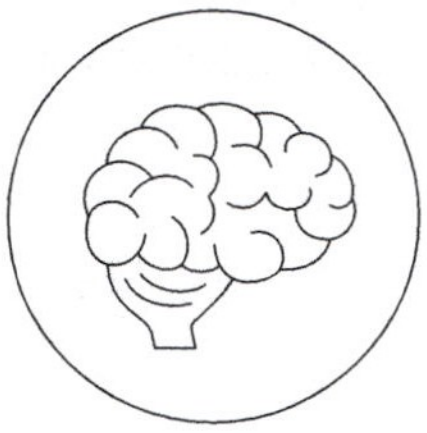

Hereditary habits

Genes control your appearance and biochemistry, but do they also influence your behaviour?

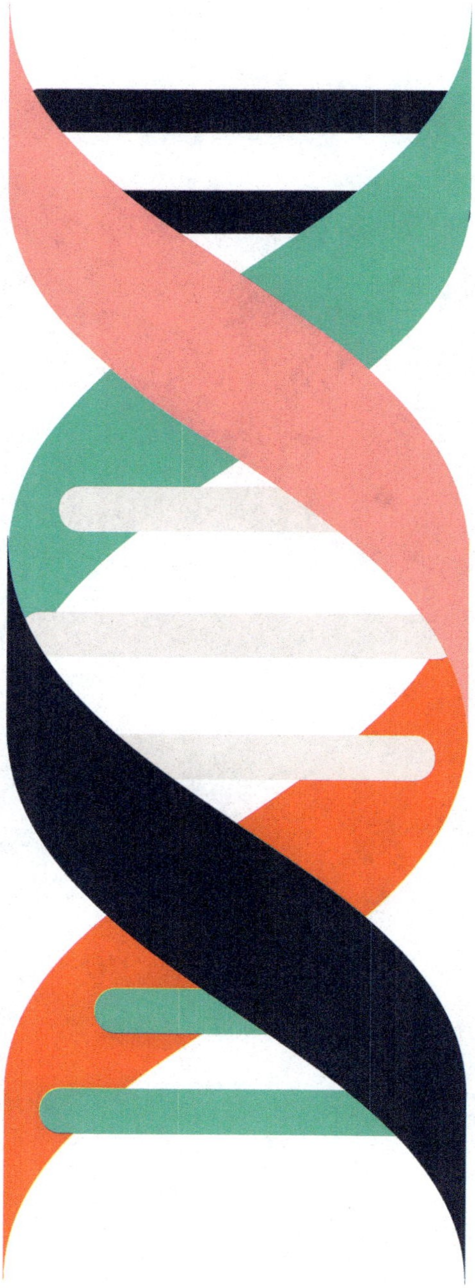

The relative influences of 'nature versus nurture' are widely debated in relation to many aspects of human behaviour. Ever since the discovery of DNA as the genetic material that dictates our biological makeup, scientists have pondered the question of just how much our genes control aspects of our personality – is there a direct link or is our environment the dominant influence? This question has significant consequences when concerning such things as our judicial system. Are the actions of a criminal truly his or her fault, or are they an inevitable product of either their genetics or upbringing?

The heritability of habits and personality traits is an area of study that is growing at an accelerating pace. With modern genetic technologies we're able to isolate and identify individual genes in a person's DNA and draw conclusions as to the apparent influence they have on specific behaviours. There is strong evidence of a direct influence of genetics on several key human characteristics, from dress sense to hobbies and interests. A large percentage of this data was collected by studying twins separated at birth, which has the potential to reveal the relative dominance of heritability over environmental factors.

An example of a behaviour studied in this way is food preference. It's not a habit that many would think has a genetic influence, but when considering the core reasons behind our eating likes and dislikes at a biochemical level, it's easier to understand why this suggests itself as a hereditary characteristic.

Our taste is controlled by receptors to different compounds in food, all of which are subject to individual differences in relative sensitivity. One person may be very sensitive to salt content, meaning they are averse to salty foods, which provide a sensory overload. Since taste receptors are controlled by genetics, these preferences can feasibly be passed down between generations.

In a study by Grimm and Steinle (2011) that focused on the genetic controls of obesity, it was concluded that people with a gene variant known as TAS2R38 were especially sensitive to bitter tastes and so were less likely to eat healthy foods, such as green vegetables, which contain bitter compounds. These people would be more prone to eating 'bad' foods – those with higher sugar contents.

Other research by Zongyang Mou et al. (2015) has demonstrated that a small mutation to a gene coding for a protein known as 'brain-derived neurotrophic factor' (BDNF), which controls when we feel full after eating, can mean less of this protein is produced. This may result in a person developing an inflated appetite, which has also been linked to obesity. If such genotypes are passed from parents to their children, then this may predispose future generations to obesity.

Another area of interest is sleeping habits. While this may be widely thought of as environmentally controlled, there is a suggested genetic influence. When we choose to go to sleep and how long we stay asleep for is moderated by our circadian rhythms – our body clock.

A study published by Jason R. Gerstner et al. in 2017 explained the role of a protein

> EVEN POLITICAL BELIEFS CAN BE PARTIALLY HERITABLE

called Fabp7 in sleep cycle control. The study found that a mutation in the gene coding for the protein resulted in fragmented sleep in humans and other mammalian species. From this we can infer that if the mutation is passed between generations, then this could not only predispose children to poor-quality sleep but could result in unhealthy family routines. A cycle of nature (heritability) and nurture (household behaviour) influence is created.

Similarly, Patke et el. (2017) discovered that so-called 'night owl' behaviour – sleeping and waking late – was influenced by the mutation of another gene called CRY1. When this fails to work correctly, proteins that activate our circadian rhythms are inhibited, slowing our internal clock. Once again, since the cause is genetic, there is the chance that the habit of failing to get up in the morning could be passed from parents to offspring.

Amazingly, even our political beliefs can be partially heritable. For example, while genetic influence has long been ignored in studies of voting behaviour, voting turnout may actually be due to ancient genetic controls of behaviour. In the past, genotypes that encouraged social conformity may have offered survival advantages, and today these appear as a choice to vote. This theory is supported by the fact that most people either always vote or never vote – a fixed pattern of behaviour. Young adults are more likely to vote if their parents do, which, while previously explained in social terms, strongly suggests a heritable behaviour characteristic.

WORDS Peter Fenech

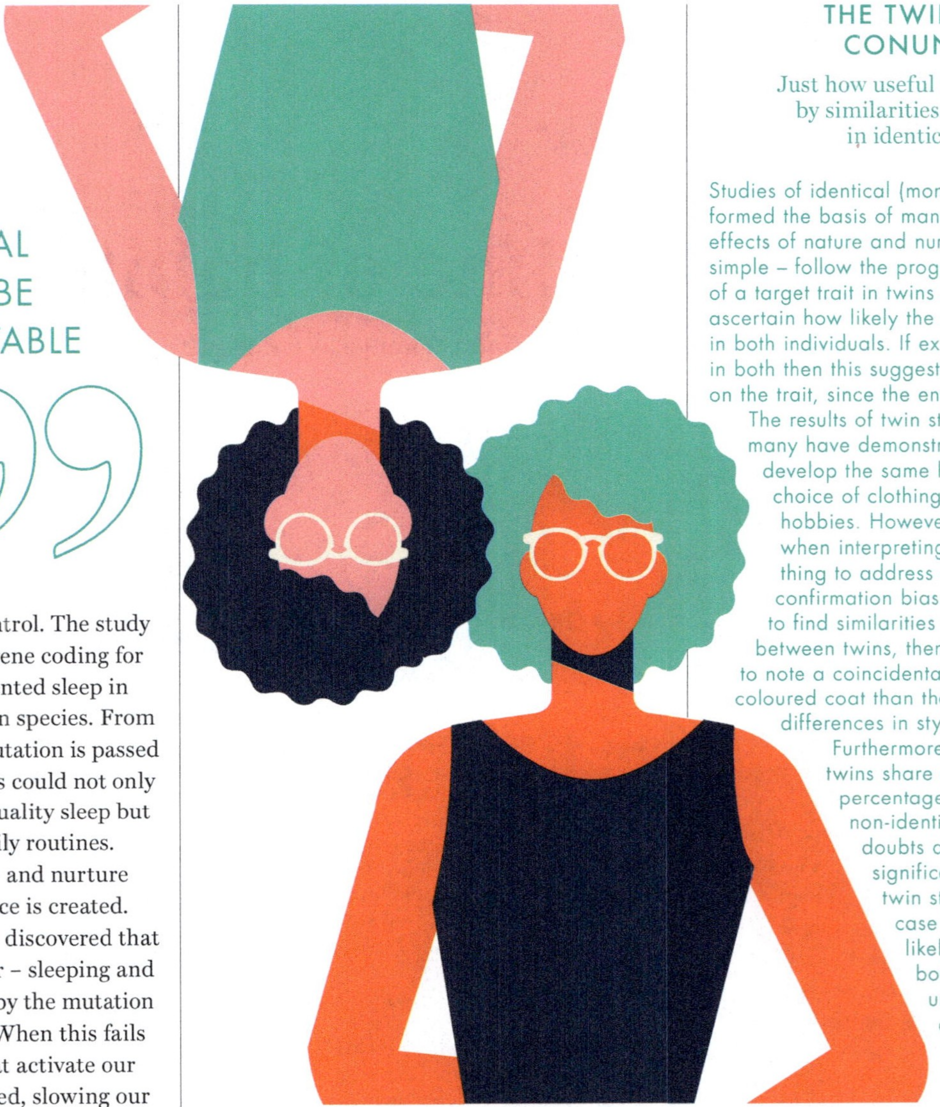

THE TWIN STUDY CONUNDRUM

Just how useful is data obtained by similarities or differences in identical twins?

Studies of identical (monozygotic) twins have formed the basis of many studies on the relative effects of nature and nurture. The concept is simple – follow the progression of development of a target trait in twins separated at birth to ascertain how likely the same traits are to occur in both individuals. If expression is concurrent in both then this suggests a genetic influence on the trait, since the environments are different.

The results of twin studies are exciting as many have demonstrated how twins often develop the same habits, down to their choice of clothing, haircuts and even hobbies. However, there are difficulties when interpreting the data. The first thing to address are the effects of confirmation bias. If investigators expect to find similarities in fashion sense between twins, then they are more likely to note a coincidental choice of a similarly coloured coat than they are obvious differences in style.

Furthermore, since monozygotic twins share a far greater percentage of their genes than non-identical siblings, there are doubts about the real-world significance of findings in twin studies. Traits – in this case habits – are far more likely to be expressed in both twins than two unrelated members of the population, exaggerating apparent hereditary influence.

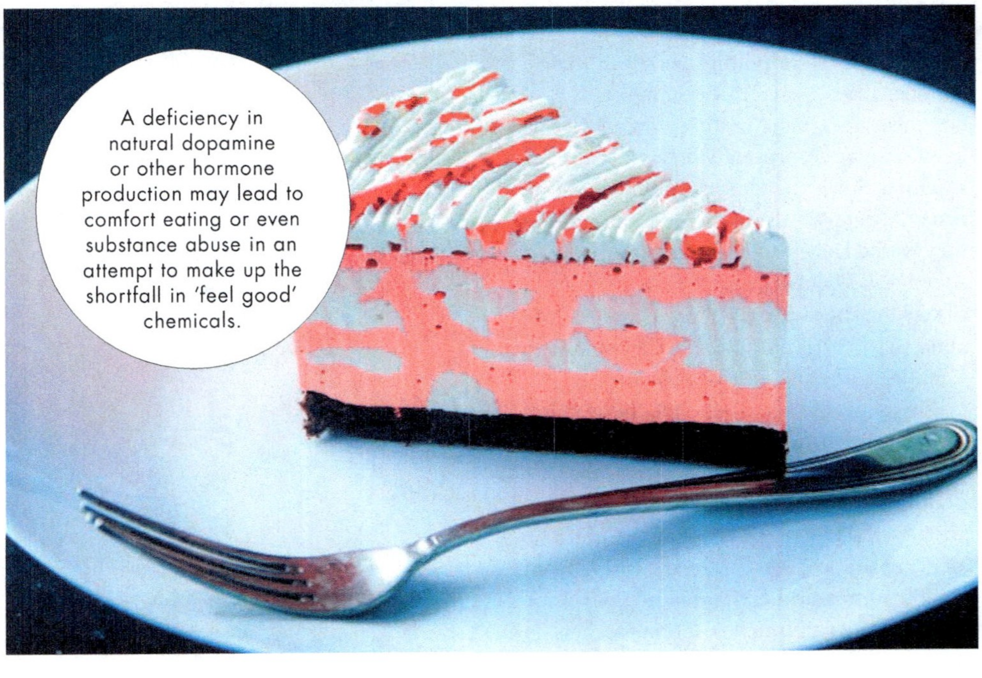

A deficiency in natural dopamine or other hormone production may lead to comfort eating or even substance abuse in an attempt to make up the shortfall in 'feel good' chemicals.

IMAGE SOURCE Getty Images, Pexels

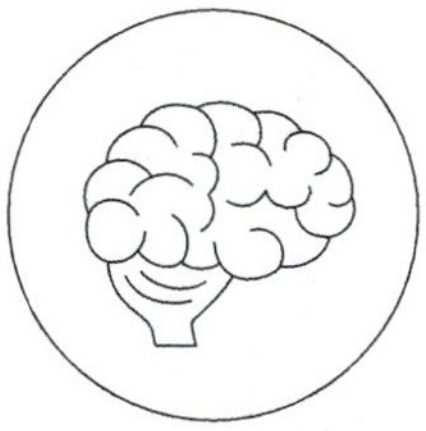

A lifetime of habits

How do our habits change as we grow?

As babies, we all had some instincts of how to act, but for the majority of our behaviour we need guidance. We first develop habits by observing what's going on around us and being led by our parents and guardians. When a child is placed in a cot, at first it won't understand what it is meant to do there, but, given a routine, it soon develops the habit of sleeping, establishing a bedtime.

While it is possible for children to pick up positive habits from those around them, sometimes parents are unaware of the problematic mannerisms young people can also copy. Some childhood habits naturally fade, while others require more discipline and practice to get rid of.

Generally, you don't encounter many adults sucking their thumb as they make their way down the street, or pulling eagerly at their earlobes like a baby. However, in some circumstances, more mature versions of these habits can arise, especially in a stressful situation. Surfacing for self-comfort, these acts can take people back to their childhood, when they worked as go-to coping mechanisms. Albeit less frequently, adults can be prone to sucking the end of a pen, or playing persistently with their hair as they deal with a challenging email or a time of anxiety.

Why is it more acceptable for children to exhibit these behaviours, yet they are frowned upon when displayed by adults? Children's minds and bodies evolve as they grow. Social behaviour is one of the main qualities that changes in the transition from childhood to adulthood, providing people with more insight into acceptable actions.

AGE-CONSCIOUS ADULTS

How does ageing lead to us enforcing healthy habits?

One major difference between adults' and children's approaches to habits is their ability to be identified. A child could continue to suck a dummy for comfort indefinitely, as they don't realise the impact of habits or even acknowledge that this has become a dependence. They either need to wait for the habit to fade or rely on an adult to help them move on from it.

Adults, on the other hand, are fully aware if they have got into the habit of biting their nails, for example. They can choose to try and stop this. As well as being more likely to try and end habits, they are also more likely to try and enforce a new habit on themselves.

As we age, we become more conscious of it. Whether in denial of old age or just more aware of health risks, anything that will help us stay healthier for longer becomes important to many adults. Researchers at Harvard University pinpointed five habits, which when all followed are thought to be able to add a decade onto your life. These were healthy eating, controlling weight, regularly exercising, not smoking, and drinking only in moderation.

For many health-conscious adults, studies like this are enough to make them enforce new habits, whether that be cutting down on processed meat on certain days of the week, replacing smoking with a new distraction, or making a habit of after-work walks.

Though it is still possible to change once in adulthood, the majority of temporary habit adaptations take place before puberty. Habits made as babies, toddlers and children can change more fluidly as the body changes. Entering adulthood, we remain more consistent in the morals we have learned and the kind of behaviours we display. The way we will act tomorrow is usually very similar to the way we have acted today. It takes more hard work and dedication to change our adult behaviours.

Some of the behaviours we practise during early adulthood form the foundations of positive habits, while others can have more negative consequences. In both cases, repetition makes them more permanent aspects of an individual's lifestyle. When choosing to try sport as a young adult, for instance, people become more used to incorporating exercise into their daily schedules. Then, before they know it, something that comes easily to them naturally induces positive impacts on both their mental and physical health.

Contrastingly, bad habits can start to occur as teenagers, when we adopt a sense of freedom and independence. As a stage between childhood and adulthood, teenage

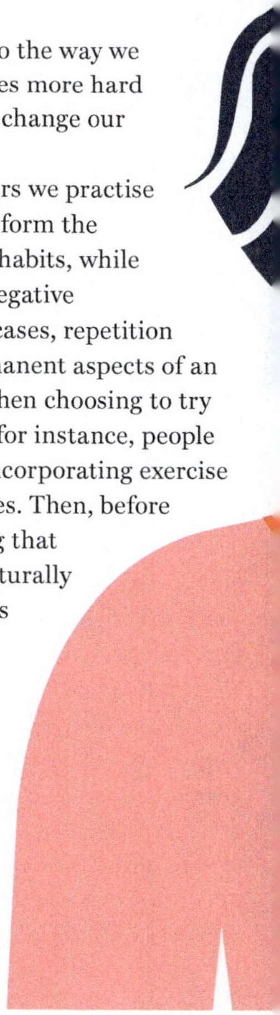

habits can be harder to break than childhood habits. No longer constantly looking towards our parents for guidance on what is good and bad, our teenage stage is when we begin to choose what we do. Late teenagers begin to leave home and – becoming the boss of themselves – they may start to test the water.

Quitting when things get difficult, lying without a higher control to answer to, or even attempting to get away with cheating – none of these life choices have desirable outcomes. Although most young adults know they are in the wrong, once a bad act has been committed it becomes easier to repeat this with less weight on the conscience. After all, how bad can it be just one more time? Like any habit, it becomes more cemented the more it is repeated and can even become an addiction.

Whether as a child or a fully grown adult, there are ways to enforce positive habits that create a more fulfilled life. Fuelling yours and your child's body with an abundance of healthy food is easier to do once you get into a habit. Many of us like a sweet treat and can be tempted to buy unhealthy snacks. Some children will choose sweets over anything, and it is the adult's job to enforce the early habit of achieving their five a day. For adult health, changes often come in the form of diets, when we try enforcing strict rules for ourselves in the hope it will eventually become less forced and more a way of life.

One of the most common causes of new habits is stress. With age comes responsibility, and with more responsibility comes more stress. Children undoubtedly experience this feeling too, over a huge range of things that we later deem as adults to be comparatively irrelevant. To children, not finding a favourite toy might seem like the be-all and end-all of everything they know. Less able to comprehend situations rationally, childish habits may include tantrums in such scenarios. These are easier to drop once emotional maturity evolves and they realise better ways to cope with minor downfalls.

Outwardly, adults cope with stress in more subtle ways. Knowing that screaming the roof down won't actively put an end to the stressful situation, nail biting, lip chewing or head scratching are examples of subtler habits that may take its place.

WORDS Ailsa Harvey

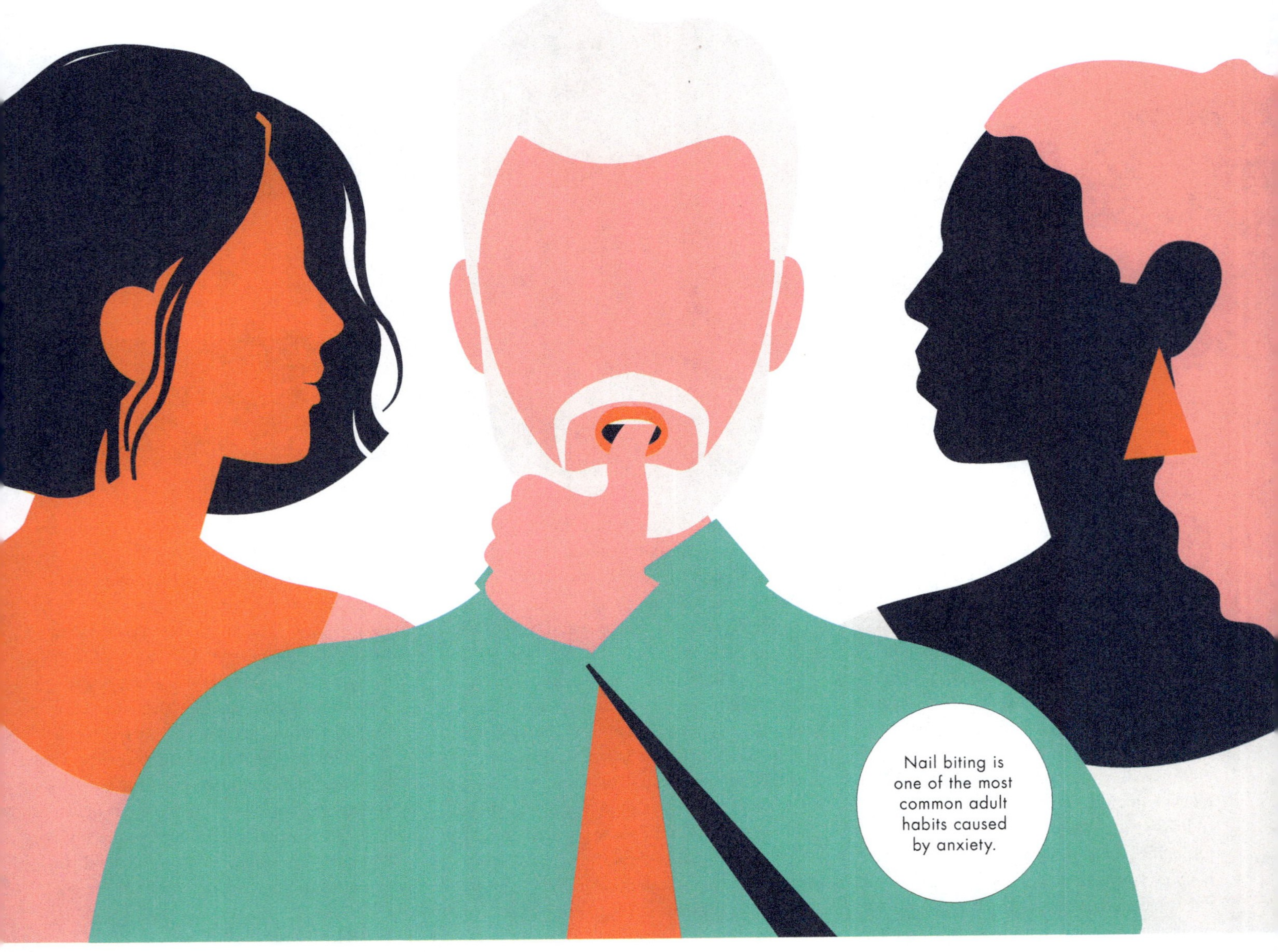

Nail biting is one of the most common adult habits caused by anxiety.

IMAGE SOURCE Getty Images

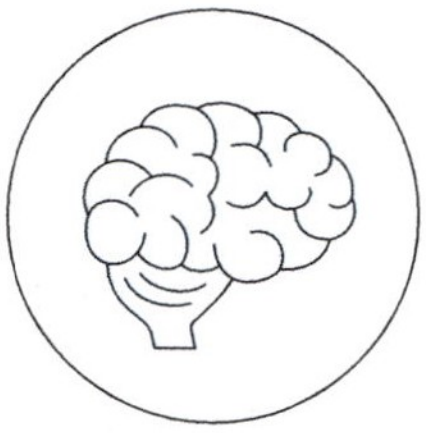

Getting into good habits

Change is hard, but it's possible to form beneficial new habits if you go about it the right way

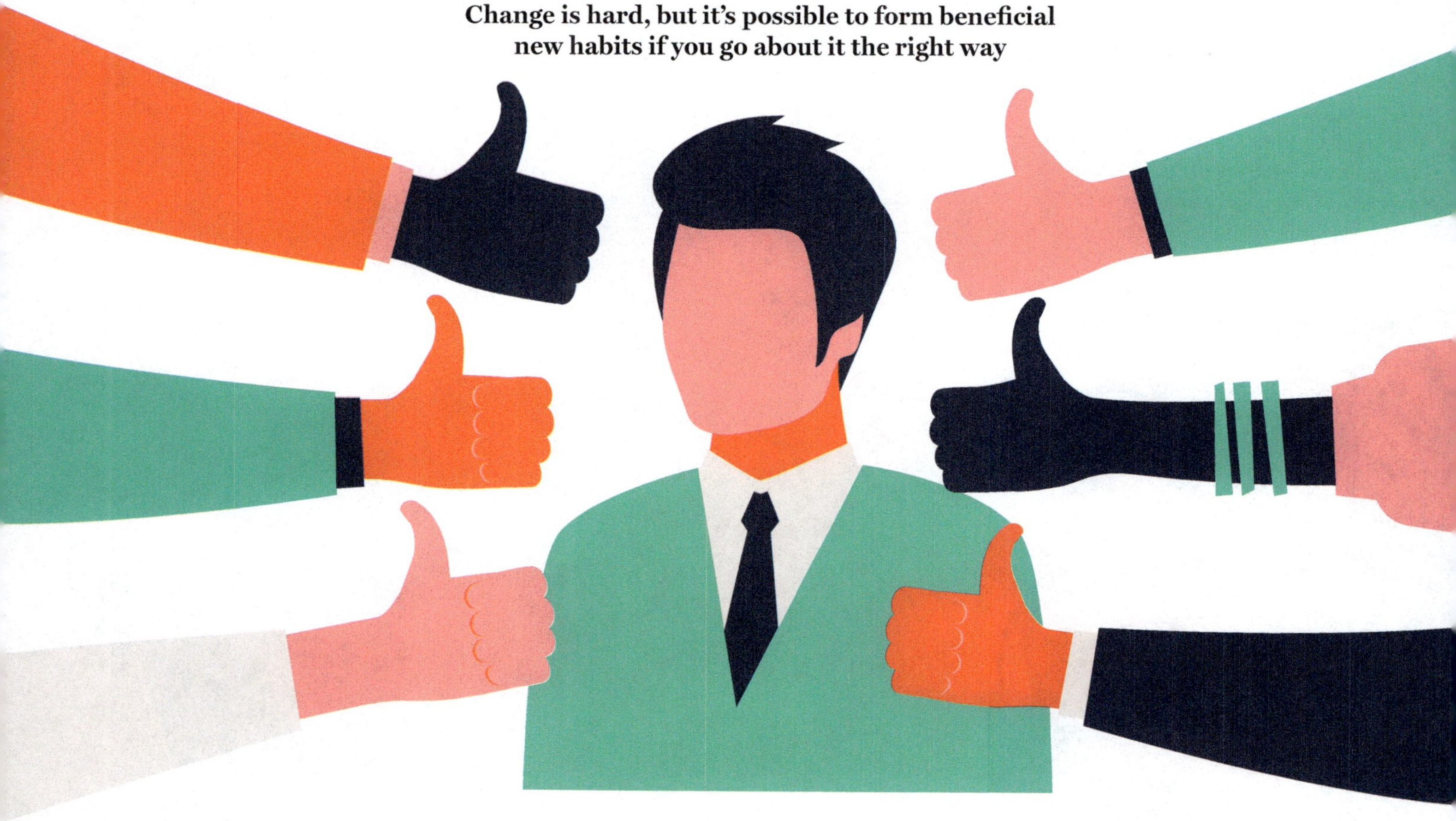

Good habits are formed by creating new habit loops: neurological loops that cycle from cue to routine to reward and back round again. Start with the routine and decide on the new habit that you want to introduce. The more specific you can be, the better; 'I want to cook five dinners a week from scratch' is much easier to work towards than 'I should make dinner at home more.'

Research shows that it's best to introduce a new habit after a routine or behaviour that's already established, so identify a specific part of your day or week that can become your cue. It can be as simple as deciding that after work on Tuesdays and Thursdays you will drive from work to the gym instead of going straight home, or that as soon as you wake up every morning you're going to go to the kitchen and drink a large glass of water.

Once you've chosen a cue and worked out the routine that should follow it, you're on your way to forming a new habit. However, the brain needs an incentive to strengthen the link between the two and remember it in the future. This is where the reward part of the loop comes in. Every time you complete the new routine you should receive a small, relevant reward; for some people, it might be that the post-exercise buzz or satisfaction of completing a task is enough, but if you're finding it difficult in the beginning you could promise yourself a reward, such as a healthy snack, a small break or some time doing an activity you enjoy.

One of the most important factors in forming a good habit is being realistic. While your ultimate goal might be to go running five days a week or get eight hours of sleep every night, it's much easier to start with something a little smaller. This way you won't be overwhelmed by the challenge you've set yourself and will still get the reward you need to reinforce the habit loop. As the connections are strengthened you'll need to put in less and less conscious effort to complete the routine, and once it becomes habit at this level you can take another step towards the big goal.

WORDS Victoria Williams

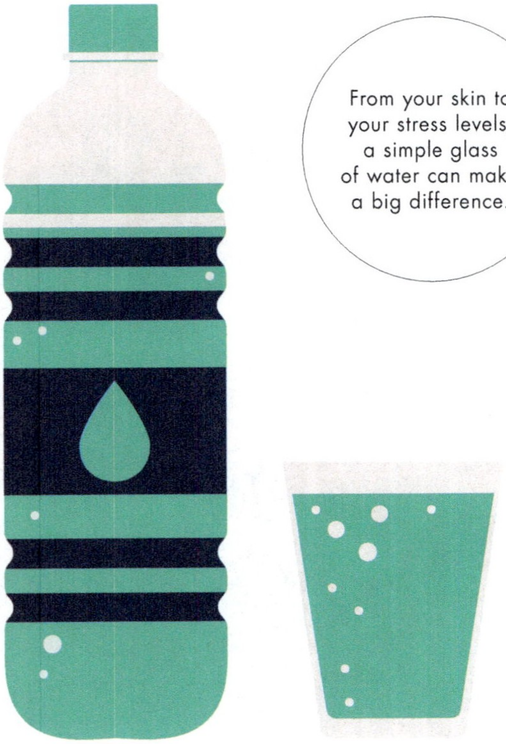

From your skin to your stress levels, a simple glass of water can make a big difference.

Drinking more water

It's common knowledge that we need to drink water, but its importance is often underestimated. More than half of the human body is made of water, and it's vital for organ health, joint lubrication, temperature regulation, digestion and clear thinking among many other things. Dehydration makes it harder for the body and mind to function and can cause long-term damage, so drinking enough water is an important habit to develop.

The best way to get into the habit of drinking more water is to carry a water bottle with you. Fill it up before you head out in the morning, then refill it wherever you can throughout the day. The easier and more convenient it is for you to drink, the more likely you are to do it.

If you find that carrying a bottle isn't enough, put a sticky note on your desk, on your bathroom door, on the fridge – wherever you're likely to spot it more than once a day. You could even set reminders on your phone or in your work calendar. If water on its own isn't to your taste, make your new habit more palatable with low-sugar squash or herbal tea.

Getting up on time

Dashing out of the door in the morning – half-eaten toast in hand, shoelaces untied – isn't the best way to start the day. Getting into the habit of waking up with enough time to do everything you need to means you'll begin the morning in a much more relaxed and organised way, setting you up to be more productive and focused for the rest of the day.

If you're a serial snoozer, try to resist that button so you're less likely to drift off again and oversleep. If your phone is your alarm clock, put it on the other side of the room so you have to get up to turn it off. Once you're up, turn on a light or open the curtains. If you don't trust yourself to stick to that plan, buy a sunrise alarm clock so the light levels in the room gradually increase and you wake up with less of a start.

Make your mornings as easy as you possibly can. The night before, as you're preparing dinner or clearing away, put out a glass and a bowl for the morning. Pick out what you're going to wear so your groggy future self can climb into an outfit without having to think about it. Keep your keys, glasses, bag, wallet and other important things in the same place so there's no panicked rummaging.

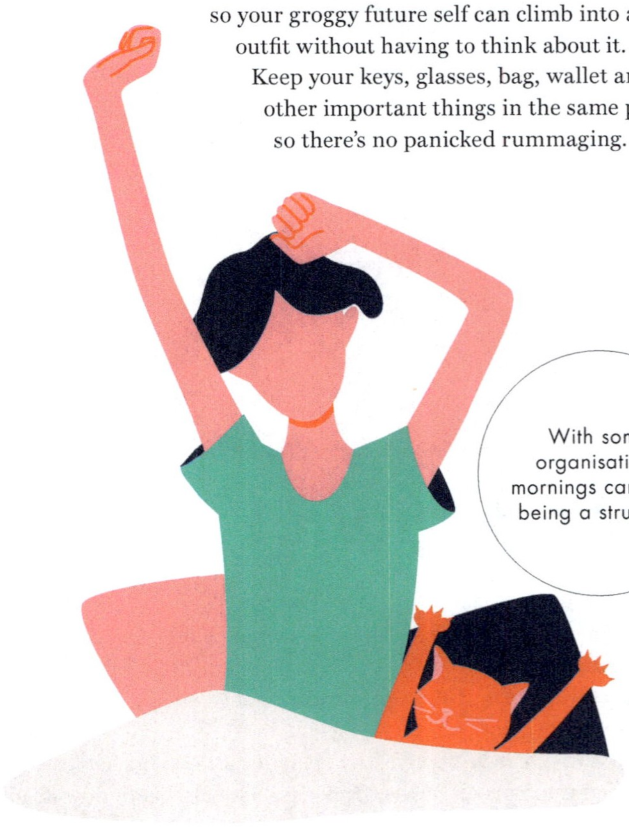

With some organisation, mornings can stop being a struggle.

"TO GET INTO THE HABIT OF DRINKING MORE WATER, CARRY A BOTTLE WITH YOU. THE EASIER AND MORE CONVENIENT IT IS FOR YOU TO DRINK, THE MORE LIKELY YOU ARE TO DO IT"

IMAGE SOURCE Getty Images

Eating healthily

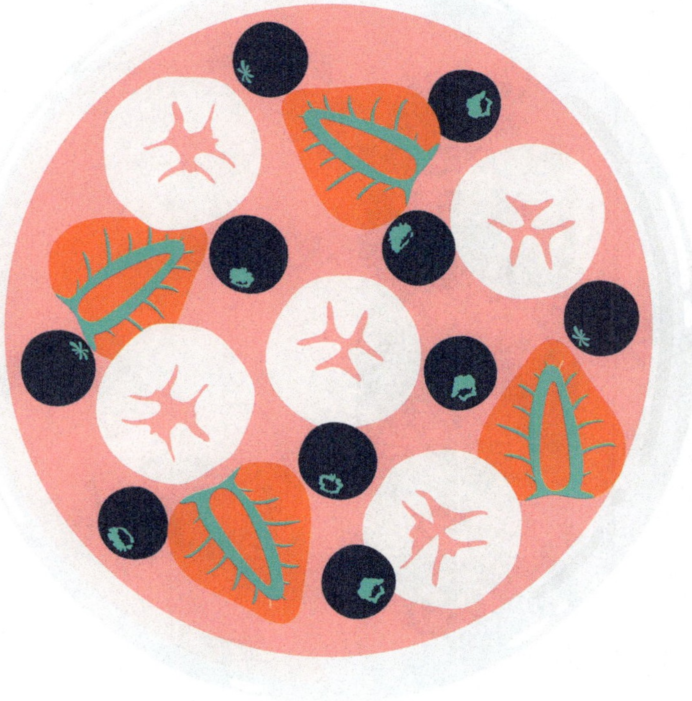

Eating a balanced diet is important for both physical and mental health, preventing diet-related illnesses and giving you the energy you need to make the most of the day. However, with so many appealing yet unhealthy options available, it can be hard to stick to good food and recommended portion sizes.

If you struggle to maintain a healthy diet, the first step is to do some research. Find out what you should be eating and compare it to your current diet. Once you've identified the main problem areas you can figure out some simple swaps and changes. There are hundreds of books and online guides, so you can find the foods and recipes that appeal – it's almost impossible to stick to healthy eating if you're forcing yourself to eat things you don't actually like.

One of the best food-related habits to establish is regularly eating breakfast. Many people skip the first meal of the day, but a big, nutritious breakfast powers your body through the morning and reduces cravings. Keep healthy options like fruit, nuts and yoghurt to hand in case you do need to snack, and over time you should feel less of a draw to sugary and fatty foods.

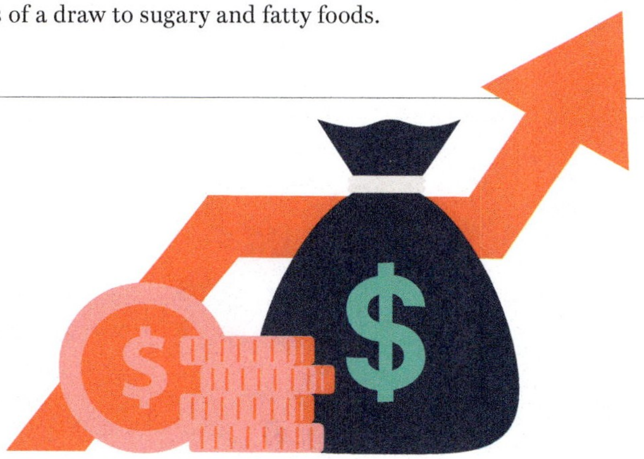

Saving money

Money can be a big source of worry for a lot of people, and saving doesn't come naturally to everyone. Small amounts really do add up, so it's worthwhile changing your spending habits and putting a little bit away whenever you can.

The first step to developing better spending and saving habits is to understand your current habits. Draw up a spreadsheet or download an app that shows you where you spend your money – you might be surprised. Once you've realised that you're impulse buying crisps more often than you thought or spending more than you'd like on taxis, you can start working out how to change your behaviour.

One of the easiest saving habits is rounding up what you spend. Say you spend £4.50 on lunch – round it up to £5 and put the 50p in a jar (physical if you're a cash person, or in a savings pot in an app if that's more your thing). On a bigger scale, try to put anything left in your current account at the end of the month into a savings account so you're not tempted to carry it over and spend it.

Time away from screens

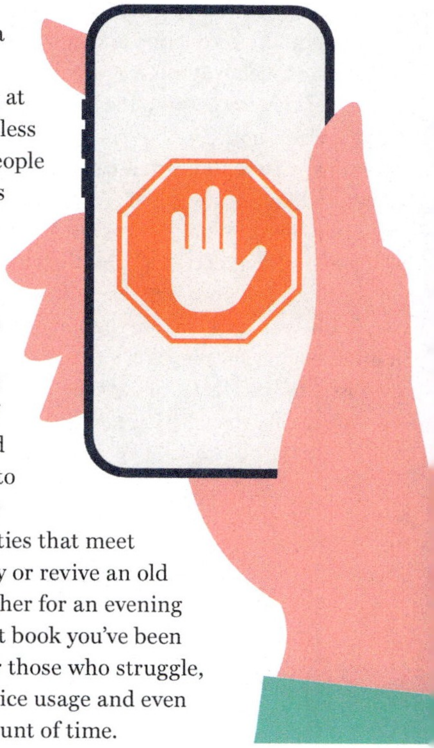

Desk jobs, great TV series and the draw of social media mean that we're spending more time than ever looking at screens, but blue light, mindless scrolling and seeing other people living seemingly perfect lives can take their toll both physically and mentally.

If you spend time with screens because it's your job, take full advantage of your lunch break and use it to get out into the fresh air, even if it's just taking a walk around the building. If you're glued to screens for entertainment or connection, find other activities that meet these needs. Try a new hobby or revive an old one, bring your friends together for an evening 'offline' or make time for that book you've been wanting to read for ages. For those who struggle, there are apps that show device usage and even lock other apps for a set amount of time.

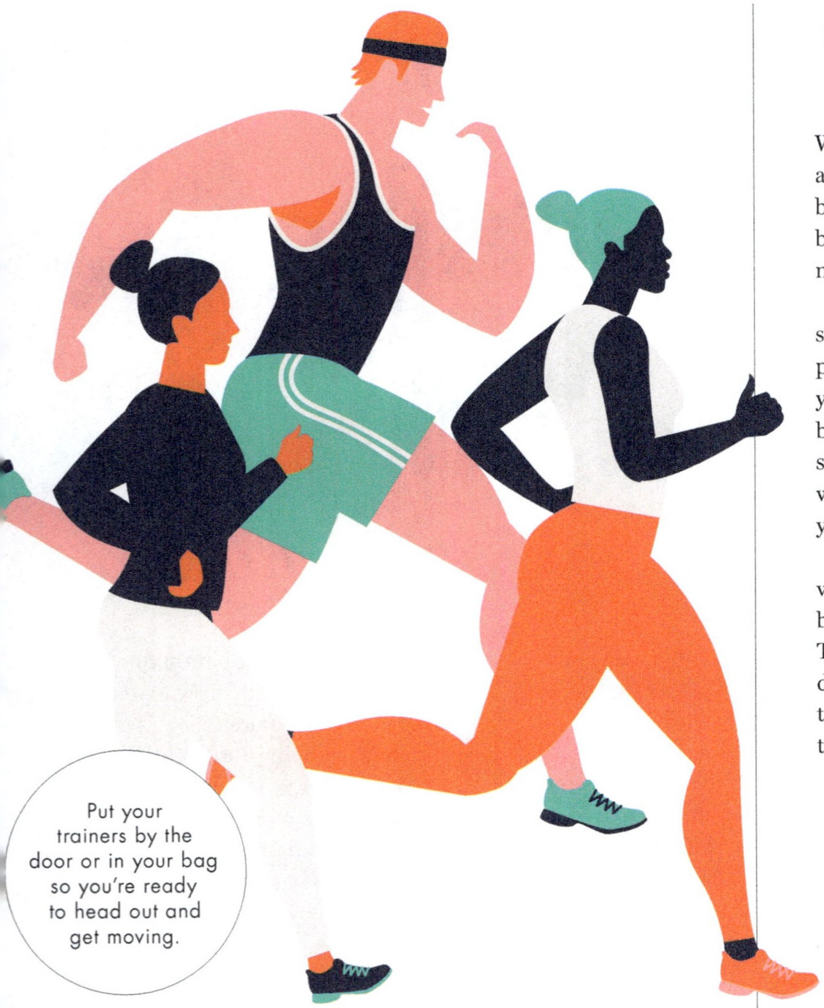

Put your trainers by the door or in your bag so you're ready to head out and get moving.

Being more active

Exercise is one of the most important habits you can develop – it's free, improves your life almost immediately, reduces the risk of major illnesses such as stroke and heart disease by up to 50 per cent and lowers the risk of early death by as much as 30 per cent.

You don't have to start marathon training or weightlifting to feel the benefits of a more active lifestyle. Anything you can do to move more is a step in the right direction; just taking the stairs every day instead of the lift is enough to reduce the risk of premature death by 15 per cent for people who spend most of their day sitting down. Find ways to fit activity into your day, such as parking further away than normal, cycling to work, going for a walk at lunchtime instead of staying at your desk, or doing a few squats while you're waiting for the kettle to boil.

If you want to start doing more intense exercise regularly, put your workout clothes out the night before so you have less of an excuse to back out the next day. Try booking onto fitness classes or joining a club – it's often easier to stick to a new habit if there's a set time and place and you've made a commitment to show up. It's even easier if you arrange to meet a friend there and get fit together.

Good posture

With so much time spent on uncomfortable seats, slouched on sofas and hunched over computers, modern life puts a real strain on the back. Correct posture is important not only for the spine but also for blood flow, confidence, relaxed breathing and the health of nerves, muscles and ligaments.

First, analyse your current posture. Think about how you sit and stand, and take a moment to consider whether you can feel any pain, pressure or discomfort in your neck or back. Next, make yourself as tall as you comfortably can and roll your shoulders back and down. Find points in your daily routine where you can slot in these checks and adjustments – maybe when you sit down with your first coffee of the day, when you get in the car or when you leave a building to walk somewhere.

Check that your environment isn't impacting your attempts to work on your posture. Any chair you sit in for long periods should be comfortable, supportive and adjusted to the right height for you. Try to wear comfy shoes that cushion your feet. If your routine demands a lot of time spent in one place or position, take breaks to move around, stretch and shake out your limbs to release any tension that's built up.

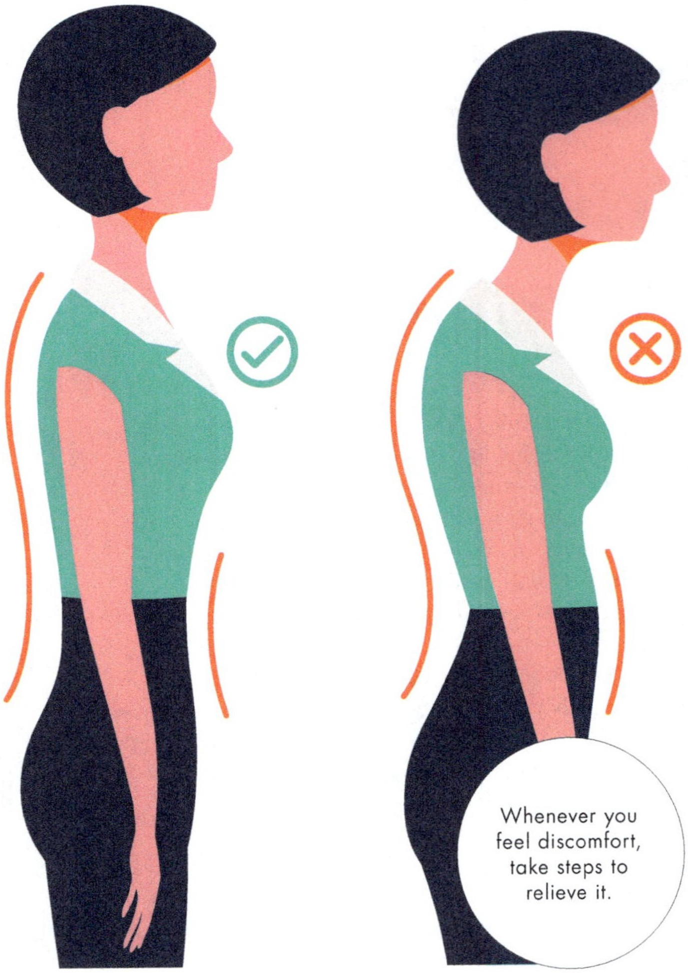

Whenever you feel discomfort, take steps to relieve it.

IMAGE SOURCE Getty Images

Flossing

Many people are told by their dentist that they should be flossing more. It's a task easily forgotten when tooth-brushing feels like it does the job on its own, but flossing gets rid of food between the teeth that a toothbrush can't reach. Good oral hygiene is vital for strong white teeth, fresh breath and healthy gums, so it's worth taking a few extra seconds each morning and evening to floss.

Remember, it's much easier to form a habit by tacking a new behaviour onto the end of an existing routine, so keep your floss next to your toothbrush and aim to floss after you've brushed. If you find you're still struggling to remember, put a note on your bedroom door – 'Did you floss?' Eventually you'll start to associate it more strongly with your bathroom routine and you won't have to try so hard to remember.

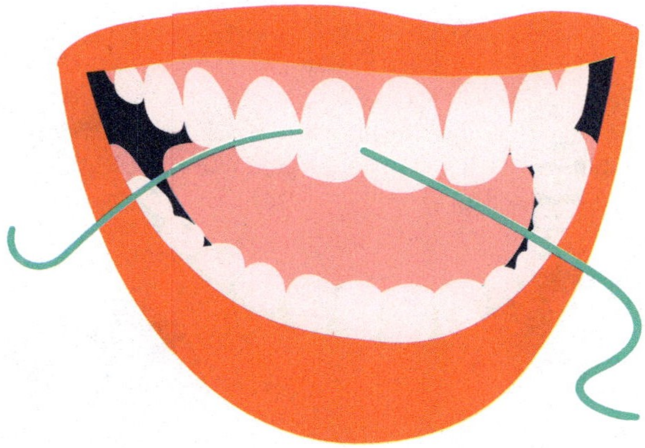

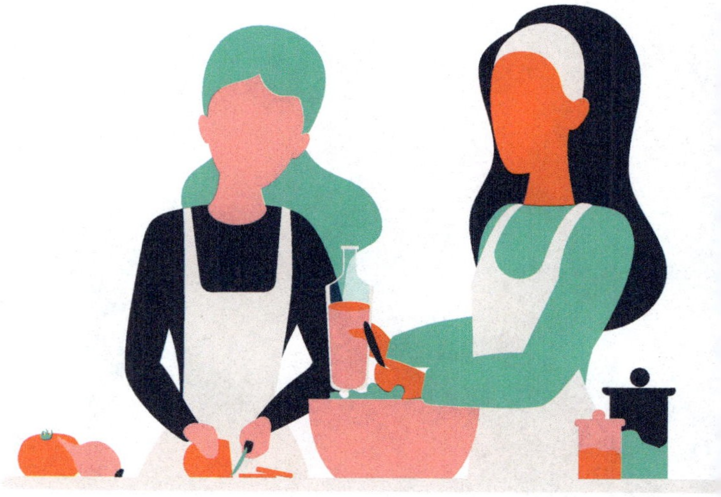

Cooking at home

After a long and hectic day it sometimes seems easiest to order food rather than cooking, but studies have shown that the more home-cooked meals a family eat the better their overall diet. Cooking and eating together has also been shown to reduce stress.

The best way to get into the habit of cooking is to make sure you always have ingredients for quick meals in the fridge and the cupboards – things like pasta, tinned tomatoes, grains, beans, eggs and vegetables. Print out or learn five to ten simple recipes so that you can throw together something speedy and nutritious even when you don't feel like cooking.

Tidying

There's truth behind the saying 'tidy house, tidy mind'. A 2010 study found links between a messy home and higher-than-normal levels of the stress hormone cortisol, and research carried out in 2011 revealed that clutter can overwhelm the brain and make it harder to concentrate.

Take a few hours to sort out the belongings you don't really need or want anymore, then sell, gift or donate them. If you've not worn that top in the last year, are you really likely to wear it again? The less unnecessary stuff you have, the easier it is to get into the habit of staying tidy. After that, it's a case of making small changes that are easy to maintain, such as making your bed in the morning and putting things away as soon as you've finished with them.

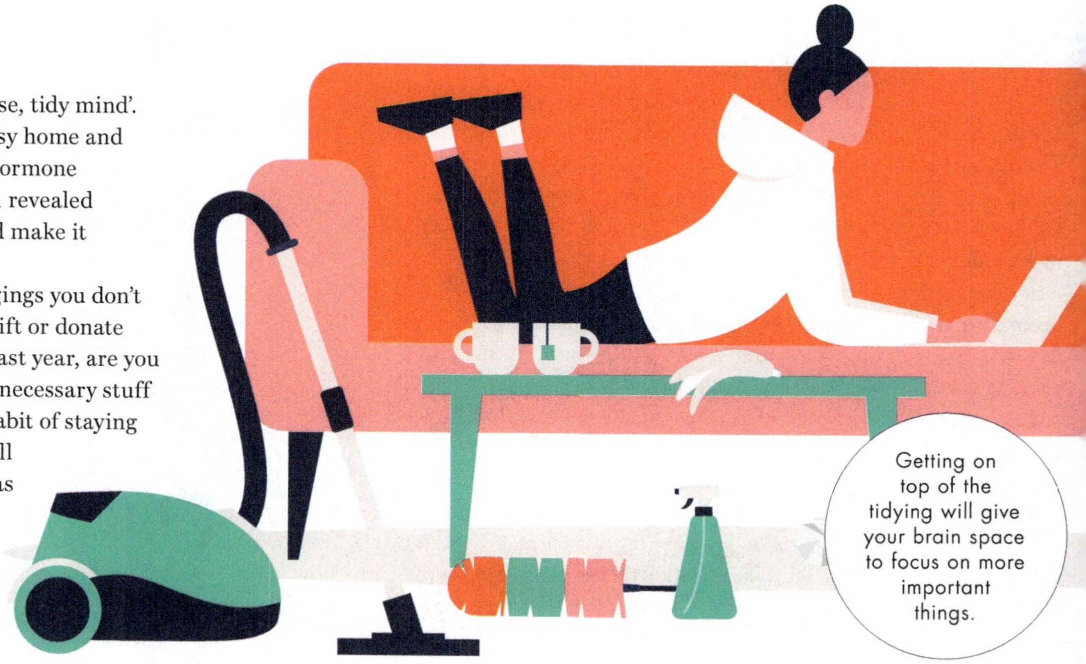

Sleeping better

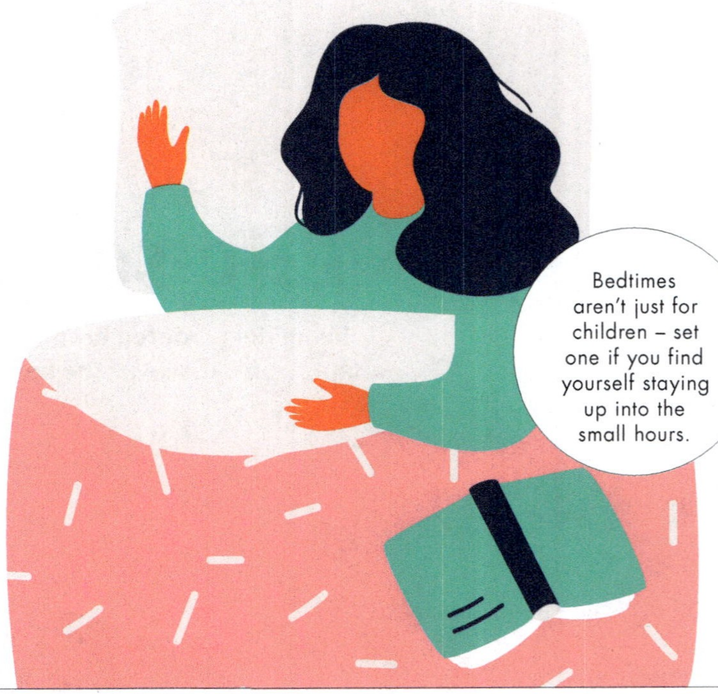

Bedtimes aren't just for children – set one if you find yourself staying up into the small hours.

Although the purpose of sleep isn't completely understood, scientists have established that it's vital for maintaining normal brain function and good physical health. Regularly getting less than seven hours of good-quality sleep a night has been linked to an earlier death, and even in the short-term a lack of sleep takes its toll; people who don't get enough rest struggle to focus, become irritable and overwhelmed more easily and can even drift into dangerous 'micro-sleeps' at work or behind the wheel.

In order to start creating a better sleep routine, it's vital to consider your environment. Keeping a bedroom tidy, cool and free from potential distractions sets things up for a good night's sleep. Work and study in other rooms so the bedroom is associated only with sleeping. Try to establish a consistent bedtime so your body feels sleepy when you want it to, and set a reminder to turn off screens and bright lights an hour before.

FOCUSING ON THE POSITIVES IN LIFE IS A HEALTHY HABIT FOR BOTH MIND AND BODY; JUST RECALLING A HAPPY MEMORY CAN BOOST YOUR MOOD AND RELIEVE STRESS

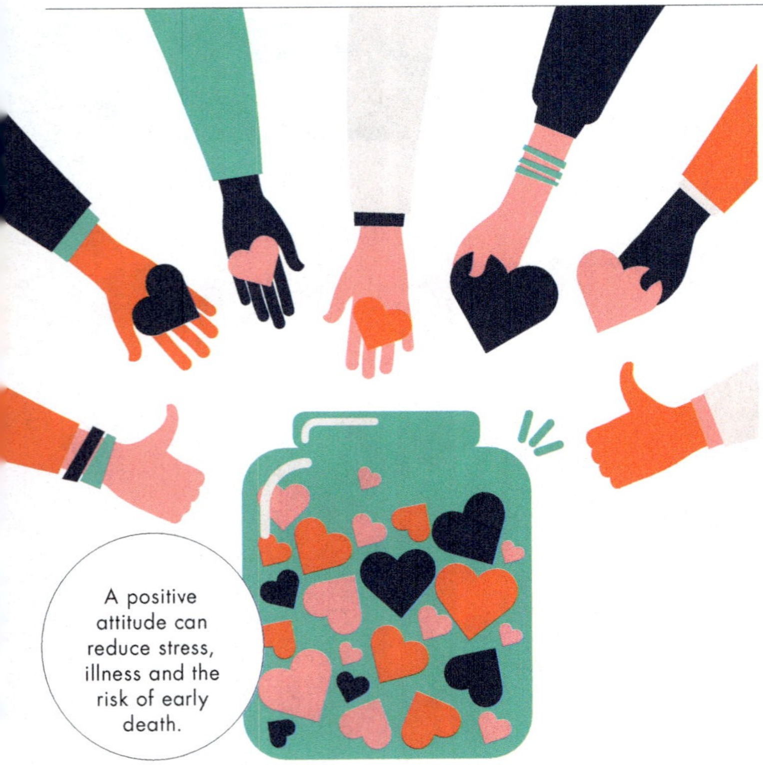

A positive attitude can reduce stress, illness and the risk of early death.

Focusing on the positives

Research by Harvard Medical School has linked a positive outlook to a longer life, and a study of coronary bypass patients found that those who were more optimistic were 50 per cent less likely to end up back in hospital in the six months following their surgery. Focusing on the good is a healthy habit for both mind and body; just recalling a happy memory can boost your mood and relieve stress.

One way to kick-start a change in outlook is journalling. Jotting down a couple of lines before bed every day about an accomplishment (however small), a funny thing that happened or something that made you smile can help you refocus if you tend to dwell on the negatives. Another important step is to challenge negative thoughts; every time you find yourself complaining or worrying about something, stop and ask yourself how important it really is or how likely it is to happen.

IMAGE SOURCE Getty Images

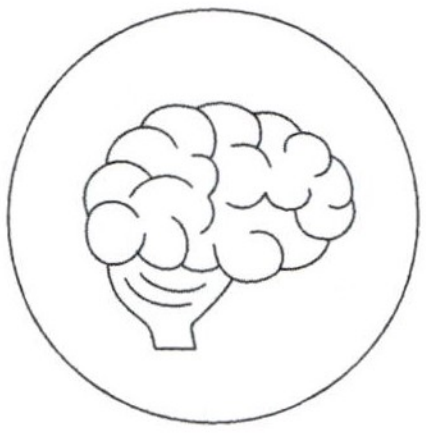

Life-saving habits

From deep-rooted human instincts to modern-world adaptations, discover the habits that are keeping you alive

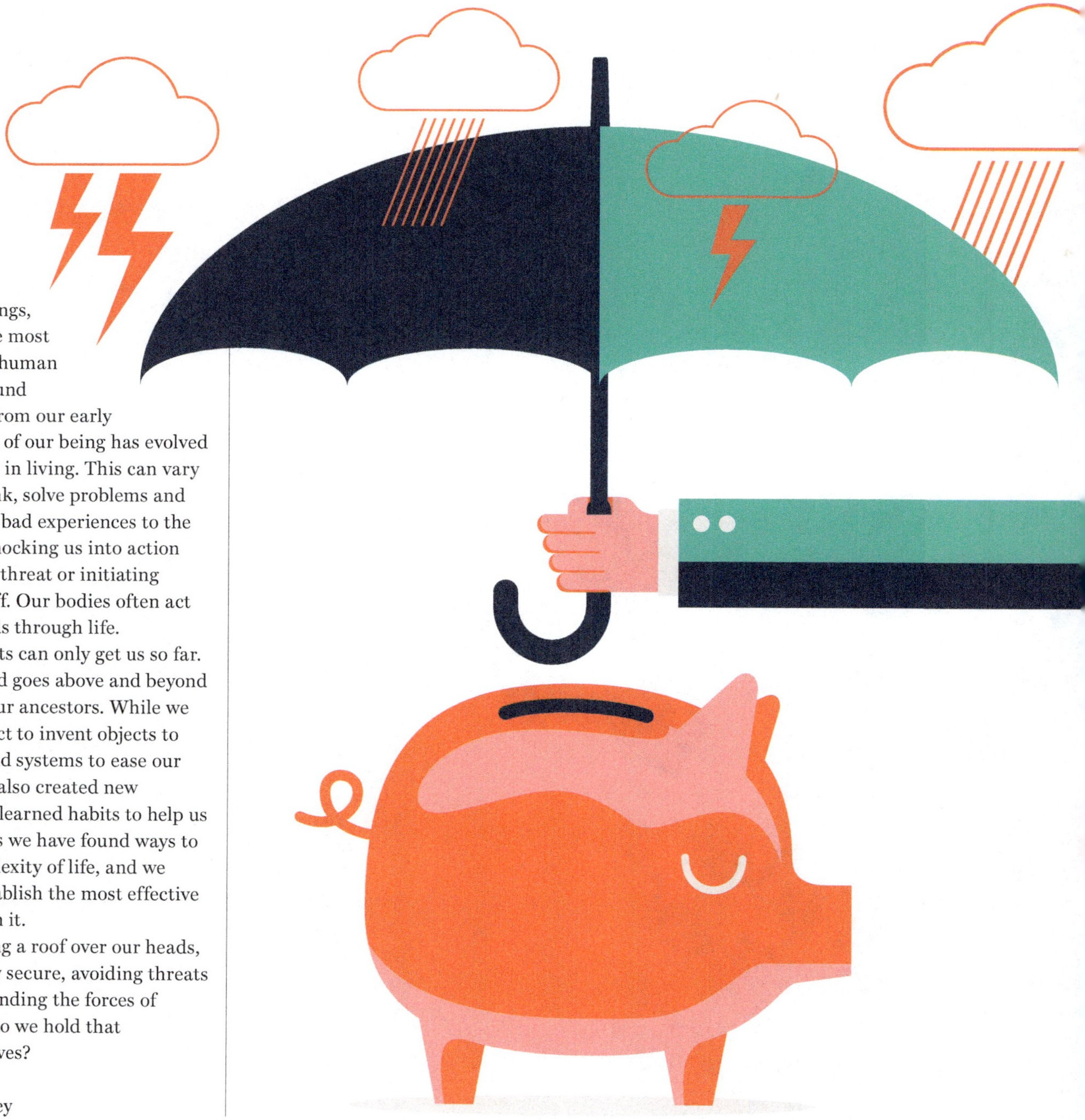

As living beings, some of the most important human instincts revolve around survival. Passed on from our early ancestors, every part of our being has evolved over time to assist us in living. This can vary from the way we think, solve problems and learn from good and bad experiences to the emotions we feel – shocking us into action when experiencing a threat or initiating disgust to warn us off. Our bodies often act as our security guards through life.

But human instincts can only get us so far. Today's modern world goes above and beyond the simpler lives of our ancestors. While we have used our intellect to invent objects to assist our survival and systems to ease our ways of life, we have also created new dangers that require learned habits to help us navigate. As a species we have found ways to adapt to a new complexity of life, and we must continue to establish the most effective methods to survive in it.

Whether it's keeping a roof over our heads, remaining financially secure, avoiding threats to health or understanding the forces of nature, what habits do we hold that ultimately save our lives?

WORDS Ailsa Harvey

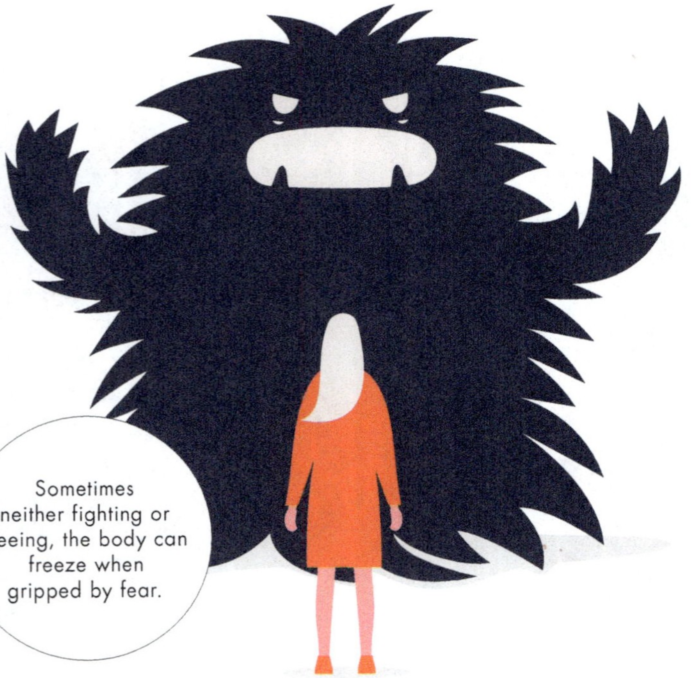

Sometimes neither fighting or fleeing, the body can freeze when gripped by fear.

Fight or flight

Life-saving ranking 1 2 3 4 **5**

As a habit of our bodies, when faced with danger or anything we perceive as a threat, we are quick to respond. Called fight or flight, the dramatic alterations in our bodies is the most important instinctive habit formed by us and other animals in times of immediate and life-threatening danger.

The rapid and automatic reaction is caused by the brain, which induces the production of adrenaline, steroids and pain relievers. Our hearts begin to beat faster, keeping us on high alert, while breathing increases to bring oxygen to our cells. When on this adrenaline high our bodies are prepared to deal with the worst and most treacherous scenarios. Whether we need to physically fight the danger or flee from the situation, this gives us the best chance of survival.

Embracing the Sun

Life-saving ranking **1** 2 3 4 5

Many of us love a holiday, searching for locations with maximum sunshine. When the Sun comes out during summer days, a lot of people adopt a habit of sitting where the rays will reach them. To an extent, a bit of sunbathing is good for our health and can enhance our lives. Sunlight exposure releases a hormone called serotonin into our brains, lifting our moods and keeping us calm and concentrated. Without enough sun, serotonin levels can dip, sometimes causing severe depression to set in.

A love of being in the Sun has many health benefits, but too much time in the Sun is dangerous. Establishing the habit of applying sun cream saves us from developing skin cancer while continuing to reap the benefits of a summer's day.

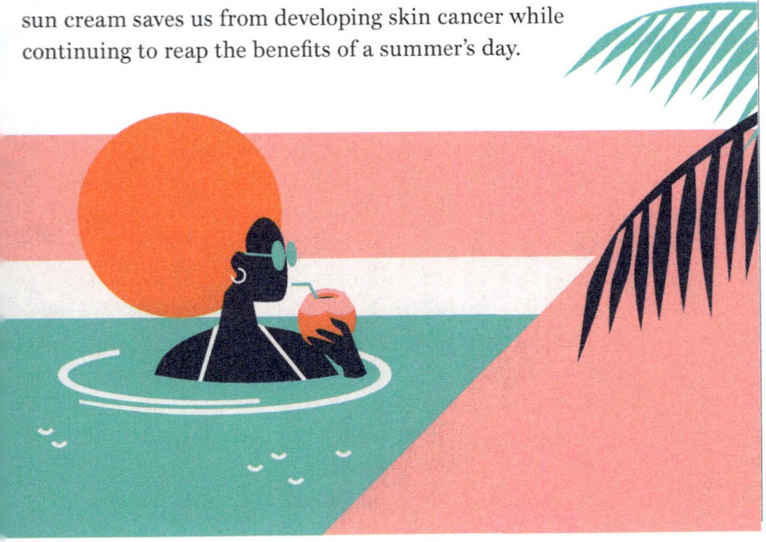

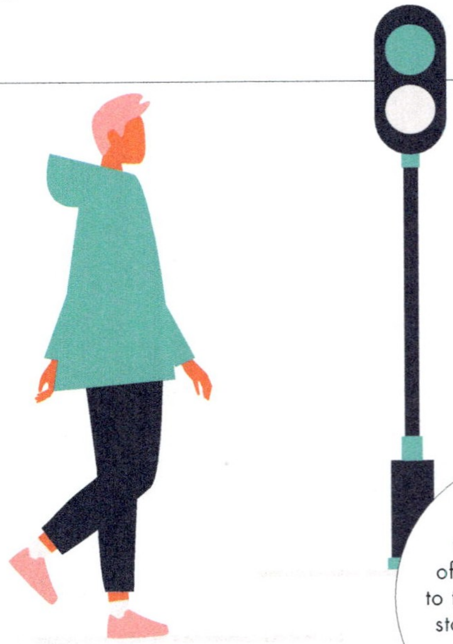

Modern technology is one of the biggest threats to this life-saving habit, stopping people from seeing their surroundings.

Observation

Life-saving ranking 1 2 **3** 4 5

What's the first thing you do before your foot steps off the curb to cross a busy road, or when you begin to drive off in your car? Chances are you will look around you for danger without even thinking about it. The risk of traffic is taught to us from an early age, and the act of stopping, looking and listening as a vulnerable pedestrian on a crowded road becomes a life-saving habit early on in your school days.

This habit of using your eyes and the vital sense of sight they provide have ensured survival for millennia. Danger rarely arises right before you, and spotting danger before it gets closer gives you time to judge a situation and act.

IMAGE SOURCE Getty Images

Smelling the perfect partner

Life-saving ranking (1) (2) **(3)** (4) (5)

We may not be able to control the genes we have been gifted with, but can your habits benefit your children's genes? You might think there's a type of person you are attracted to based on their appearance or personality, but would you consider scent to be up there on the list?

Some studies have shown that as a species we have formed a habit of choosing our partners based on a specific cluster of genes that determine our immune function. Not only this, humans may also use their noses to choose partners with the most different genetic make-up to their own. This means that any children born with this mixture of genes will have the genes to fight more threats to their immune systems.

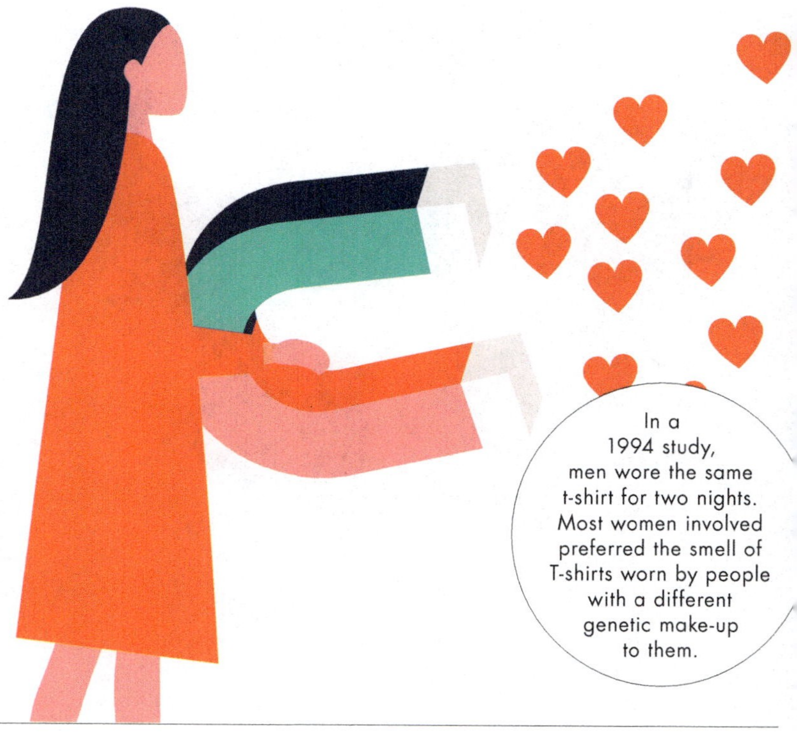

In a 1994 study, men wore the same t-shirt for two nights. Most women involved preferred the smell of T-shirts worn by people with a different genetic make-up to them.

> SOME STUDIES HAVE SHOWN THAT AS A SPECIES WE HAVE FORMED A HABIT OF CHOOSING OUR PARTNERS BASED ON A SPECIFIC CLUSTER OF GENES THAT DETERMINE OUR IMMUNE FUNCTION

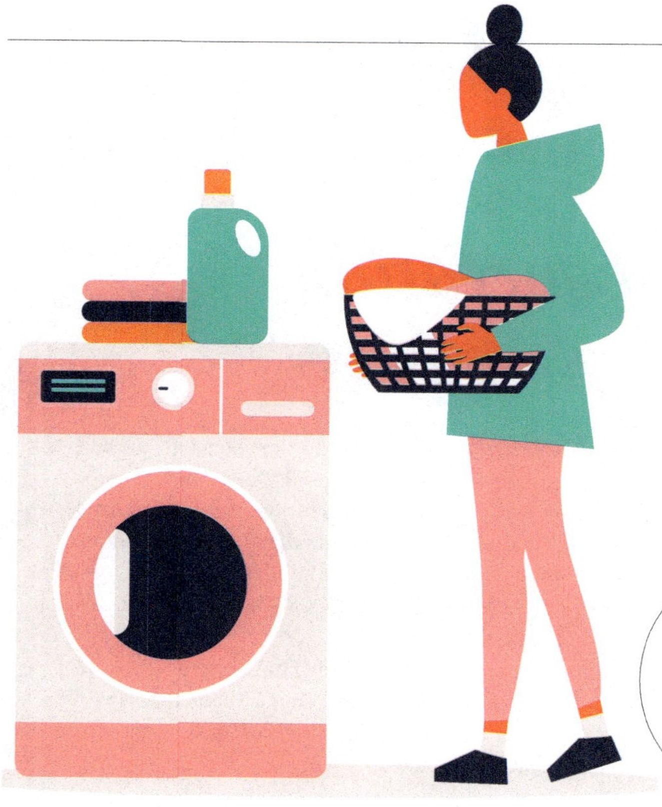

Hygiene rituals

Life-saving ranking (1) **(2)** (3) (4) (5)

However desperately you want to be in bed, there are a few hurdles to get over first. Without brushing your teeth, washing your face and changing from the day's clothes, sleep simply can't happen. That's the way it's been since childhood, and it is one of the best routine habits we have for our health. And these hygiene rituals don't stop at our bodies.

Keeping our surrounding environments germ-free by regularly cleaning surfaces with bleach or anti-bacterial wipes ensures that we stay healthy and happy in our homes. It's also important to wash clothes regularly – not just when they start to smell bad – as well as keeping bedding and towels fresh and drying them in a clean, warm environment to stop mould forming. Hoovering regularly is another good household habit to help keep dust at bay.

Washing maintains a successful balance between good and bad bacteria, preventing infection.

Cry babies

Life-saving ranking 1 2 3 **4** 5

We first enter the world when we are in our most vulnerable state: small in size, under-developed, immobile and lacking words to communicate. One thing babies are experts at, however, is crying. A baby's habit of crying when uncomfortable, hungry, in pain or in any situation that they deem to be a threat is crucial.

Crying is a baby's only way to signal to a parent that something isn't right. This high-pitched, loud and unsettling noise can't be ignored and more often than not forces the parents to work out the problem, alerting them to any threat to their newborn's wellbeing.

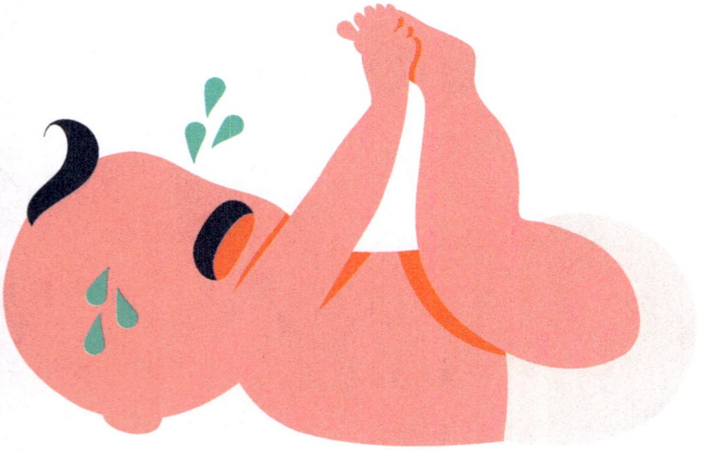

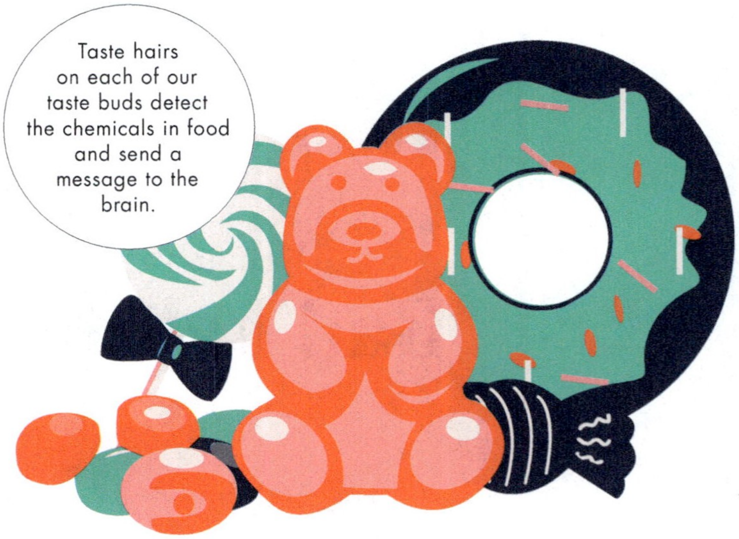

Sweet tooth

Life-saving ranking 1 2 3 **4** 5

The habit of indulging in sweet treats might lead to some of us becoming unhealthy, but being in tune with our taste buds can protect us from poison. Favouring sweet and savoury foods helps us to steer clear of bitter and rotten foods. By creating a sense of disgust and negative responses, our taste buds keep us in the habit of eating the safest delicacies. If poisonous or rotting foods didn't evoke such strong reactions, we would continue to eat bad foods, which could make us severely ill – or even kill us.

Sleeping and napping

Life-saving ranking 1 2 **3** 4 5

Keeping to a consistent sleep routine helps us to get the recommended seven hours or more of sleep a night. To function at our optimum, remaining alert and productive while keeping our energy levels up gives us the best quality of life. We are more likely to make mistakes when we are sleep-deprived.

One of the most explored consequences of sleep deprivation is dangerous driving. All it would take is to miss a night's sleep for you to take to the wheel and veer unintentionally off the road.

Sleeping has been proven to make us physically healthier beings in a range of ways. Lowering the risk of heart disease, improving mental health and strengthening our immune system are just a few of the benefits that come with the habit of a good sleep routine.

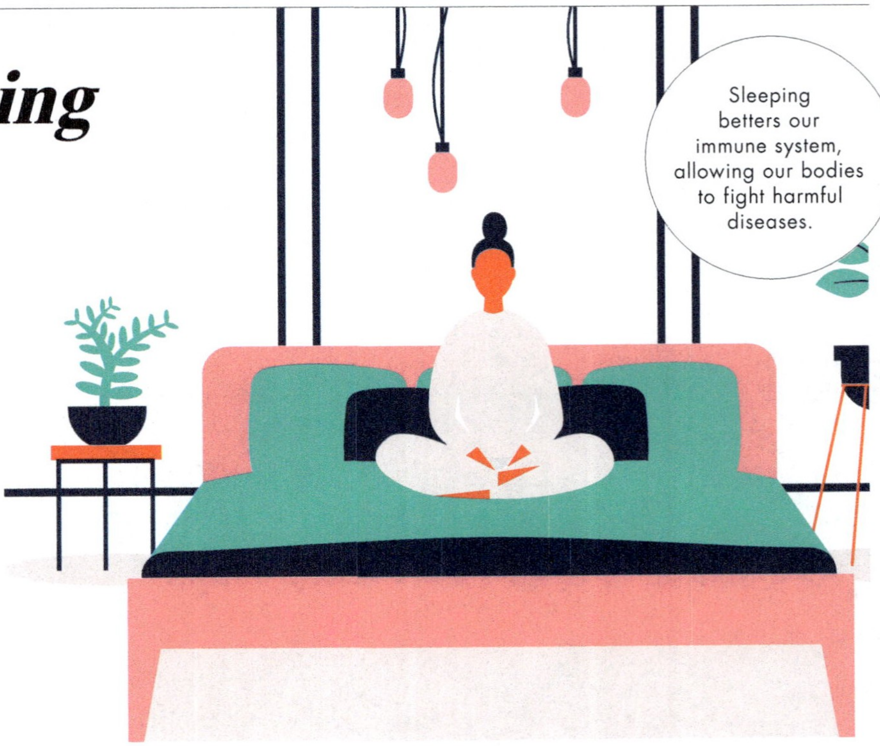

IMAGE SOURCE Getty Images

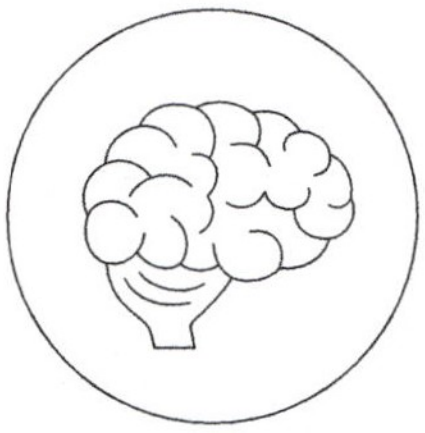

Bad habits

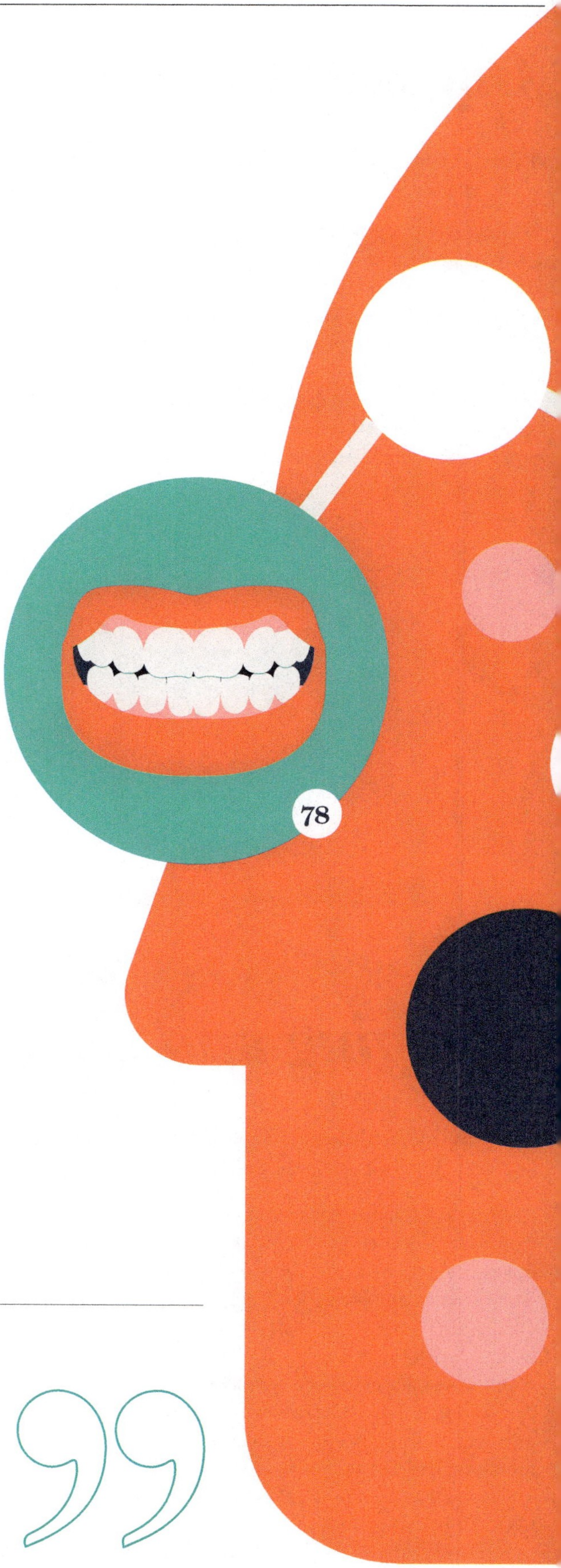

"COGNITIVE BEHAVIOURAL THERAPIES CAN BE EXPLORED TO UNDERSTAND THE EMOTIONAL ROOT OF THE HABIT AND SEEK TO REMEDY THE UNDERLYING PROBLEM"

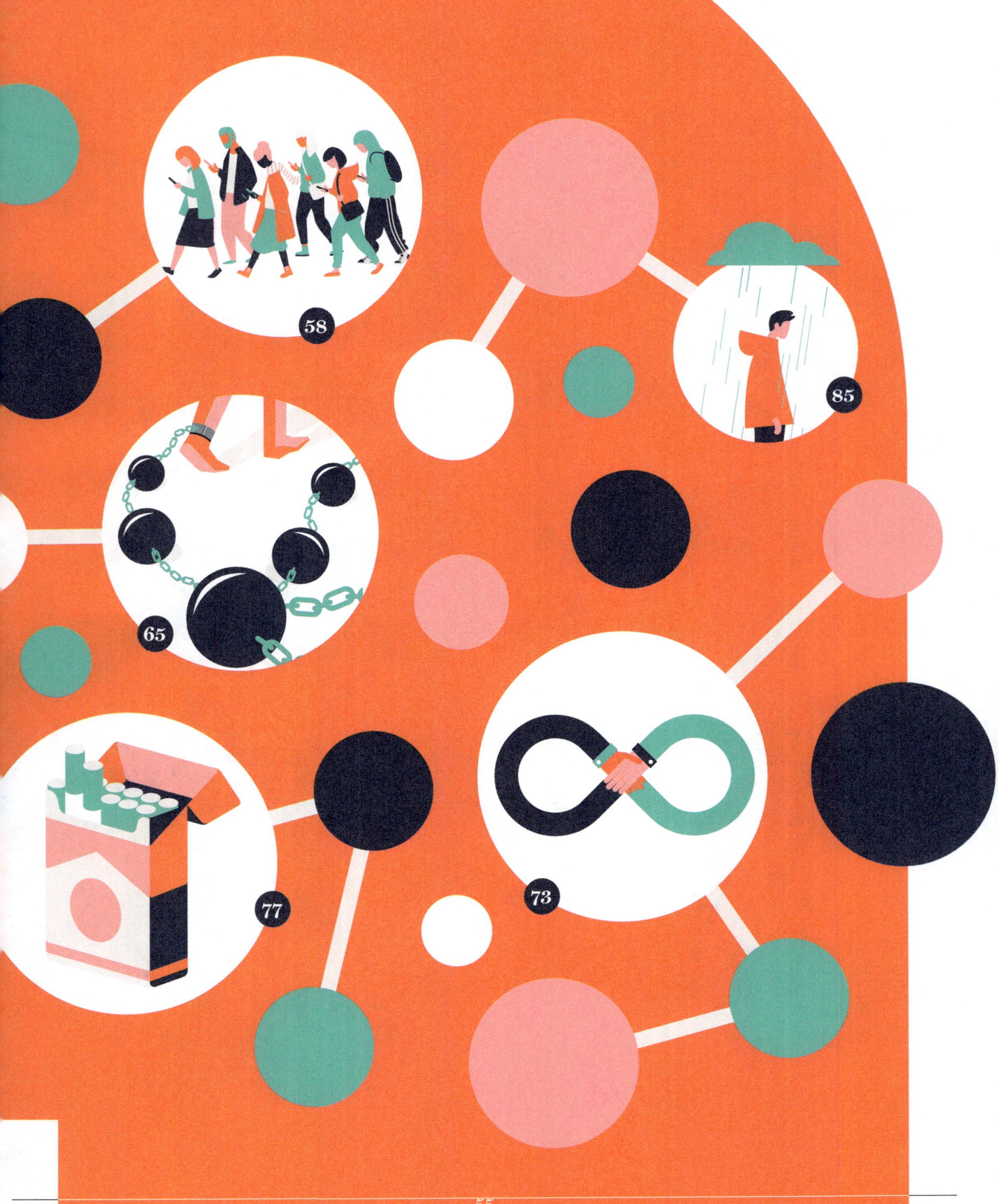
58
85
65
77
73

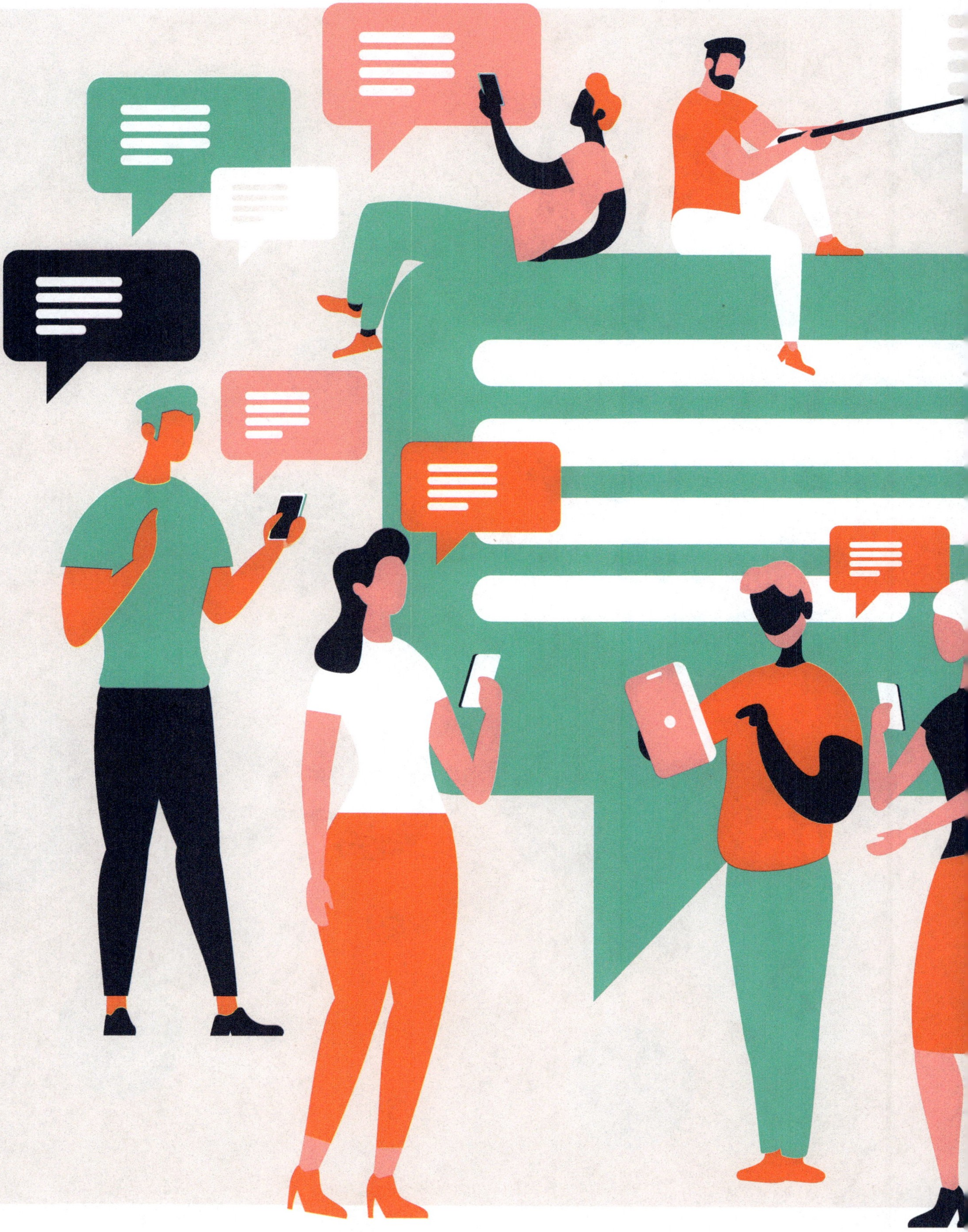

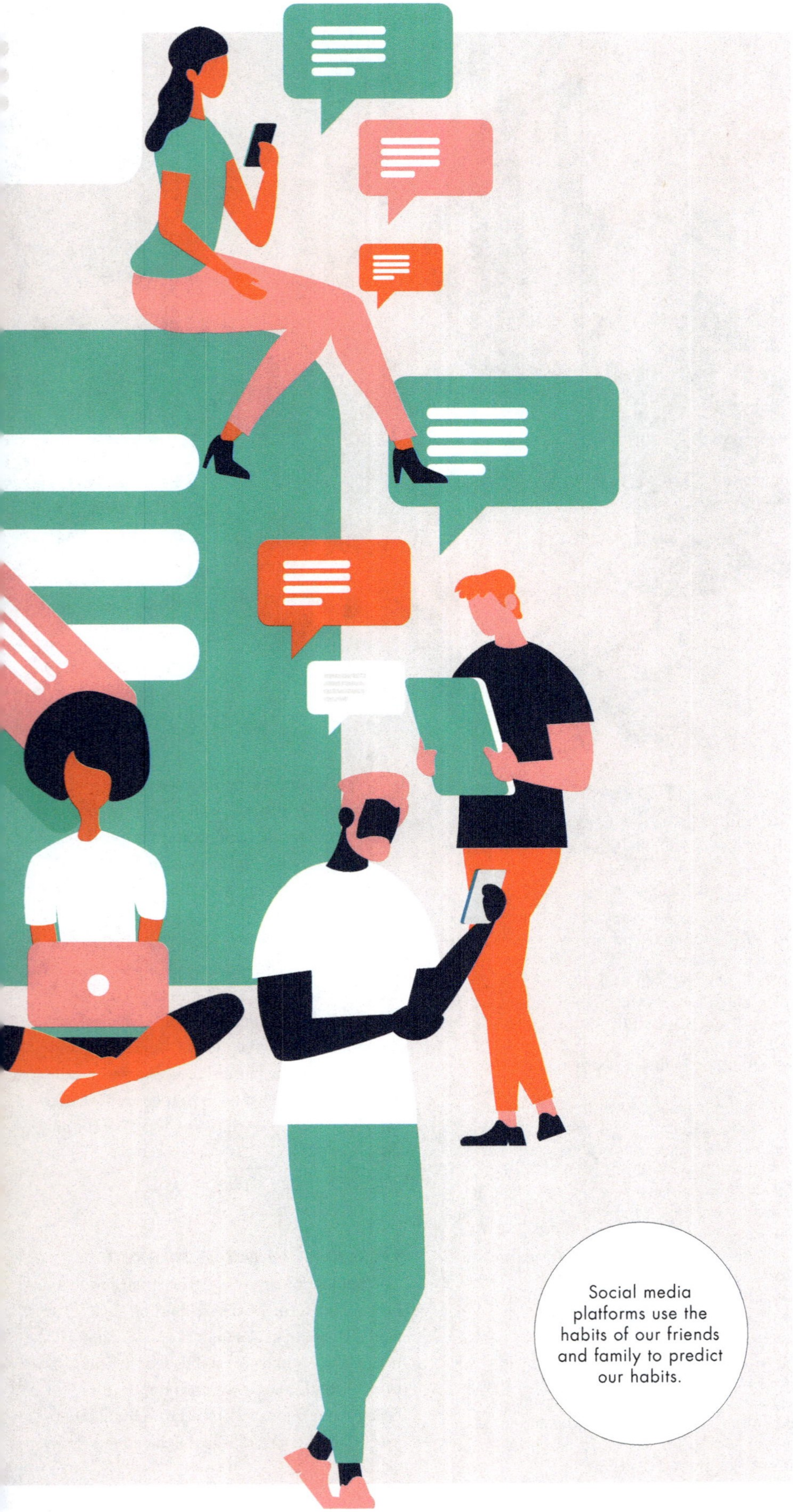

Social media platforms use the habits of our friends and family to predict our habits.

When good habits turn bad

Are we fighting an uphill battle against bad habits or do we just lack the willpower to get our behaviour under control?

Habits are an essential feature of our biology: the brain makes them to save time. If we encounter a situation and a behaviour gets us a reward, it's natural to want to repeat that behaviour again and again. But weighing up whether the reward is worth it every time is a waste of processing power. The more we repeat the same action and get the same reward, the more the brain relaxes. Eventually it stops asking whether the reward is worth it, and a habit is formed.

From then on, whenever we encounter the trigger situation, the brain sets the habit in motion. Often it doesn't even bother to check whether we got the reward or not; it just finishes the habit and moves on to the next thing.

For good habits, like flossing or eating a piece of fruit, that's great; even if we don't really enjoy the process, we'll keep automatically performing the habit anyway. But for bad habits, like mindlessly scrolling through social media when we're supposed to be spending time with friends, or popping into the local takeaway when we're supposed to be on a diet, our automatic behaviours conflict with what we actually want. So why do we make them in the first place?

IMAGE SOURCE Getty Images

Reflect or reflex?

The brain has two conflicting systems that fight it out over bad habit behaviour. In his book, *Thinking, Fast and Slow*, Nobel Prize-winning economist Daniel Kahneman called them 'system one' and 'system two'.

System one is fast, instinctive and driven by emotions. It runs on reflexes and it doesn't need any working memory to operate; it just sees a trigger and sets off an automatic response. It doesn't demand much of the brain, using little in the way of processing power or attention, and it can do more than one thing at once.

System two is slow, logical and driven by rational thought. It uses the parts of the brain involved in future planning and goal setting to monitor the current situation, match it up with the desired outcome for the future and work out the best course of action right now. It's powerful, but it can only do one task at a time and it demands our full attention.

To save bandwidth, the brain breaks any repetitive system-two tasks down into automatic system-one tasks. It's so efficient at doing this that it can handle between 40 and 95 per cent of our choices without us even needing to think. But sometimes the process goes wrong.

We often make habits without even realising, and habits we made in the past don't always match up with our goals right now. And once behaviours start running on autopilot, they're hard to switch off. System two does have the power to override system one, but it takes serious willpower.

When good habits turn bad

It's not the brain's intention to hardwire bad habits; we form habits because they seem likely to be beneficial in the long run. But many feel-good behaviours can have unintentional side-effects.

Take smartphones as an example. We have computers in our pockets with a million times more working memory than the computer that took astronauts to the Moon. Smartphones have put the sum total of human knowledge at our fingertips and connected us across the globe like never before. But this incredible technology has its downsides.

Our phones are always with us, and they make a huge number of demands on our attention. According to stats collected by the RescueTime app, we pick up our phones an average of 60 times a day. Most of those interactions last less than two minutes: we're constantly checking.

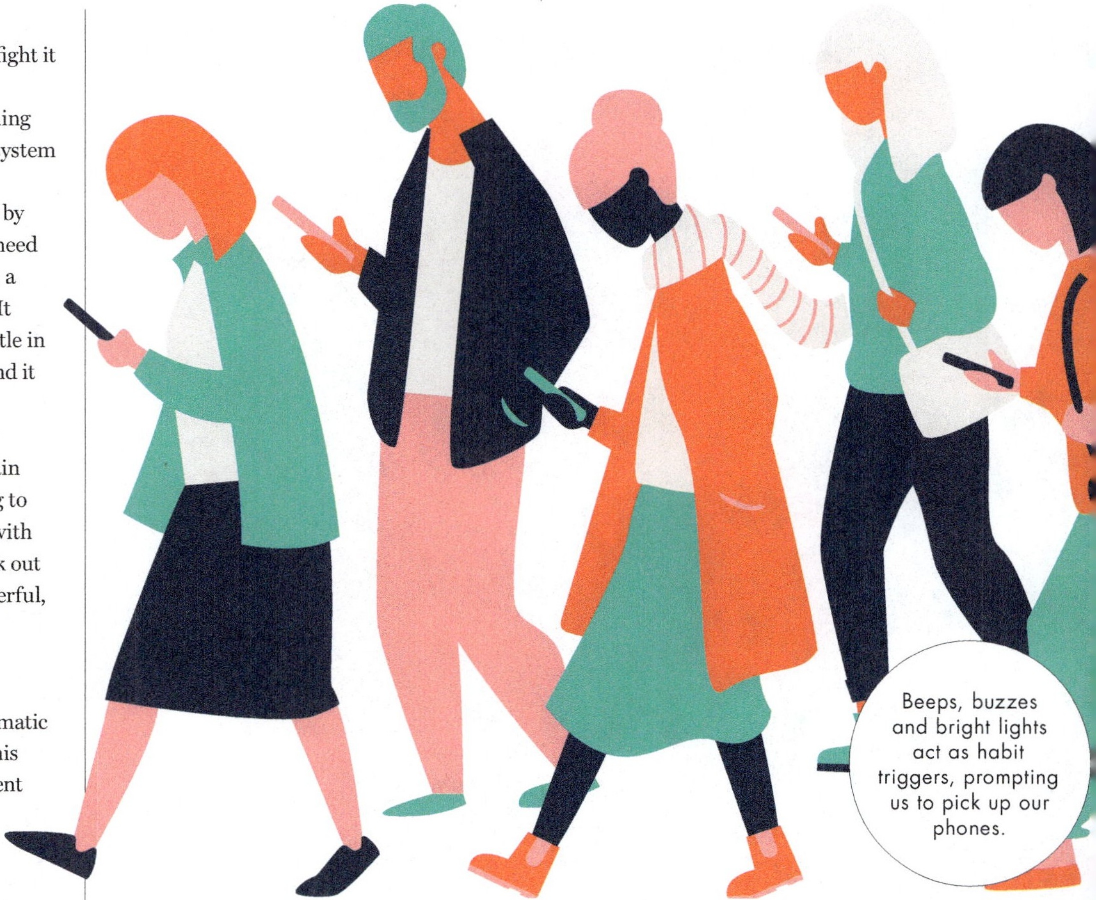

Beeps, buzzes and bright lights act as habit triggers, prompting us to pick up our phones.

BAD HABIT OR ADDICTION?

Addictions are more than just bad habits: they hijack the brain's reward system

Addictions start in a similar way to habits: we try something, we get a reward and we try it again. With repetition, addictive behaviours become automatic. This is partly because addictions affect the striatum, a key part of the brain involved in habit formation. But it's made worse by the impact addictions have on the brain's reward system.

The brain has built-in reward circuits that evolved to make us feel good when we perform survival behaviours, like eating high-calorie foods. These circuits use the neurotransmitter dopamine: the brain's reward chemical.

Addictions activate the brain's reward circuits artificially, supplying an instant dopamine hit followed by cravings and withdrawal symptoms. At the same time the excess dopamine hijacks habit circuits, helping to make the sequence of behaviours needed to get the next fix to become automatic. This combination is what makes addictions so difficult to overcome.

Once a habit is formed and we start performing a behaviour on autopilot, we'll still do the actions even if the reward goes away. Even after someone gets over withdrawal from an addiction, unexpected triggers might still reactivate old habits, making it more likely for them to become addicted again.

Beeps, vibrations, notifications and even our own boredom all act as triggers for subconscious mobile habits. Add it all up and we spend an average of 3 hours and 15 minutes looking at our screens: scrolling, watching, gaming, liking, listening, messaging.

These automatic habit behaviours affect our concentration, sleep and social interactions. But like most things, smartphones aren't all bad. To break unwanted mobile habits we need to monitor our behaviour, judge every action and work out which habits are good and which we want to change. That takes immense effort, and even if we have iron willpower, we're not the only ones in control.

Designed to get us hooked

Companies don't want us to use their product just once – they want us to keep coming back for more. And if they can get us to do it on autopilot, all the better. Once a habit is established they don't have to offer continuous rewards and incentives, because our brains switch off the circuits that assess whether our repeated behaviour is really worth it.

There are a variety of tactics that companies use to help establish habits in their customers. For app and game developers, these include a trick called a 'core loop'.

The loop has three components – action, reward and progression – which loosely correspond to the three parts of habit formation – trigger, reward and repeat. The action might be to kill a monster, the reward a random item and the progression an achievement or level up that encourages us to repeat the loop again.

Habits settle in fastest if behaviours are quick and rewards are immediate, so habit-forming apps and games tend to open up in seconds and can be dropped at any moment. If a user can get into an app, complete the core loop and get out again in the time it takes to queue for a cup of coffee, the app is onto a habit-forming winner.

Take *Candy Crush Saga*, for example. This mobile game now has more than 270 million logins every month. Since it launched in 2012, its player base has clocked an unfathomable 8.3 million years of play time. Although it's free to play, people can choose to buy power ups with real money, and in 2018 it made more than £700 million (approximately $909 million).

Candy Crush Saga encourages us to form habits because it's got short loops with instant rewards and loads of opportunities for progress: there are more than 5,000 levels to play.

Habits are most sensitive to rewards while they are first forming, so many games bunch early milestones close together and offer lots of instant rewards, like loot crates and upgrades, to reinforce the habit behaviour. Once a habit is formed, which only takes about two months, the rewards can start to drop away.

Just one more episode

Habit-forming tricks don't just work for quick-fix apps – they can keep us hooked on the same activity for hours. Streaming services like Netflix use algorithms to recommend our next binge watches based on data gathered from tens of millions of customers. The data includes not only what, when and where we watch, but small details like our browsing habits, how long we left between episodes and where we pressed the pause button. These algorithms constantly update themselves as new information comes in, working out which content to recommend to keep us coming back for more.

According to Netflix, those recommendations have just 90 seconds to catch our attention.

> COMPANIES DON'T WANT US TO USE THEIR PRODUCT JUST ONCE – THEY WANT US TO KEEP COMING BACK FOR MORE

The cover art that we see when we log in is no accident; it's the result of careful testing and data-driven design, optimised to encourage us to click through.

User testing has revealed that, in general, we're more likely to choose a show if the picture we see has recognisable characters with emotional expressions. But the same images don't work for everyone. In fact, the thumbnails you see are personalised to your account. They are customised to your viewing history, showing you the same titles as your friends but with different featured actors, expressions, text and ambience, all designed to keep you watching.

These kinds of techniques can even get us to do things that don't induce such an obvious feel-good reward as films or games. According to an exposé in the *New York Times*, taxi firm Uber uses a combination of Netflix-style technology and game-design techniques to encourage drivers to keep driving during busy hours and in popular locations. These include awarding achievements and badges when drivers reach particular milestones and an app feature called 'continuous ride', which queues up the next passenger before the current one has even left the car.

A 2018 study found that there are 1.67 billion households with TVs globally.

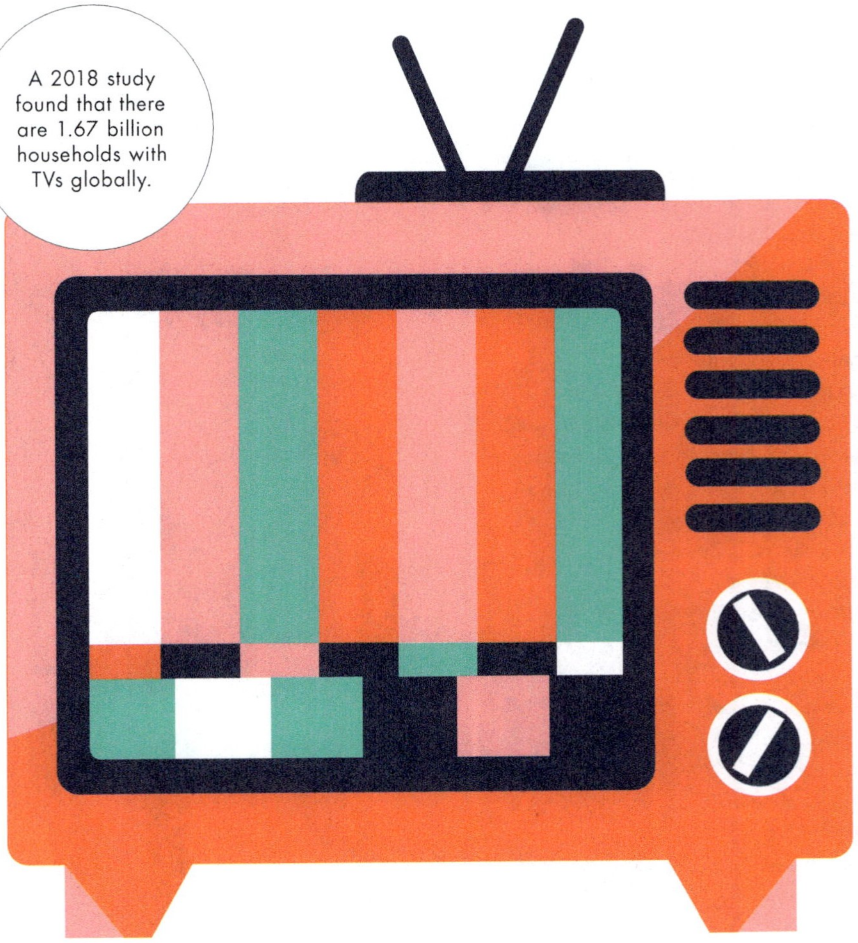

IMAGE SOURCE Getty Images

My habits or yours?

Big companies aren't the only ones influencing our habit formation. Our friends and families have a huge role to play in the habits we make and struggle to break. The people who influence us most are those we share very close relationships with, and it's more than just peer pressure; our friends and family can change our habits without us even realising.

Some of the habit similarities between family members are down to genetics, especially among parents and siblings, but not all of our shared habits can be explained away by biology. Studies to find out the health habit similarities between parents and their children revealed something unexpected. While there are similarities between mothers and daughters and fathers and sons, there is also habit crossover within couples. What's more, these similarities increase over time.

Couples tend to share similar diets, similar body weights and similar patterns of smoking, alcohol and drug use. The effect is so striking that it creates a noticeable impact on their mental and physical health, which doctors know as 'health concordance'. Researchers think it's likely that the close bond between couples, and the amount of time they spend together, is partly responsible.

This kind of social habit sharing is partly down to how our species evolved. We're social animals, and gathering together to share with our companions has been crucial for our survival.

Throughout human history, making and sharing food has been a powerful way of bonding as a group. When we came together to eat in the past, it made sense for everyone to behave in the same way. If one person always ate all of the food, we wouldn't do well as a team, but if everyone behaved in the same way and we all got a fair share, it boosted our chances of survival.

It's likely that we evolved to enjoy food more when we're eating with close companions, setting off an extra reward sensation in our brains that encourages us to keep eating.

Even in the modern world we still eat more when we eat with others – in some cases up to 50 per cent more. We also eat for longer, and our food choices change. If the people around us eat vegetables, we're more likely to eat vegetables too, but if we're surrounded by sweet wrappers, there's a good chance we'll indulge.

SHOPPING ON AUTOPILOT

Do we really like the foods we pick up in the supermarket, or are we just shopping out of habit?

A single supermarket can contain 50,000 different products. If we had to make a conscious choice about whether to buy every one of them, we'd never get our shopping done, so we make habits and choose our groceries on autopilot. There's even a term for it – brand loyalty – and it's big business.

Food shops are the perfect places for habit formation because we visit them so often. Grocery brands go out of their way to get us to buy their products without considering the competition. They trigger our habit loops with recognisable branding. They encourage us to keep coming back again with consistent quality, special offers and discounts. And they keep our interest in the long term with new products and loyalty rewards.

At first we might choose a product for rational reasons, but over time habit loops set up and the rational parts of our brains go offline. This is good for business and for our busy schedules, but it can be bad for our health and our bank balances if we become locked into purchasing unhealthy or expensive items when we'd really rather switch to something else.

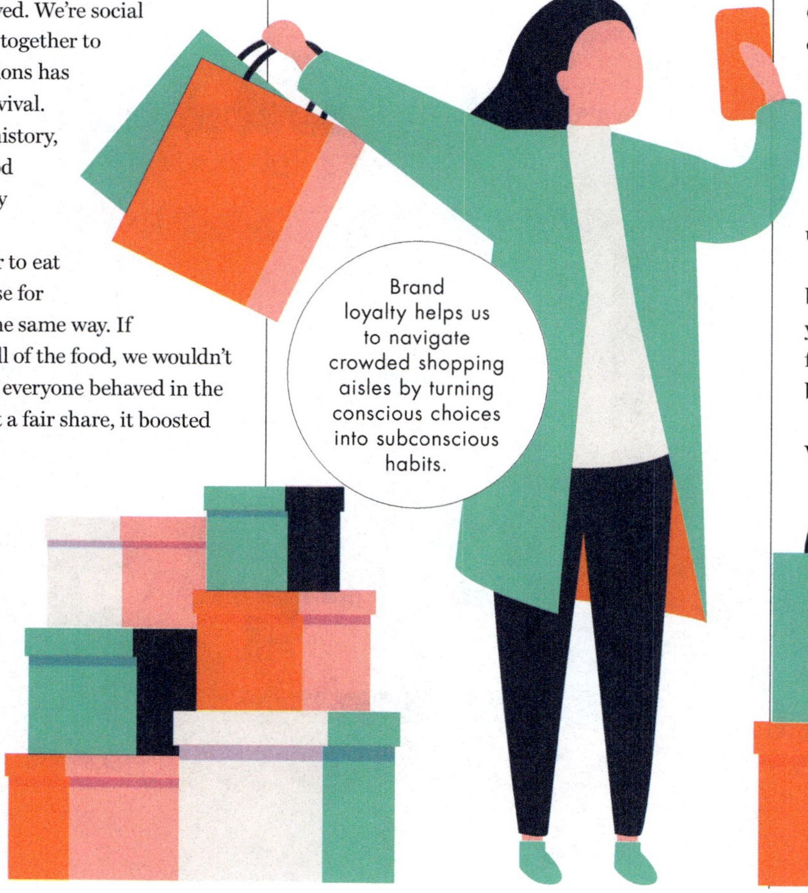

Brand loyalty helps us to navigate crowded shopping aisles by turning conscious choices into subconscious habits.

Sharing habits in the digital age

Our social connections don't just affect our habits when we're together. They feed back into our digital lives, affecting our online habits, shopping habits, entertainment habits and much more.

Social networks and search engines collect vast quantities of data from our likes, clicks, shares, comments, connections and impressions. They know our location, past searches, age, gender, interests, job, relationship status, friends, family, health, fitness habits, the apps we use and the videos we watch. And they can access our webcams, our microphones, our contacts, our emails, our calendars, our messages and our photographs once we've allowed it.

Seven out of ten apps share data with third parties, and they don't necessarily need our explicit permission to do so. For example, if a friend gives permission for an app to access their address book, your details will be shared too. Given that we tend to share likes and dislikes with our social groups, even a small amount of data provides a huge amount of information.

That data, combined with the data from friends and family and other users with similar interests, can help companies to work out what we want and how best to encourage us to make using their products a habit.

So next time you're beating yourself up for that bad habit you're struggling to change, give yourself a break: your biology, environment and friends could all be helping to reinforce your behaviour. Changing a habit is no mean feat.

WORDS Laura Mears

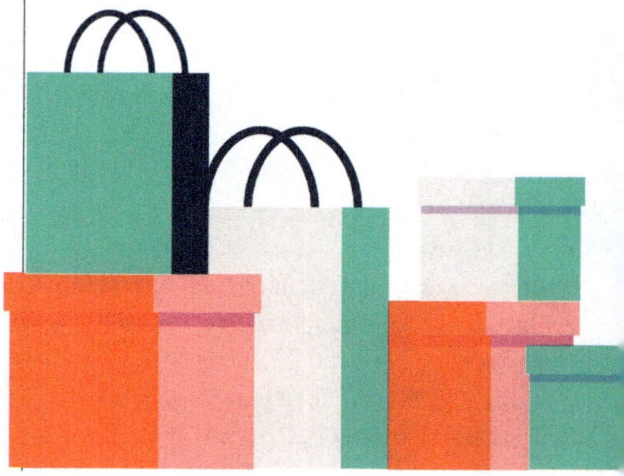

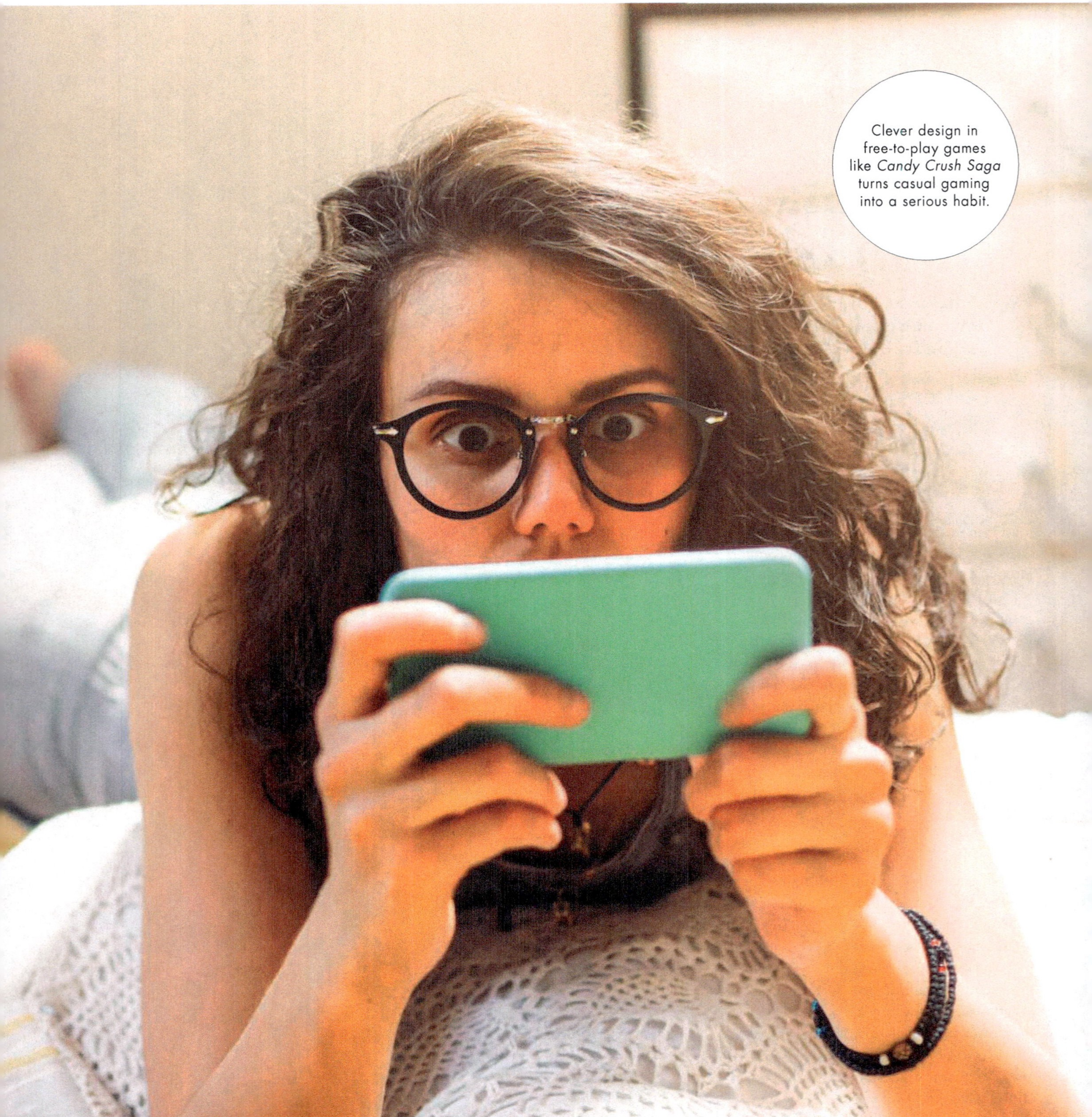

Clever design in free-to-play games like *Candy Crush Saga* turns casual gaming into a serious habit.

IMAGE SOURCE Getty Images

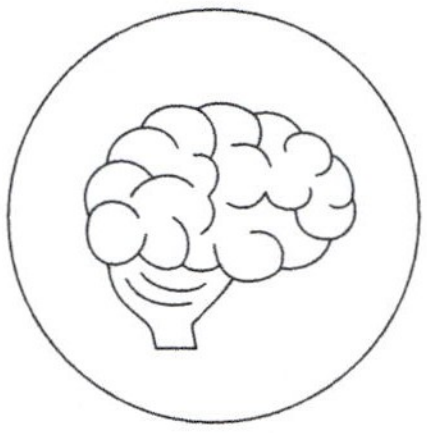

Criminal habits

What makes a habitual criminal? How some crimes can be as addictive as hard drugs

On 7 February 2010 Detective Sergeant Jim Smyth of Ontario Provincial Police (OPP) brought a man into interview room 216: Colonel David Russell Williams, the commander of a nearby airbase, CFB Trenton. He wasn't arrested; it was just a chat in relation to a spate of violent assaults on local women, including the murder of 27-year-old Jessica Lloyd and 37-year-old corporal Marie-France Comeau.

These women had been attacked and bound in their homes before being murdered. The colonel was helping with enquiries. The detective sergeant almost apologetically pointed out where the cameras and microphones were, and they spoke to each other on first-name terms. It was friendly, relaxed. Williams chewed gum and flashed an easy smile at the ceiling camera as Smyth laid out another mic, asking Williams whether he'd ever been interviewed in a police station before. "Never," Williams replied, then paused and said, "The closest was when I was interviewed by NIS for top-secret clearance." He was reminding Smyth exactly how important he was and that it was in the detective sergeant's interests not to upset the apple cart. What he didn't know was that Smyth belonged to OPP's Behavioural Science Unit and that Williams was already being set up for a drastic fall. He went into that interview room a decorated, high-ranking airman who had once been trusted to fly the Queen and Prince Philip across Canada: nearly ten hours of

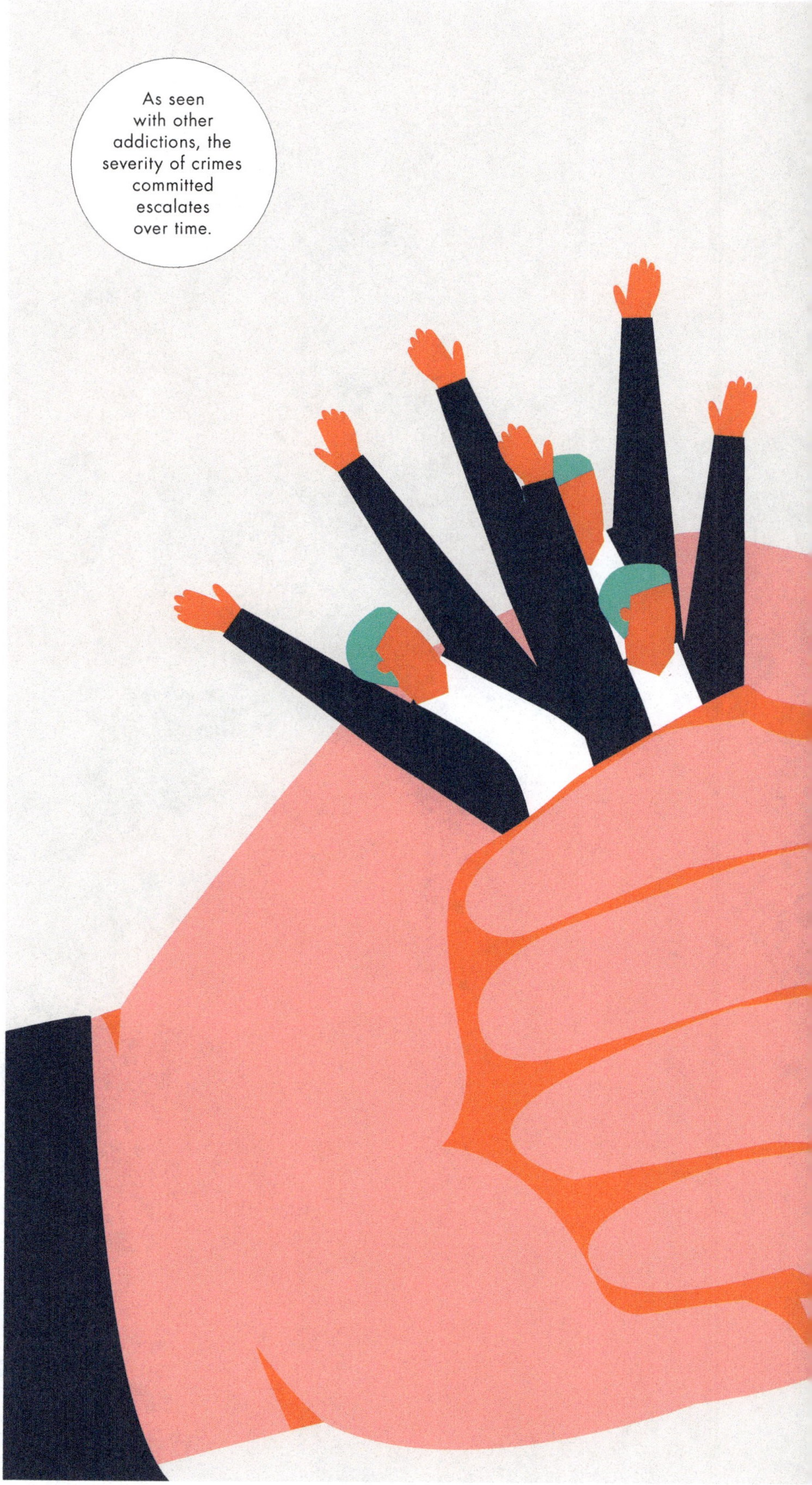

As seen with other addictions, the severity of crimes committed escalates over time.

> WHAT WILLIAMS DIDN'T KNOW WAS THAT SMYTH BELONGED TO THE OPP'S BEHAVIOURAL SCIENCE UNIT AND HE WAS BEING SET UP FOR A DRASTIC FALL

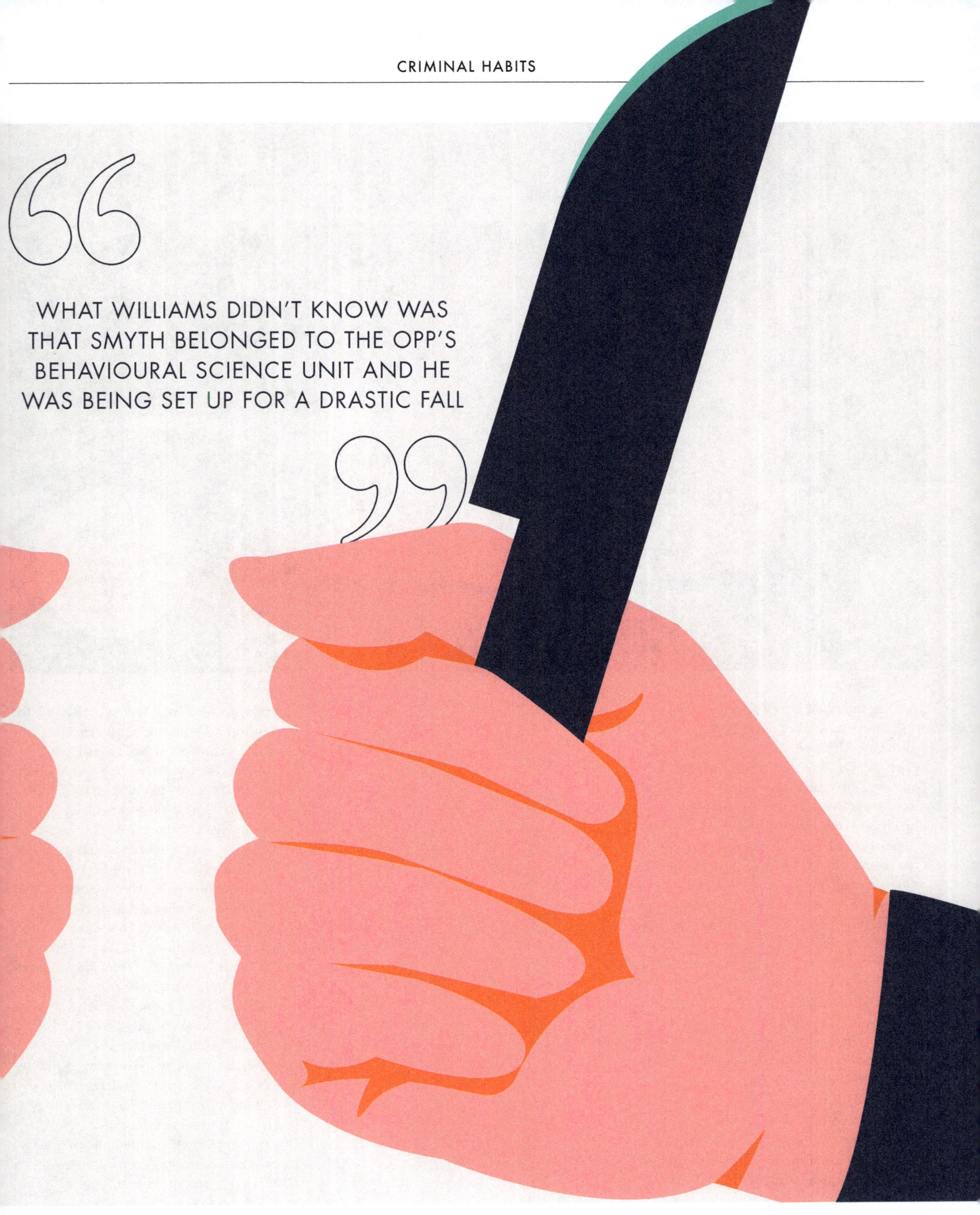

IMAGE SOURCE Getty Images

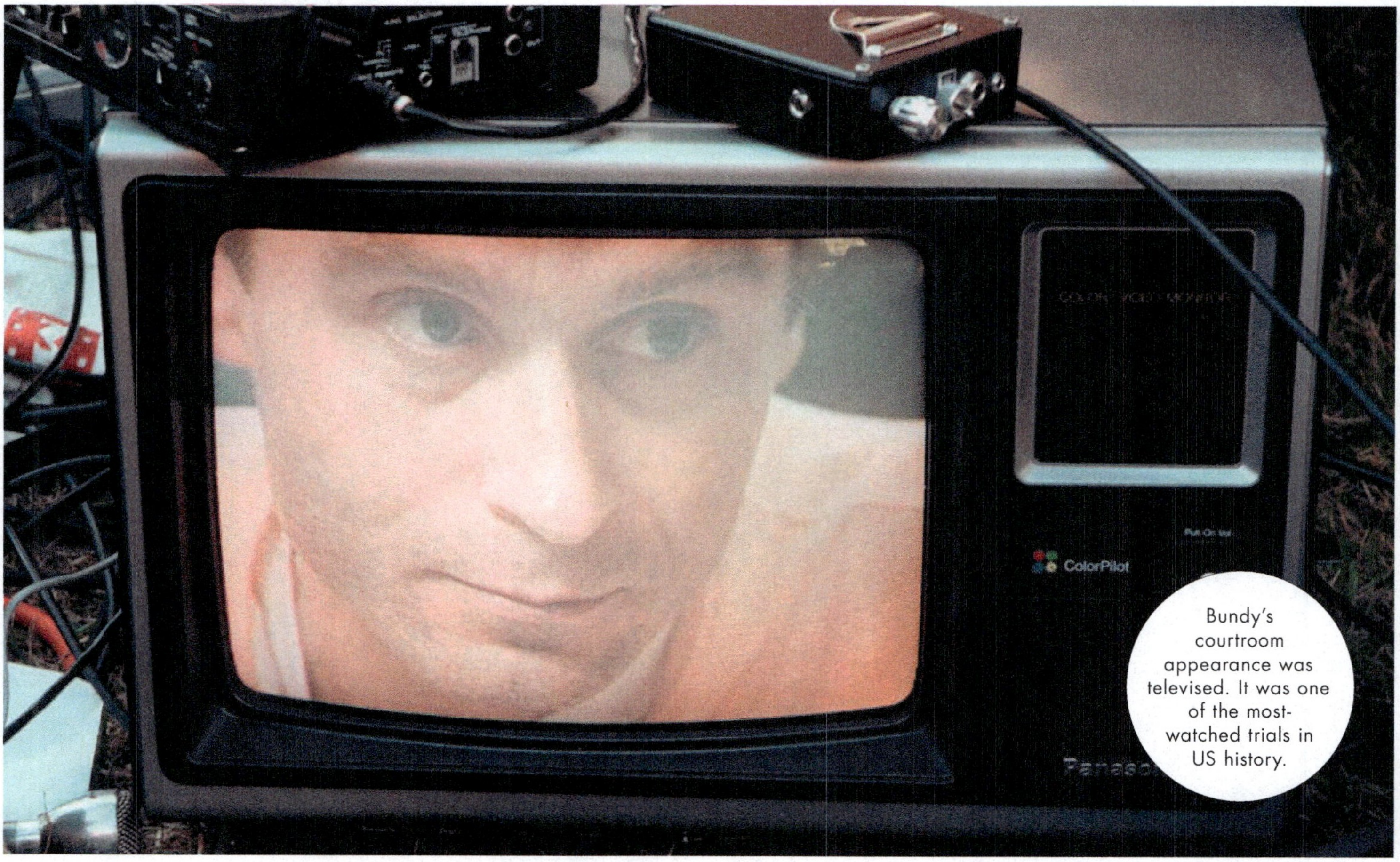

Bundy's courtroom appearance was televised. It was one of the most-watched trials in US history.

gruelling interview later a sexual sadist and serial murderer walked out, a broken man now facing a life sentence.

The investigation had given Detective Sergeant Smyth the upper hand in the interview before it had even started. The OPP already had compelling evidence that the colonel was at Jessica Lloyd's house on the evening that she had vanished: the distinctive wear and tread on the tyres of his Nissan Pathfinder SUV matched the tracks left in the deep snow outside. But it was only with Smyth's considerable interviewing experience and a profile of this suspect that he was able to extricate a confession from him.

David Russell Williams pleaded guilty to all charges in October 2010, which included two counts of first-degree murder, sexual assault and forcible confinement, plus 82 counts of breaking and entering: Williams had worked his way up to the murders over several years. A cycle of deviant offences – sexual in nature – began with him stealing women's underwear from clothes lines and houses. From the hundreds of lurid photos, videos and audio tapes discovered in the colonel's Ottawa house, OPP was able to build a picture of how this had escalated. He seemed contrite as he faced the judge in October the same year, telling justice Robert F. Scott that he was "indescribably ashamed" and saying, "I know the crimes I have committed have traumatised many people... I deeply regret what I have done and the harm I know I have caused to many."

It's hard to believe he felt genuine remorse for the pain he'd inflicted, but he certainly had a lot to lose from this conviction besides his freedom - not least of all his reputation, career and his marriage. Even if he had given no thought to his victims or their families he must have, at some point, considered what he was putting on the line personally for the sake of this habit. And gradually the compulsion became so overwhelming that he simply had to repeat the cycle, regardless of what it might cost him. Whatever positive psychological feedback the colonel was experiencing from these criminal acts, the payoff was diminishing each time. And each time, the only way for him to be fully gratified was to take it to the next level.

BUNDY'S 'PORN ADDICTION'

Even in the hours just before his execution, manipulative serial killer Ted Bundy was trying to shirk responsibility for his crimes. In his final prison interview on the afternoon of 23 January 1989, he told psychologist and anti-porn activist James Dobson that he'd had a wonderful, healthy childhood with loving parents. But Bundy alleged that it was his discovery of pornography that set him on a dark path.

"I'm not blaming pornography," he said, telling Dr Dobson exactly what he wanted to hear. "I'm not saying it caused me to go out and do certain things... The issue is how this kind of literature contributed and helped mould and shape the kinds of violent behaviour. I've lived in prison for a long time now, and I've met a lot of men who were motivated to commit violence. Without exception, every one of them was deeply involved in pornography – deeply consumed by the addiction."

The idea that young Theodore Bundy's addiction to porn was a stepping stone to exceptionally violent serial murder as an adult was largely debunked by another, more renowned psychologist, Al Carlisle.

Dr Carlisle considered Bundy's pornography habit too simple a reason to explain his compulsions and stated that a far more complex addiction was at play in Bundy's murders: a fantasy of power over a vulnerable woman.

This feedback loop isn't common to everyone with habitual criminal behaviours. Just because you repeatedly rob houses doesn't mean you're addicted to burglary. Perhaps your circumstances mean you feel that this is the only viable source of income – maybe you're a heroin addict and this is the quickest and easiest buck you can make. But this cycle can be seen in many convicted of more serious serial crimes, where powerful emotions in the moment can be as potent as any drug.

In 1994, truck driver Keith Hunter Jesperson took his 15-year-old daughter, Melissa, to breakfast at a Denny's diner near her home in Spokane, Washington. Melissa loved her father, but he made her feel uncomfortable with some of the things he told her – like details of his sex life. Mid-meal, it seemed another one of those awkward chats was on the cusp of ruining her appetite.

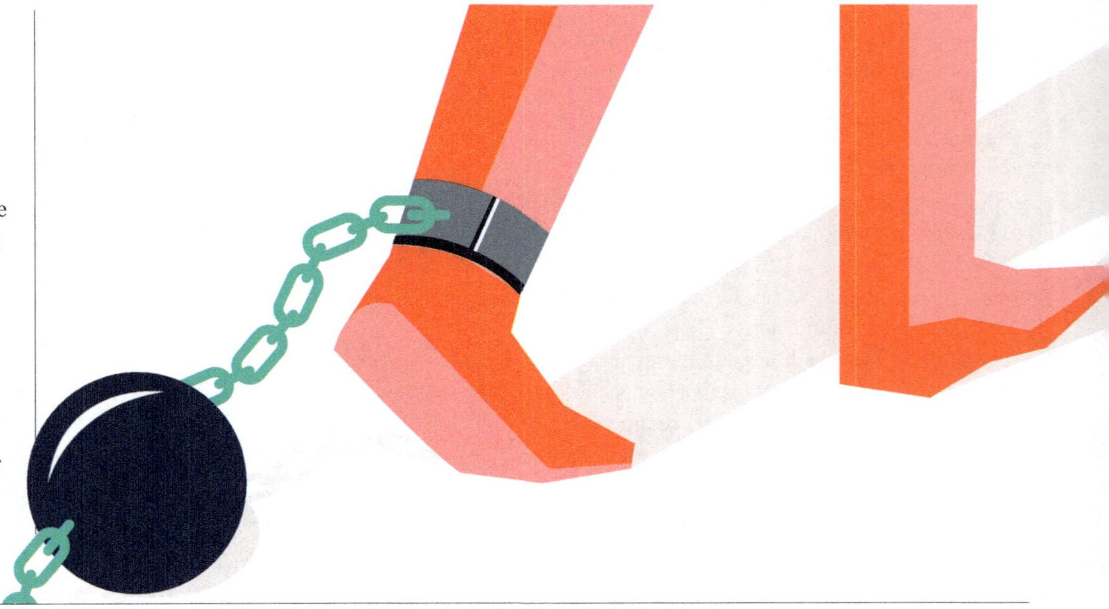

> WHATEVER POSITIVE PSYCHOLOGICAL FEEDBACK THE COLONEL WAS EXPERIENCING, THE PAYOFF WAS DIMINISHING EACH TIME. THE ONLY WAY TO BE GRATIFIED WAS TO TAKE IT TO THE NEXT LEVEL

"Not everything is what it appears to be, Missy," he said. "What do you mean?" Melissa replied. "You know, I have something to tell you, and it's really important..." A tense silence followed in which her father carefully considered his next words. "I can't tell you sweetie. If I tell you, you will tell the police. I'm not who you think I am, Melissa."

Probably even more nauseated by what was unsaid, Melissa ran to the toilet, and when she returned to their booth, her dad acted as if the conversation had never happened. What Jesperson might have gone on to tell his daughter was that he had murdered seven women and that police were looking for a serial killer dubbed the 'Happy Face Killer'. He would go on to murder again just after this pivotal moment with his daughter before he was arrested. Had he confessed to Melissa, she certainly would have told the police.

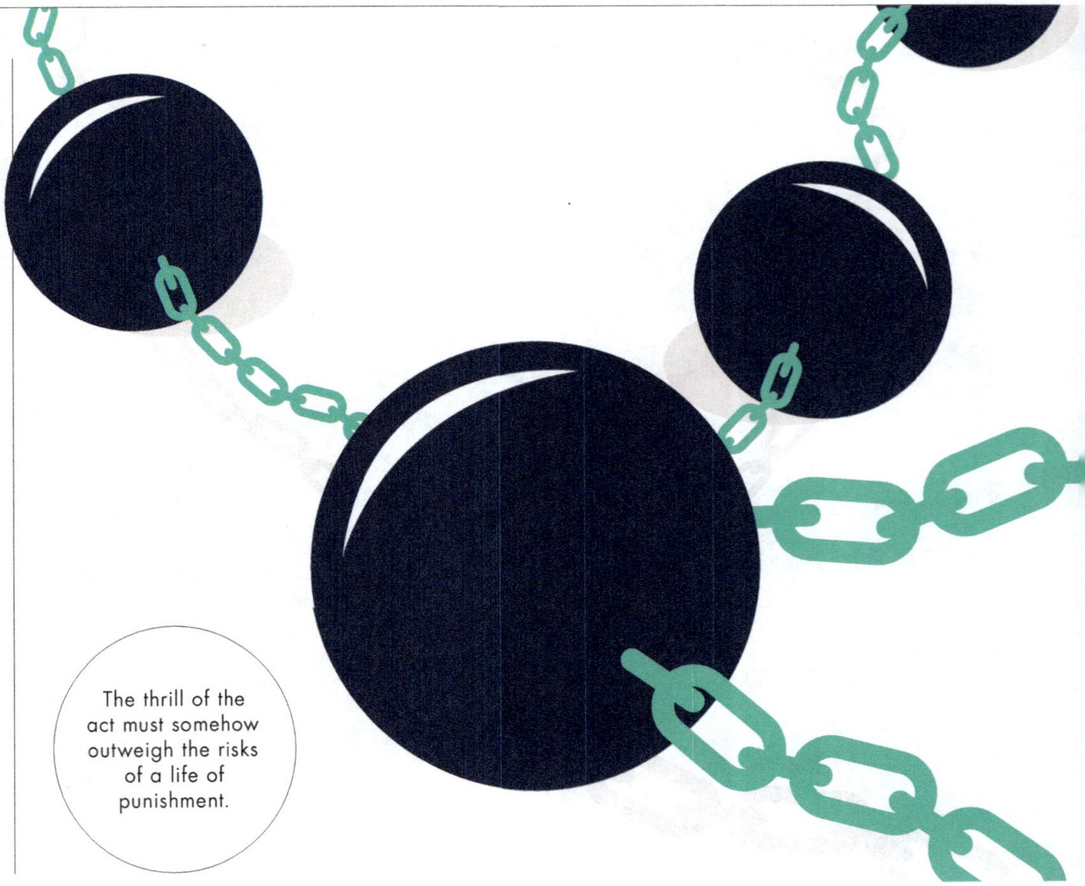

The thrill of the act must somehow outweigh the risks of a life of punishment.

IMAGE SOURCE Getty Images

Melissa reflects on her earlier memories of her father before he was arrested in her book, *Shattered Silence*, where she talks about how her father told her how he was going to be in Oregon State Penitentiary one day. This was one of many times when Jesperson's mask slipped and he half-boasted, half-confessed to his crimes. In the Happy Face Killer's case, maybe tempting fate in this way was cathartic, another aspect of his addiction to the heady thrills of murder.

Ted Bundy was as addicted to his variety of murder as Jesperson, perhaps more so, as his addiction escalated over many more murders, to the point that even this intelligent and calculating criminal threw caution to the wind. A month before his final arrest in February 1978, he entered a Florida State University sorority and became a fox in a hen house, attacking four women as they slept and killing two. The psychologist who helped evaluate Bundy at his 1976 trial for aggravated kidnapping, Dr Al Carlisle, made a damning, almost prophetic assessment of the man who, unknown to the court, had already claimed the lives of more than a dozen young women. He realised that despite none of the usual psychological hallmarks of a killer flagging up in his interview, Bundy was a dangerous man. Carlisle later developed his analysis of Bundy's criminal behaviour in his book, *Violent Mind*.

Three main processes characterised the evolution of his compulsion to kill: Bundy

DEADLY TRIAD

In a 1963 paper, psychiatrist J. M. MacDonald proposed that three distinct traits in children, when displayed beyond a certain age, could indicate a predisposition to violence: bed wetting, pyromania and cruelty to animals. The 'MacDonald Triad' was supported in later studies, including those conducted by the FBI criminal profiler John E. Douglas, of Netflix's *Mindhunter* fame. Broadly speaking, setting things alight is thought to release aggression, and animal cruelty is a kind of dry-run for violence towards humans. The subsequent shame felt after wetting the bed may then lead to animal cruelty or pyromania. These behaviours are just indicators, of course, and not everyone who displays them will go on to commit violent crime, just as not everyone who commits violent crime displayed all or any of the triad as a youngster.

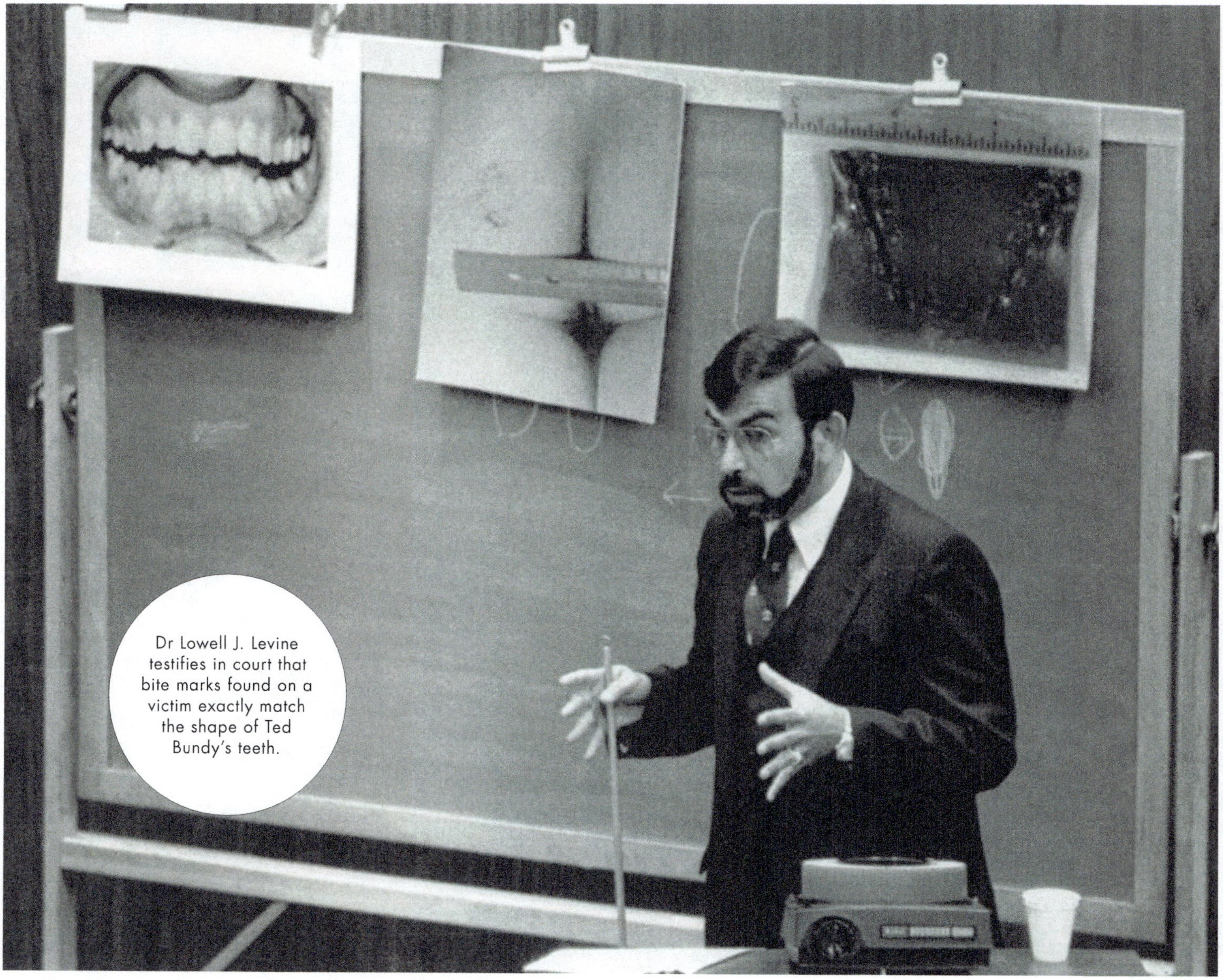

Dr Lowell J. Levine testifies in court that bite marks found on a victim exactly match the shape of Ted Bundy's teeth.

fantasised about scenarios in which he would kill, and he was able to disassociate himself from any vestige of uncomfortable emotions and memories. He also compartmentalised different ideas to separate mindsets and was able to maintain a mental distance between them, meaning that he was able to contain the killer inside - where he would nurture dark thoughts - and present an affable public face. Carlisle thought that Bundy's day-to-day life became increasingly boring or frustrating for him and he would turn to his dark fantasies more frequently, feeding them with more victims as murder became a powerful addiction.

Serial killing isn't the only type of crime from which a criminal might derive some

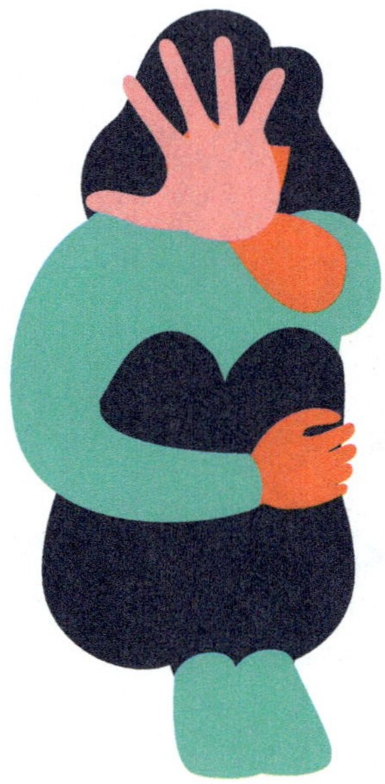

respite from their lives, or even pleasure. Compulsive shoplifters and arsonists are driven by a dopamine high they get from their criminal behaviours, a temporary but very pleasurable buzz that can make it hard to resist repeating once the association has been made. Whether it's a serial killer's first murder, a kleptomaniac's first theft, a pyromaniac's fire, gambler's win or a heroin addict's first hit, tolerance to that high they achieve builds very quickly. To obtain a similar level of ecstasy the behaviour has to be repeated more frequently and with more intensity, whether that means a more violent murder or a higher dose next time.

WORDS Ben Biggs

Q&A

CAN YOU BE ADDICTED TO MURDER?

Forensic psychologist Dr Terri Cole explains why some criminals are repeat offenders and whether the compulsion to commit crime can be controlled

Q. Could you say some serial criminals are 'addicted' to crime?

While offenders appear to have preferences, most research would suggest they are generalist rather than specialist. Many serious offenders have previous convictions for other types of crime. For example, a rapist's most likely previous conviction is for burglary. However, we are now finding that some offenders, like those who view indecent images of children online, are far less likely to have any previous criminality. The reasons offenders continue to commit crime is multifaceted: it may be they enjoy it – like serial killers – or need to – like robbers needing money for drugs.

Q. Are there other common habits among criminals of the same kind?

A. Commonalities involve experience of abuse, neglect and trauma in childhood, usually early engagement with police or other services, truancy or difficulties in school. Other general features may include diet, peers, offending family or living in poverty.

Q. Do you think a serial killer who derives some kind of positive psychological feedback from killing, rather than a hitman, for example, can switch off or suppress the urge to kill?

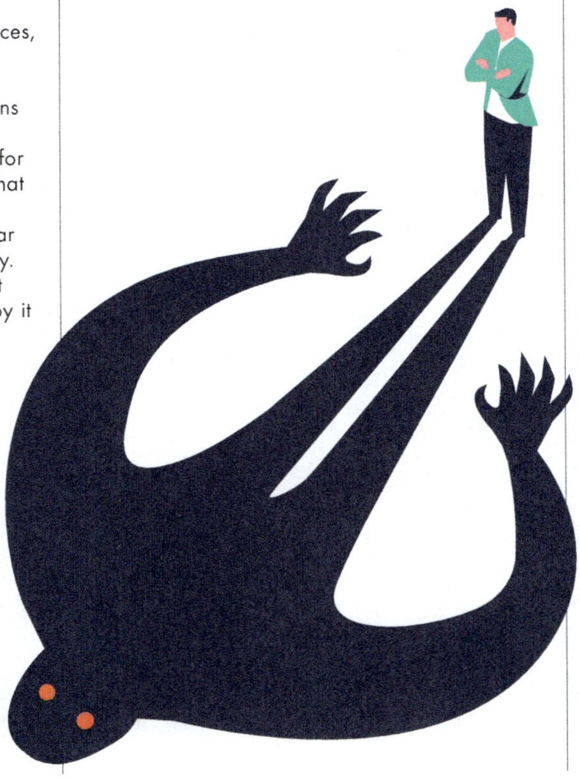

A. Probably not. Like any sexual desire, can we change it? Could we make a heterosexual person suddenly homosexual? There are methods of avoidance and cognitive behavioural strategies, but the fantasies are likely to have developed over some time and are likely to remain. They may, however, be reduced or compensated at certain times in their lives. For example, urges may get heightened in times of stress, or they may be reduced if they have access to alternative sources of enjoyment, like a consenting partner.

Q. Can criminals who repeatedly commit the same serious crime be reformed? Is there a treatment – perhaps like an alcoholic going to recovery meetings – that is effective?

A. That's the million-dollar question. There's loads of literature about what works and what doesn't. There are loads of different treatments; some generic (life skills, for example) and some specific, for aggression or sexual offending. The latest research demonstrates a need to look at making the offender want to live a 'good life'. Offenders want many of the same things we do, it's just that often they choose methods to get there that don't fit expected norms – they want money so steal, they want power and control so they rape – rather than gain money or power via legitimate means.

IMAGE SOURCE Getty Images

> OUR BRAINS TAKE SHORTCUTS TO ENABLE RAPID JUDGEMENTS – KNOWN AS HEURISTICS – WHEREBY WE PRIORITISE CERTAIN PARTS OF LARGER PROBLEMS

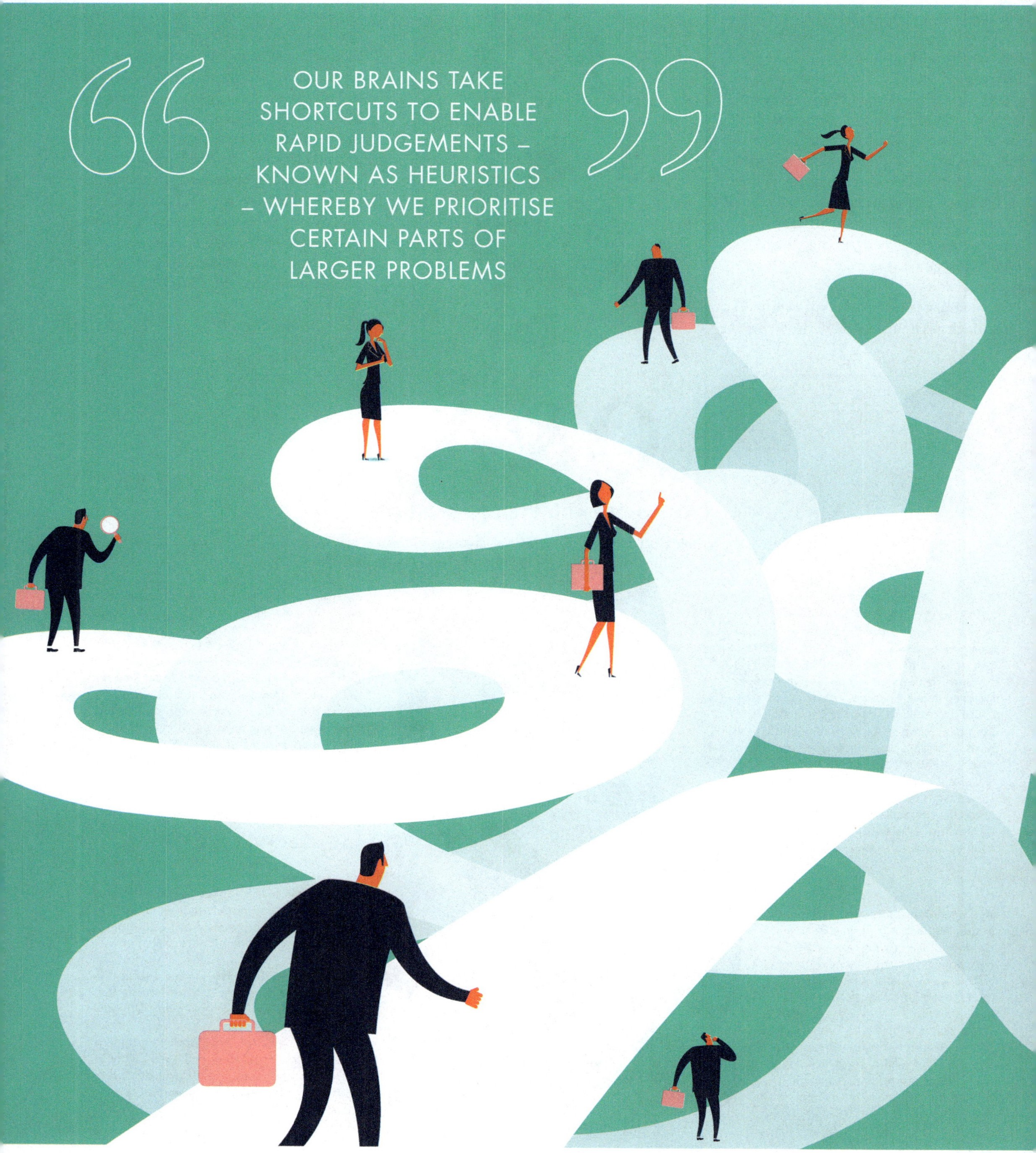

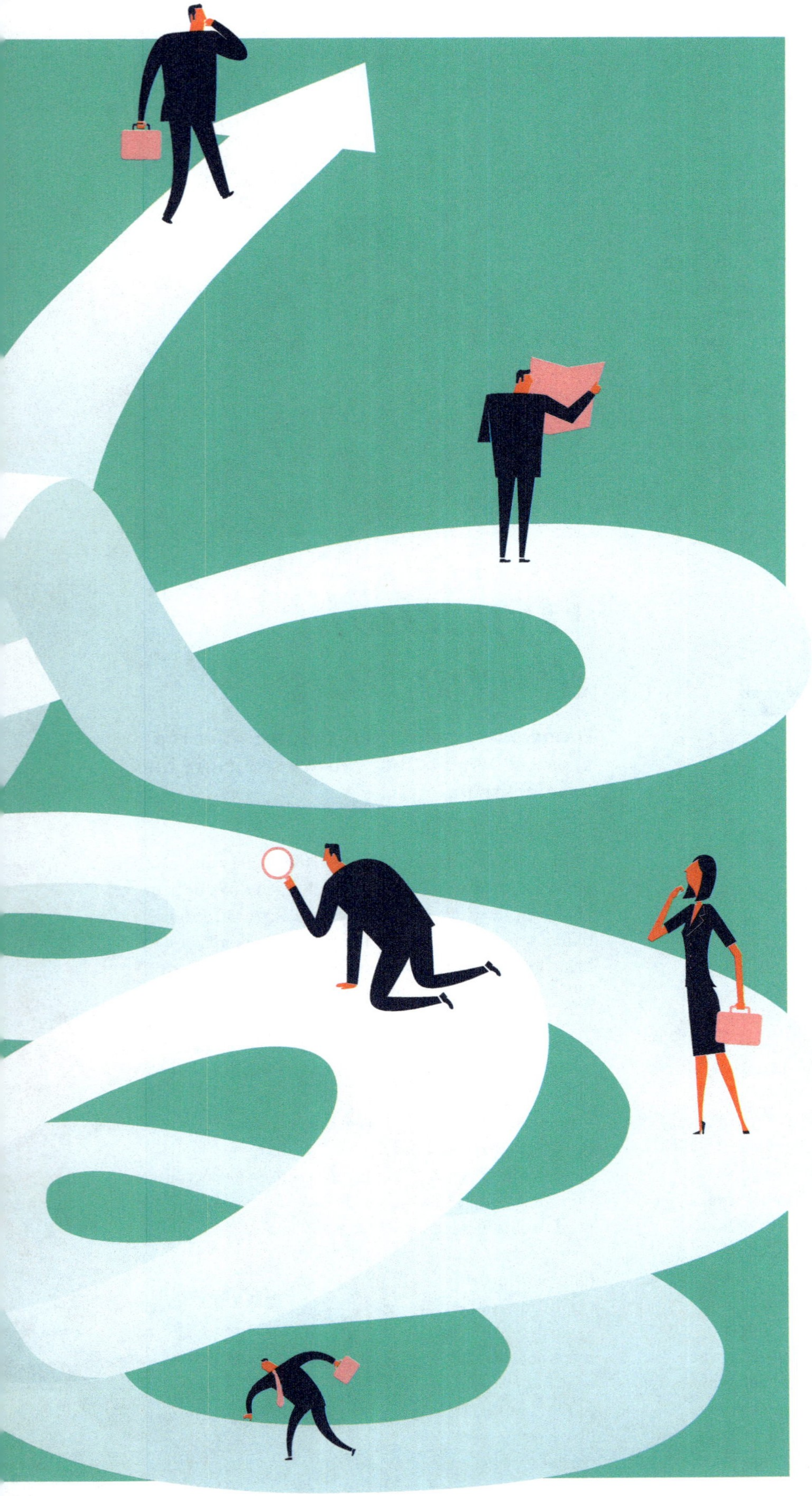

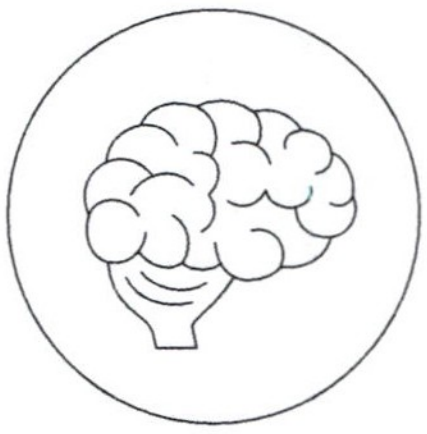

Cognitive bias

Explore how the peculiarities of human information processing influence our perception of situations and events

As humans living in an ever-changing world, we have rather a lot to think about. We make hundreds of decisions everyday, from simple choices like what to eat for breakfast to devising complex business strategies at work. As we are bombarded by sensory inputs, each providing new information to process, we must draw on previous experiences to recognise, understand and act on our perception of the world. To do this our brains take shortcuts to enable rapid judgements – known as heuristics – whereby we prioritise certain parts of larger problems over others.

While this is a critical coping mechanism to compensate for the limited processing amplitude of the human brain, it can lead to faulty thinking – errors in perception that cause us to make assessments based on subjective influence rather than real-world information. This is known as a cognitive bias – a deviation from rational, logical thinking influenced by multiple psychological and social factors.

There exists a variety of recognised cognitive biases, each with the potential to negatively impact on the economy of our real-world decisions, with consequences for our social and financial success. Here we examine ten of the most widely studied biases and how these habits impact our perceptions.

WORDS Peter Fenech

IMAGE SOURCE Getty Images

Survivorship bias

The tendency to ignore absent information and only ever plan for the best

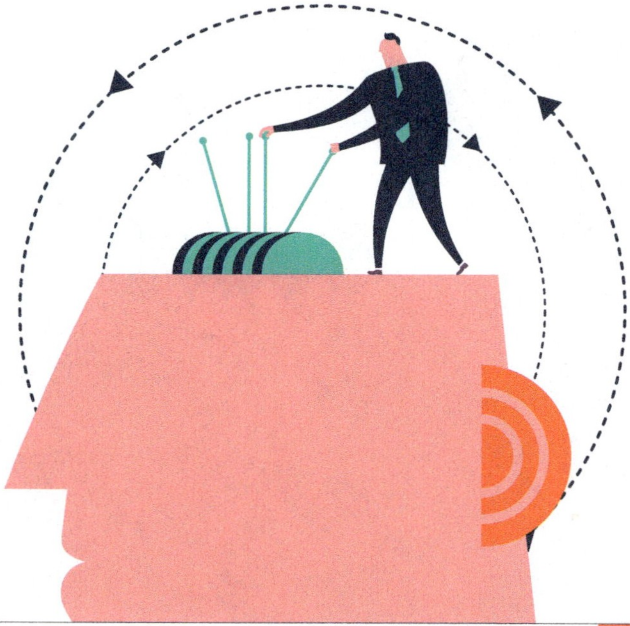

It can be a challenge to consider information that is not observable in our assessment of a situation. Where a person or object is not present, humans will naturally focus on those that we can see and form an opinion based solely on that condition.

Survivorship bias refers to situations where we make assumptions based on the apparent success of a group of objects or people but fail to recognise that our sample is not representative of subjects that have been excluded.

Looking at data on injuries sustained by car crash survivors, we may conclude the worst injuries occur when sitting in the front seats, when in fact this data does not include people who were sat in rear seats and were killed. To say better crash protection should be installed in front seats would be a common but clearly false conclusion.

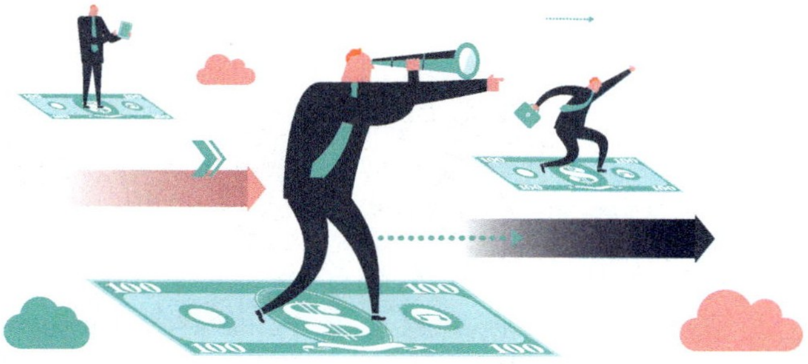

Endowment effect

The attribution of greater regard for that which we already own, independent of actual value

We can all find ourselves becoming sentimentally attached to objects, even when there is no obvious reason to value them so highly. The endowment effect describes a common situation where people place greater value in something they already own than something they are yet to acquire, due to an emotional bias.

In psychological studies, such as that by Kahneman, Knetsch and Thaler in 1990, it has been regularly observed that participants will demand a far greater price for something they perceive as their property than the amount they are willing to pay for something of equivalent value. It has been suggested that this is a form of loss aversion – as a species we experience greater anxiety in losing something than we feel pleasure from gaining an equal reward, although the motivation is unclear.

An evolutionary suggestion is that in the past natural selection favoured humans who were less willing to part with property when there was less choice of people to trade with to find a better deal. In economics this can be problematic in the modern day, as holding onto something unprofitable, such as inherited shares in a failing company, is irrational and can prove financially disastrous.

Hyperbolic discounting

Immediate rewards don't always offer the greatest benefits, but you are still more likely to select them

Willpower plays an important part in society and is often seen as a measure of strength of character by our peers. However, the choice to accept a smaller reward sooner rather than a larger return in the future is a far more complex behaviour than may be immediately obvious at first.

There is a tendency among humans to perceive future rewards as less attractive, attributing less value the more temporally distant this becomes. We make inconsistent choices over time, even when presented with the same information.

In evolutionary terms this can be explained by the choices early humans would have faced – with immediate risk, such as starving to death, it made more sense to select instant solutions. Today, however, where we need to think longer term, such as saving for a pension, this can be ineffective – worth remembering the next time that you're tempted to buy an expensive pair of shoes.

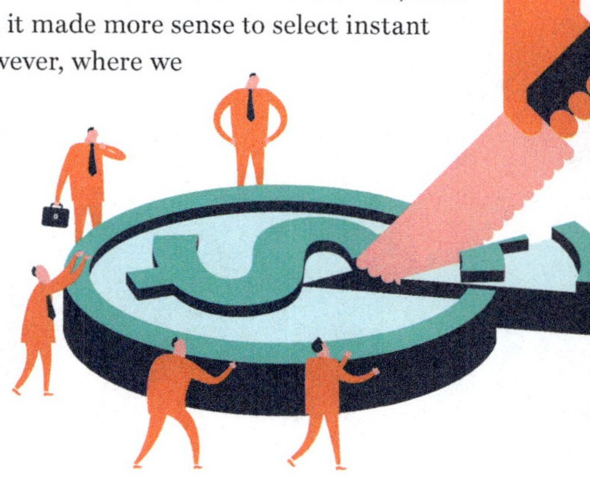

> THE CLUSTERING ILLUSION IS CENTRED AROUND THE HUMAN PREDISPOSITION TO SEE EVENTS CLOSELY DISTRIBUTED IN TIME AS RELATED

Clustering illusion

How we interpret groups of events can affect our ability to predict future probabilities

Sport and gambling are two activities that are most obviously affected by cognitive biases and are two of the most studied. This is largely due to the great influence individual perception can have on our ability to see patterns in events and predict future outcomes.

The clustering illusion bias is centred around the human predisposition to see events that are closely distributed in time as related, when in fact such events are random. The most famous example of a study of this effect is a 1985 investigation carried out by psychologists Gilovich, Vallone and Tversky, of Cornell and Stanford universities on the 'hot hand fallacy' – the belief that in basketball a player is more likely to score if previous attempts to do so have been successful.

While confidence can improve performance, this incorrect assumption is largely caused by an overestimation of our ability to predict random events, something that is actually impossible. When we have little information to rely on (a small sequence of attempts at something) we assume events will be more spread out, so when a cluster occurs, such as a string of successes, we perceive it as non-random. This makes us overconfident in predicting such a sequence will continue for future attempts.

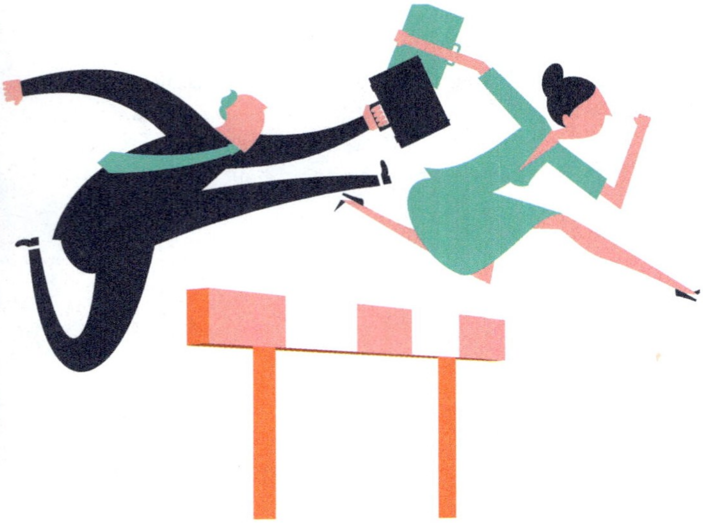

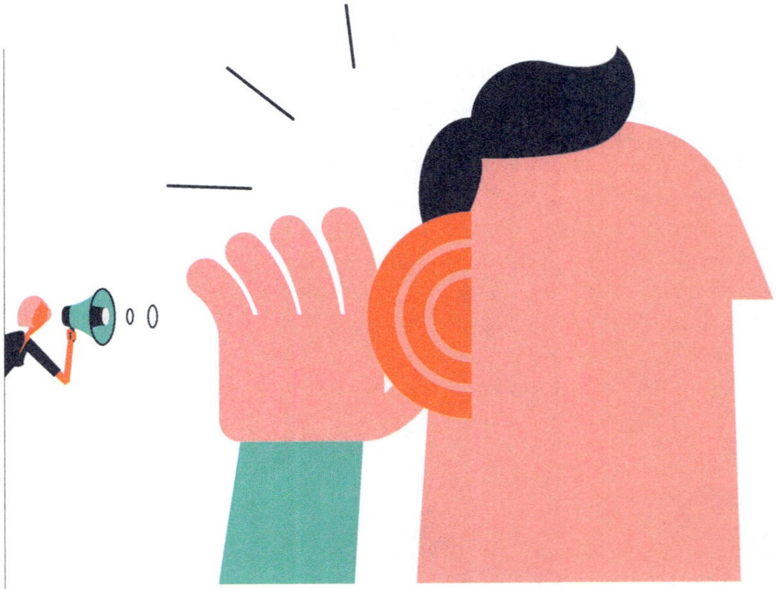

Confirmation bias

Our process of gathering information to form our opinions is not as impartial as we may believe

While we like to believe that we are open-minded and observe all of the available information on a subject before drawing a conclusion, the reality is that this doesn't always happen. Confirmation bias is a flaw in how we collect, process and recall information, which suffers from a tendency to favour that which confirms pre-existing beliefs.

Since decision-making falls back on experience and preconceived ideas, it can be uncomfortable for us to reject what we think we already know and accept a new truth. We therefore pay greater attention to data that reaffirms our beliefs and ignore facts that question them. This can have significant implications in areas such as the medical profession, where a doctor diagnosing a patient may recognise initial indicators of an illness and fail to seek, recognise and act on other diagnostic markers that may disprove their hypothesis. On the other hand, multiple doctors observing the same information but with opposing preconceived ideas may draw very different conclusions due to their unconscious choice to dismiss disaffirming facts.

With an influence in stereotyping, confirmation bias can make us see patterns in data where there are none and fail to see those that are present in new information.

Availability heuristic

The bias towards recent, easily remembered information when assessing importance and relevance in new situations

Memory recall is a critical brain function, yet we experience so much sensory input that we rely on mental shortcuts to identify familiar stimuli. The availability heuristic, first described by Amos Tversky and Daniel Kahneman, is the process of unconsciously prioritising most recently acquired information, biasing assessments of a situation towards that which is most easily recalled.

Research has shown how participants overestimate the relevance of information that they are able to easily remember, even if this is a first impression of the broader situation. The likely thought process is that we assume if information is readily available to recall it must be more important than that which does not quickly come to mind. While cognitively useful, the implications for judicial decisions, education-curriculum design and learning performance are significant, where the methods for conveying information in a lesson and then demanding recall in an exam situation are not compatible.

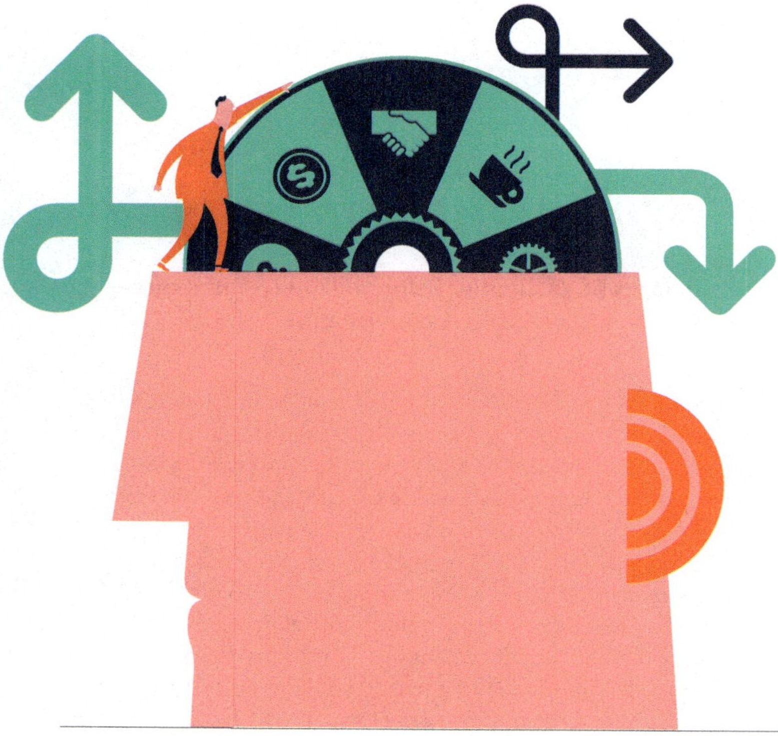

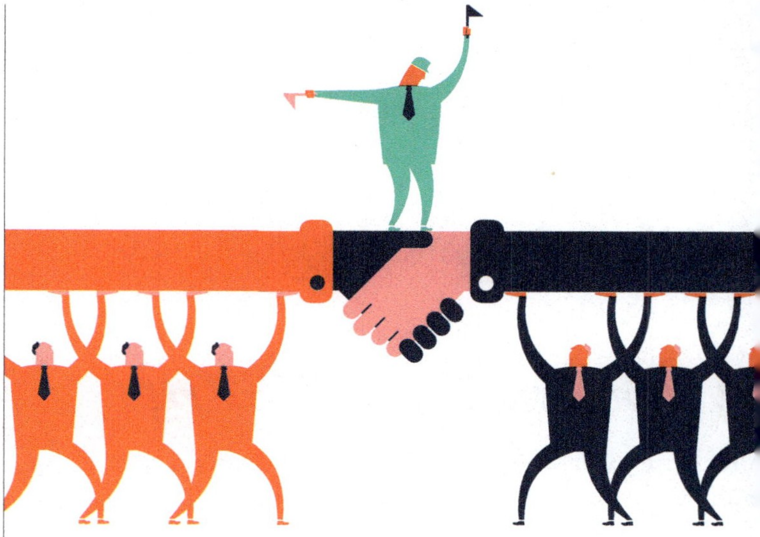

Stereotyping

While it may be associated with discrimination against minorities, stereotyping does have an innocent cognitive function

Stereotyping is one of the most recognised cognitive biases and carries with it many negative connotations. The stereotyping of people often results in the feeling of judgement within the subject group, and there are sinister implications for unreasonably assuming all members of that group are the same. However, as with many biases, there is a heuristic component that allows for the rapid identification of people, places and objects.

You might find yourself instinctively asking a person dressed in an airline's uniform for help with flight information, for example, assuming that they will be an expert. This stereotype provides a rapid solution to a potentially complex real-world problem. With such social categorisation we learn to identify people less as individuals and more as part of a social group. We may be aware of this or it may be a subconscious process – known as explicit and implicit stereotyping respectively.

As a type of confirmation bias it can be difficult to challenge our own beliefs about a group. This explains how easy it is to link emotional responses to our stereotypes (develop a prejudice) and in turn alter our social behaviour (discriminate against a group). We naturally seek characteristics that reinforce our assumptions.

> "GAMBLER'S FALLACY IS THE INCORRECT REASONING THAT AFTER A SERIES OF REPEATED EVENTS, SUCH AS SCORING RED ON A ROULETTE WHEEL, A DIFFERENT EVENT BECOMES MORE LIKELY"

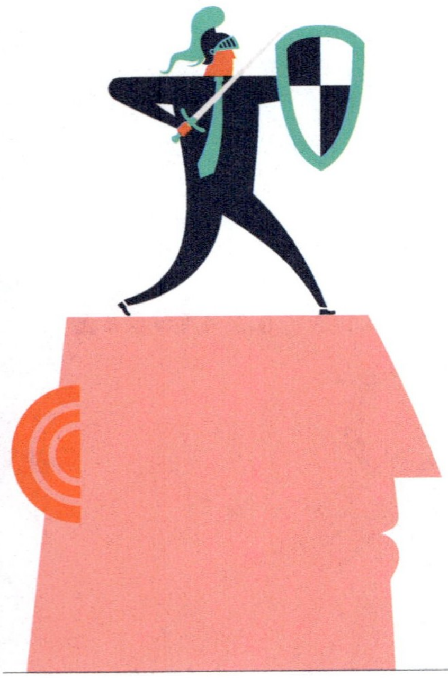

Risk compensation

Does perceived safety yield increased complacency?

Every decision we make is a process of weighing up costs and benefits. If we deem the potential costs too high to justify an action we may decide not to engage in it. Risk compensation is a hypothesised mental adjustment whereby we take greater risks when perceived safety is increased, thereby nullifying those safety measures.

Closely associated with this theory is Professor Sam Pelzman, who suggested road safety strategies are useless, since with increased protection comes increased risk taking. While this has been widely disputed, another study by Gerald J. S. Wilde noted decreased traffic deaths in Sweden after a change in driving side. However, once drivers became accustomed to right-hand driving, fatality rates increased, an effect termed risk homeostasis – the balancing of perceived and actual danger. This is likely due to our predisposition to seek actions that will yield the greatest reward with the least effort, a trait that poses a challenge in hazardous workplaces. Recurrent training is often required to maintain safety.

Knowledge of risk compensation can also help in marketing, as a safe online marketplace can encourage sales.

Gambler's fallacy

An opposite effect to clustering illusion, this bias also results in faulty expectations about future events

Gambling creates complex responses in humans. There is a clear emotional investment in the outcome of a bet, yet there are more deep-seated psychological processes at work. Gambler's fallacy is the incorrect reasoning that after a series of repeated events, such as scoring a red on a roulette wheel, a different event becomes more likely – scoring a black, for example. This is opposite, yet related to, the hot hand fallacy, arising from a misperception about small sample sizes, where we assume shorter series of random occurrences yield similar results to longer sets. Where a winning or losing streak is encountered, we expect an inverse event to create balance. Tversky and Kahneman called this the representativeness heuristic – comparison to previous experiences of event sequences.

In reality, where events are discrete, one will not affect the probability of the other occurring. Suggested biological causes for the false belief that they will are the stimulation of parts of the frontal and parietal lobes of the brain involved in decision-making, judgement and reasoning – zones attributed to increased risk-taking after experiencing a loss. The bias is sometimes dubbed the Monte Carlo fallacy after a famous night of roulette losses in 1913 in the casino of the same name.

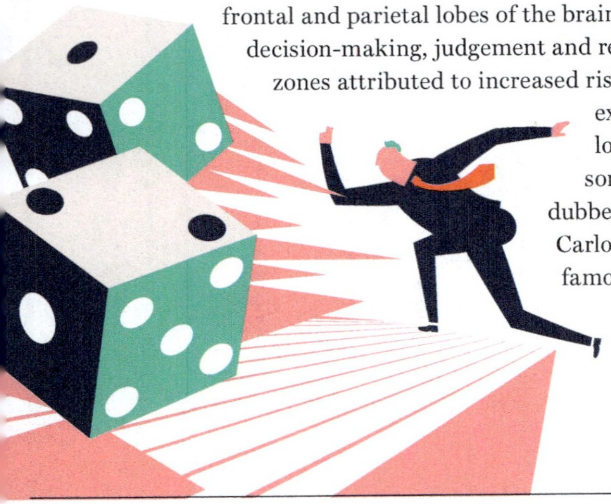

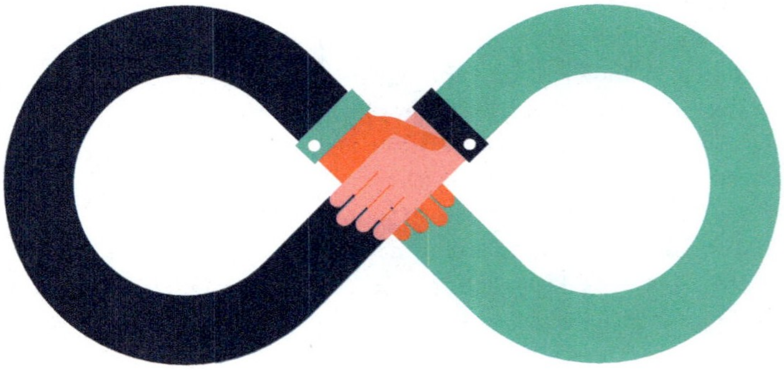

Anchoring bias

Even business-savvy people can fall foul of this bias towards initial information

As other cognitive bias examples have demonstrated, humans rely heavily on impressions of a situation in order to quickly make assessments. However, anchoring is another shortcut that can prove inefficient in the modern world. With this bias, we are prone to fixing on the first piece of information that we receive and then using this as a basis for judging all subsequent facts. The common example is being given a lower-than-expected price for a product and immediately accepting this while missing out on potential better deals elsewhere.

Another Tversky and Kahneman investigation suggested that we often incorrectly adjust expectations from the anchor, affecting our judgement. Even with experience and when armed with awareness of anchoring in action it can prove difficult to avoid, influencing multiple decisions of a financial, social or professional nature. While it is possible to illustrate the effects, it has proven a challenge to pinpoint the greatest psychological causes.

IMAGE SOURCE Getty Images

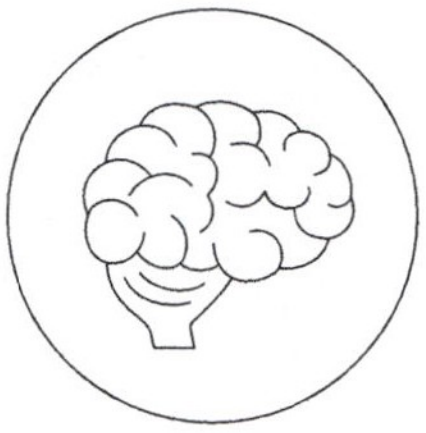

Bad habits and how to break them

Discover some of the most common repetitive behaviours that can lead you astray and how to best break the cycle

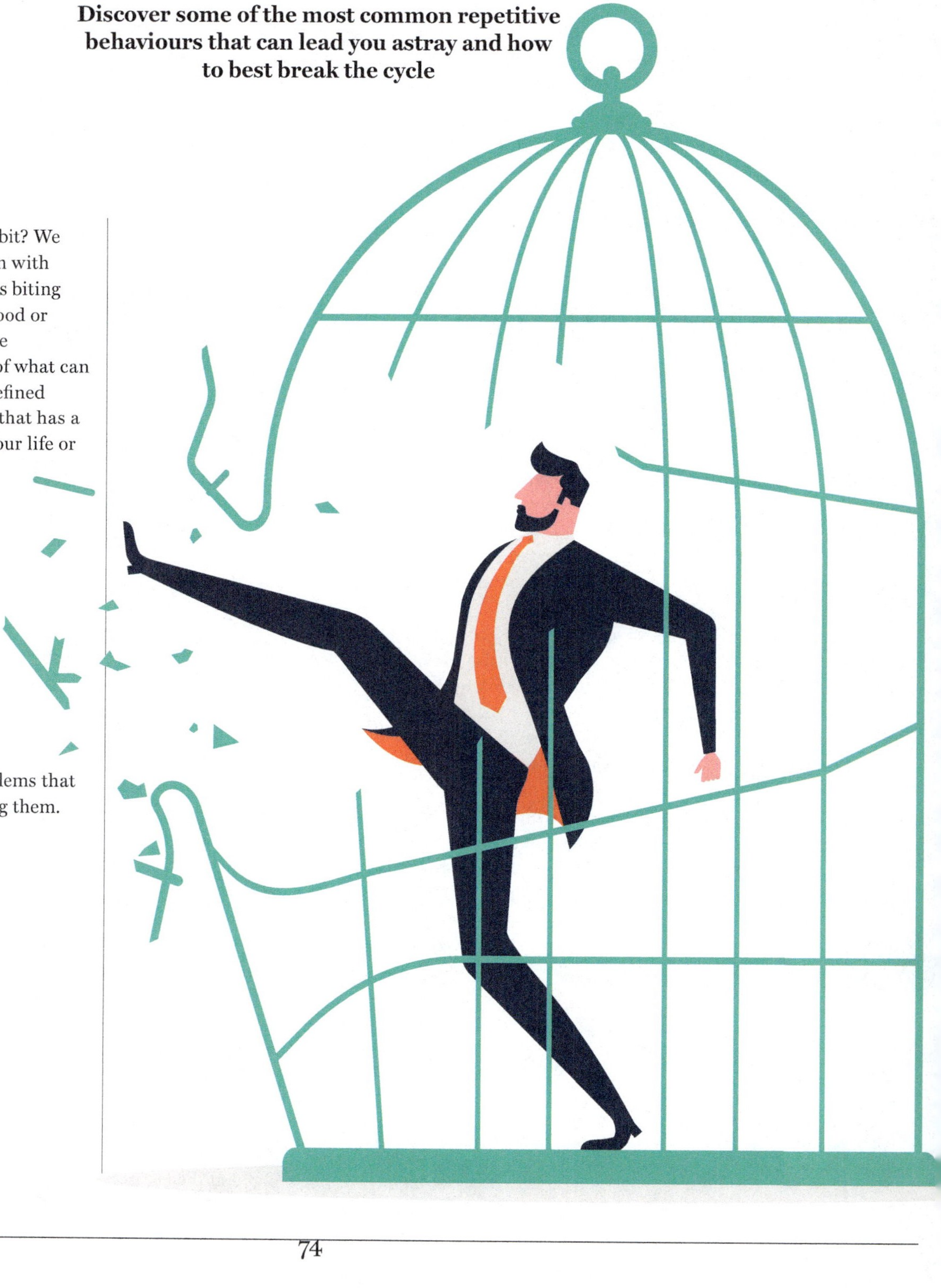

What exactly is a 'bad' habit? We often associate the term with classic examples such as biting the ends of your nails, eating fast food or smoking. While these can indeed be undesirable behaviours, the scope of what can be classed as a bad habit is vast. Defined merely as any repetitive behaviour that has a negative or detrimental effect on your life or health, bad habits can manifest in a myriad of ways. From fighting the urge to go to sleep just so you can see what's happening on social media to heading to the beach without first putting on sun protection, sometimes it's the bad habits we are unaware of that can cause the most damage. However, there are many simple ways to fight bad habits, even if you've had them for many years. Ultimately, understanding the underlying problems that trigger them may be key to breaking them.

WORDS Scott Dutfield

Nail biting

Gnawing at the ends of your nails for a lot of people manifests in moments of anxiety, stress or simply as a bad habit. As many as 30 per cent of the population bite their nails, with teenagers being the biggest perpetrators. It may seem like a harmless habit, except for leaving your nail a little jagged, but by continually chewing your nails, dirt and bacteria are being transferred into your mouth, putting you at greater risk of infections. Nailing biting is a habit that often develops as a child, so tackling it at an early age can help prevent the long-term effects.

In the past, preventing nail biting involved coating fingertips with bitter- or sour-tasting foods. However, today there are many nail polish products that have the same effect. Creating a physical barrier between the mouth and nail, such as gloves, mittens or even a mouthguard, can also help to break the habit. Maintaining short nails is also a method to alleviate the problem, preventing the habit from being able to manifest.

For the more severe cases, known as onychophagia, nail biting may have a connection to your mental health, such as anxiety or depression. In these cases cognitive behavioural therapies can be explored to understand the emotional root of the habit and seek to remedy the underlying problems.

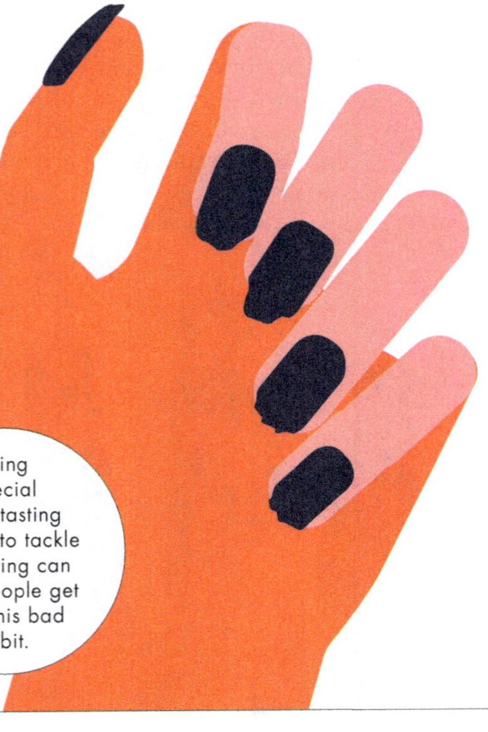

Using special bitter-tasting varnish to tackle nail biting can help people get over this bad habit.

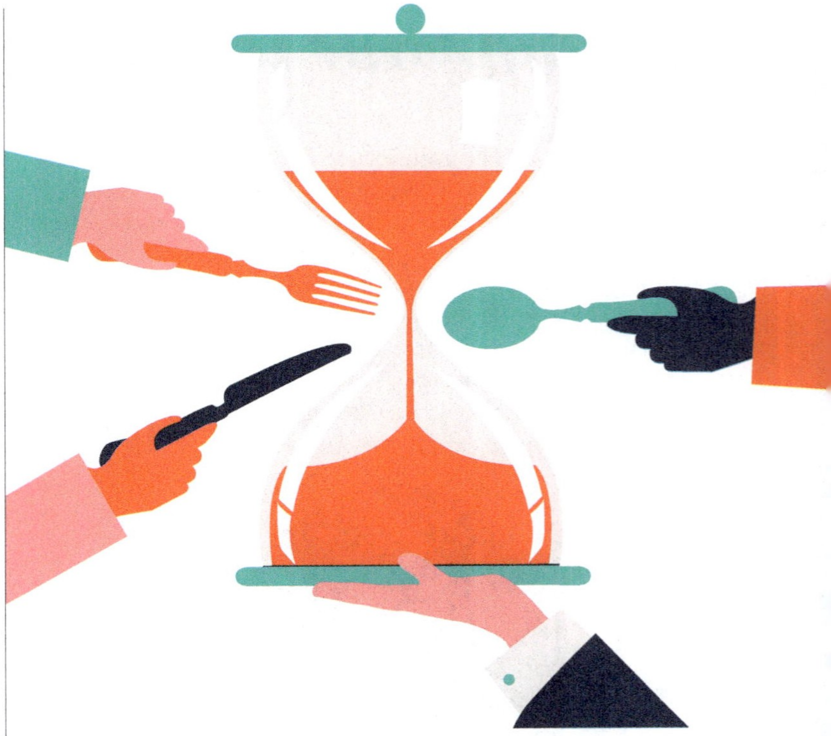

Eating too quickly

Sitting in front of a freshly delivered pizza or a gooey chocolate brownie, it's easy to get lost in the excitement of the flavour explosion that's about to follow. However, for some people it's an experience that's over in a matter of moments. Not only bad dinner party etiquette, eating too quickly can be a bad habit that affects your health. Studies have shown that those who are quick to munch on a mouth-watering meal have a greater risk of obesity and of developing metabolic syndrome, a group of conditions including heart disease and diabetes, when compared to those who take their time to chow down.

To remedy rapid eating, the solution can be quite simple: slow down and savour the flavour of your food. It's believed that it takes around 20 minutes for the stomach to signal to the brain that it's full. Therefore, to make sure you're giving your body enough time to catch up, spend at least 20 minutes on each of your meals. This isn't to say you have to spend this amount of time continually eating at your usual speed but rather increasing the time spent on your usual portion size.

“COGNITIVE BEHAVIOURAL THERAPIES CAN BE EXPLORED TO UNDERSTAND THE EMOTIONAL ROOT OF THE HABIT AND SEEK TO REMEDY THE UNDERLYING PROBLEM”

IMAGE SOURCE Getty Images

Sucking your thumb

It's a naturally occurring instinct to suck your thumb as a child, typically dissipating as a habit after the age of five. However, many adults carry the behaviour into later life. It's believed thumb sucking may release an endorphin rush, similar to that which occurs when infants breastfeed. Although it may provide a sense of comfort and relaxation to engage in this habit, it can cause problems in later life.

Often leading to the misalignment of your teeth or affecting the roof of your mouth, tackling this habit can be similar to that of nail biting. Covering your thumb with a glove or coating it in a bitter taste may help to wean you away from this bad habit.

Around one in ten adults still suck their thumb.

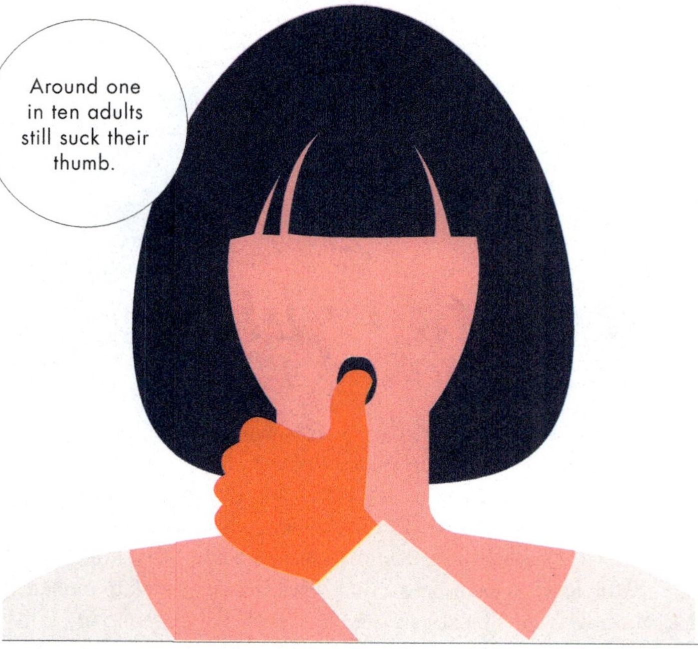

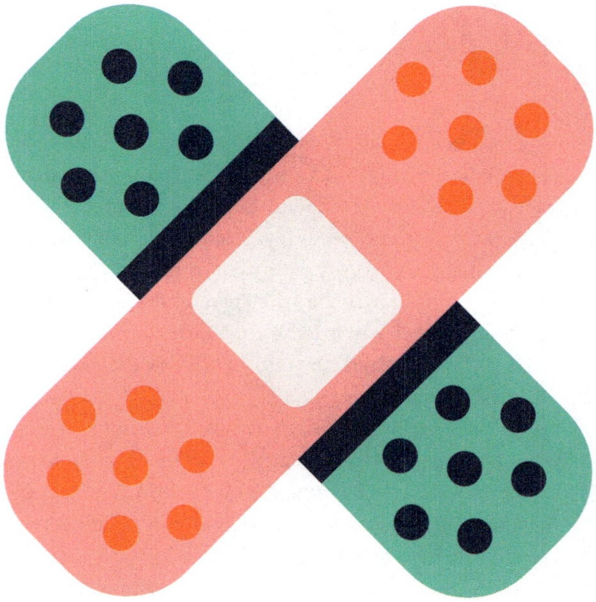

Picking scabs

There can be something satisfying about finding a scab and picking it straight off, especially when you're a child. However, there is a good reason why your mother scolded you for doing it. When the skin is cut or scraped, a scab develops to act as a protective barrier over the repairing skin beneath. By removing this layer you increase the risk of infection and the time it will take to heal. To break this bad habit distraction may be key. By preoccupying yourself with another task such as reading, drawing or grabbing a fidget spinner you can offer relief from the compulsion to pick.

Cracking knuckles

There is still a debate on whether cracking your knuckles can be classed as a bad habit due to research suggesting no connection between doing so and the development of arthritis, as previously believed. However, there are still concerns over potential injuries that can occur while self-cracking. Overall, jerking your knuckles back and forth to release the build-up of gas bubbles between your finger joints may lead to the weakening of your grip or even promote swelling.

Occupying your hands may offer some relief against the compulsion to crack, for example squeezing a stress ball. It has also been suggested that putting an elastic band around your wrist, pulling it back and releasing it to snap against your skin when you feel the need to crack may create a negative association with the consumption and train you to stop. This method can also be used with a range of bad habits, such as nail biting.

Using a stress ball may help to prevent you from cracking your knuckles.

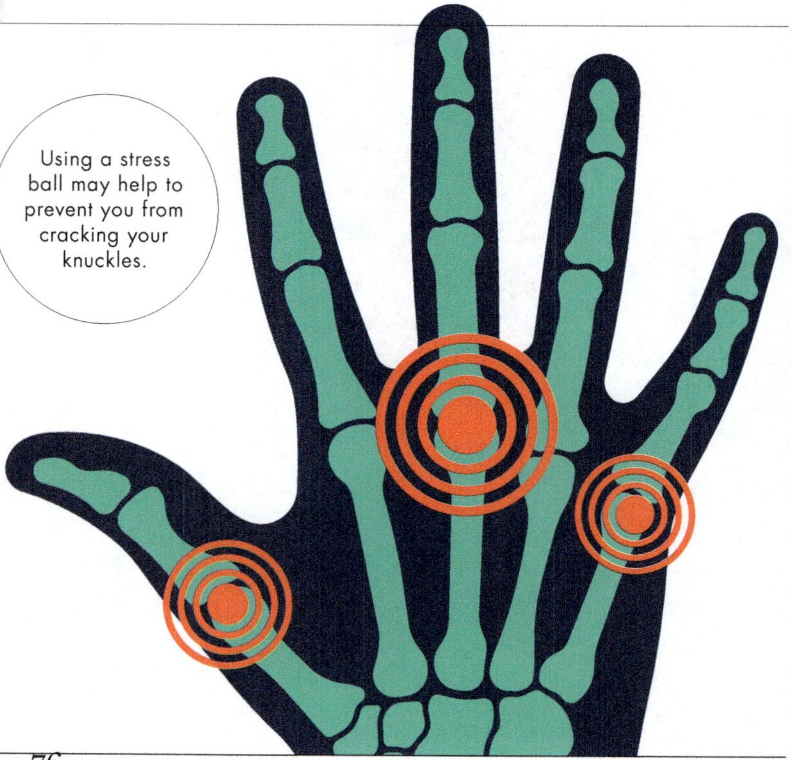

ONE OF THE REASONS SMOKING IS SO DIFFICULT TO GIVE UP IS THE EXPERIENCE OF DAILY TRIGGERS THAT MAKE YOU WANT THE TEMPORARY RELIEF A CIGARETTE MAY PROVIDE

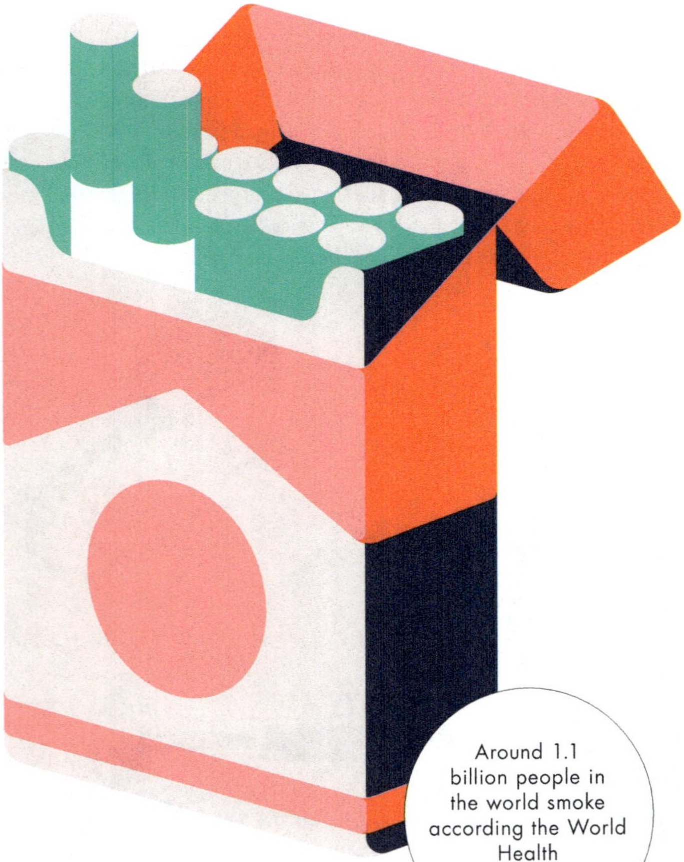

Around 1.1 billion people in the world smoke according the World Health Organization.

Smoking

Arguably one of the worst routines to develop, smoking can lead to a host of problems. A nicotine-fuelled addiction, smoking is more than a bad habit – it's been linked to several health concerns including cancer, heart disease and respiratory conditions.

Unlike solving some bad habits, there isn't one single way to quit smoking. Tackling both addiction to nicotine and the behavioural practice of lighting a cigarette can be difficult. That being said, many alternative products such as patches and gums have been proven to satisfy the need for nicotine without ingesting the harmful chemicals within a cigarette.

One of the reasons smoking is so difficult to give up is the experience of daily triggers that make you want the temporary relief a cigarette may provide. These triggers can include stress, anxiety, boredom and socialising with other smokers. Addressing the root of the triggers may also alleviate the craving to smoke.

Using a smartphone in bed

We can all be guilty of scrolling through social media while tucked up in bed. However, staring at your smartphone before sleep can be a bad habit. The blue light emitted from your phone has been found to suppress the production of a night-time hormone melatonin. As part of our body's natural 24-hour cycle, the setting of the Sun signals that the time to sleep is near, and so our bodies produce melatonin to relax the muscles and dull the nervous system to ease us into a deep slumber. However, the light emitted from our phone hijacks that signal and delays melatonin production, resulting in a disturbed sleep cycle. This can lead to tiredness and insomnia.

To prevent this bad habit disturbing a good night's sleep, allow for one hour between updating your online profile and hitting the hay. Of course, smartphones aren't the only perpetrator for interrupted sleep: tablets and TVs can have the same effect. If the temptation to log on is too much, leave your smartphone in another room and use a digital alarm clock to keep your schedule.

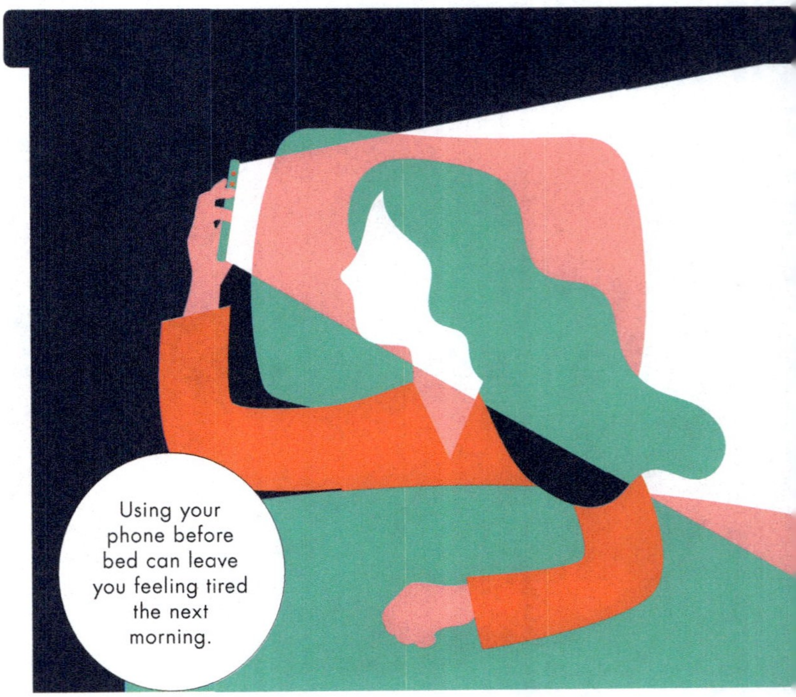

Using your phone before bed can leave you feeling tired the next morning.

IMAGE SOURCE Getty Images

Money worries have been linked with several serious health concerns, with overspending being a large culprit.

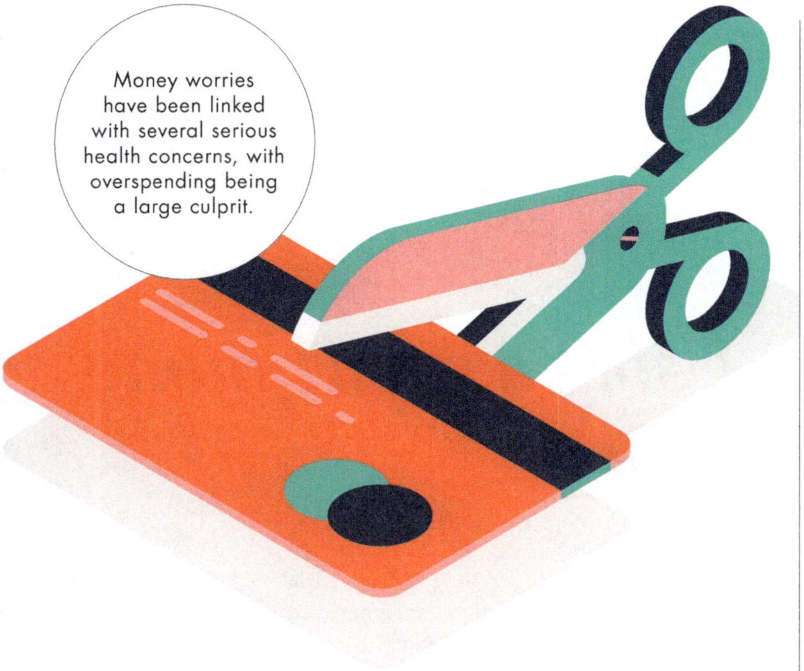

Overspending

Financial stress can have serious health consequences, from high blood pressure to depression, so spending outside your means when you should be budgeting can have a bigger effect on your life than a low bank balance. Overspending is a bad habit that can be a tricky one to confront because the only way to overcome it is with self-discipline. Creating and sticking with a budget can help keep you in the black. In extreme cases, overspending can lead to racking up large amounts of debt. By freezing your credit cards, you may be able to nip the problem in the bud before it gets out of control.

Slouching at your desk

In a world where everyone is sitting in front of a computer or smartphone for the majority of the day, it's easy to find yourself hunched over a keyboard. Poor posture can lead to back pain, circulation issues and fatigue.

To get you on the straight and narrow while seated at your work desk, sit so your knees are parallel with your hips and raise your computer screen to your eye line with a straight back. Making sure you have a chair with a supportive backrest will also help to prevent you slouching forward. While you are hunched over tension builds between your back muscles and causes discomfort. Taking time to get up and walk around will relieve some of that tension.

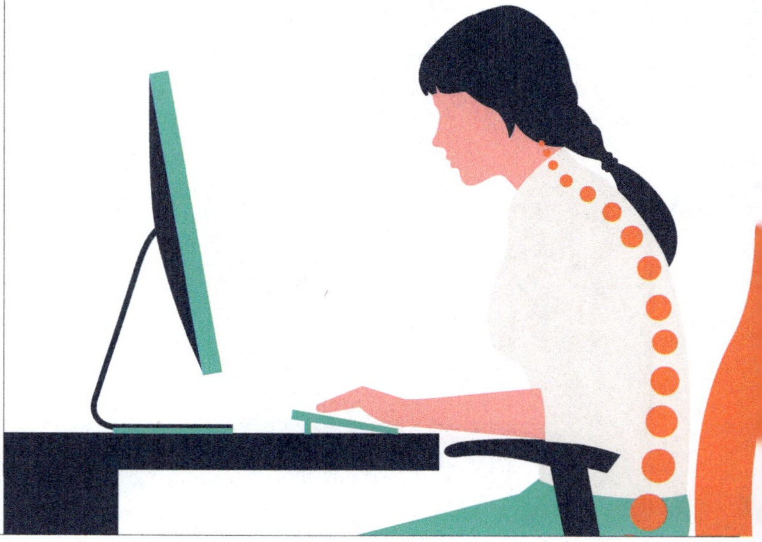

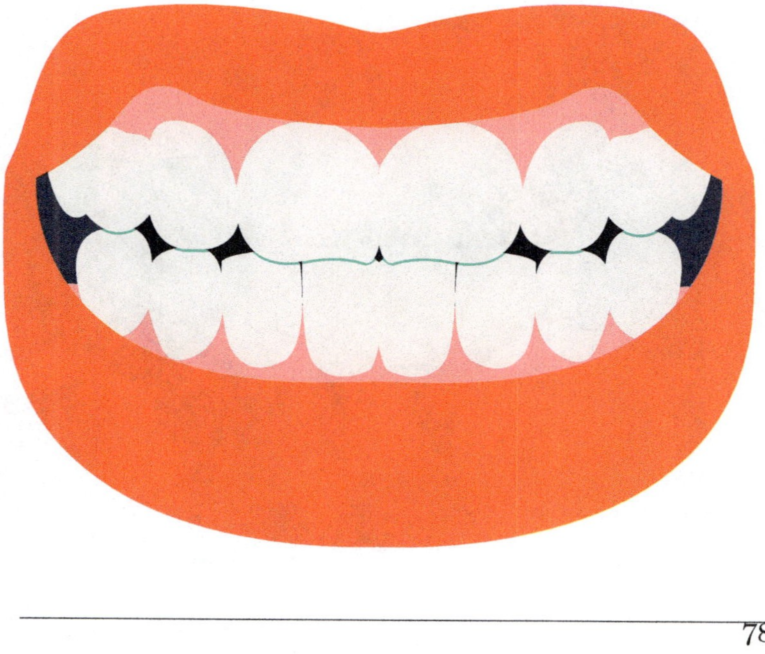

Grinding your teeth

In moments of stress and anxiety, many people have adopted the habit of tightly clamping their jaws together and grinding their teeth. Aside from wearing down your teeth, this bad habit can lead to headaches, jaw stiffness and even earache. In many cases the person exhibiting this behaviour isn't even aware they are doing it. Often occurring during sleep, night grinders wake up with jaw pain and no recollection as to why.

To tackle teeth grinding, first addressing the root of the problem may be the solution. Meditation, therapy and exercise for the release of endorphins may help to keep your stress and anxiety levels in check and in turn keep your teeth from coming to blows. However, for the unconscious sufferers, using a mouthguard while you sleep will help to prevent the damaging effects of teeth grinding.

Procrastination

Whether it's washing the dishes, answering a work email or writing that school essay that's due tomorrow, procrastination is a bad habit that can affect many different aspects of your life. Other than the stress and anxiety caused by rushing to finish a task you've put off completing, procrastination can lead to you challenging your self-worth, producing poor-quality or incorrect work, and fatigue.

To prevent putting tasks off until the last minute, set yourself a daily schedule, listing six or so of the most important things you need to achieve that day. Also, be realistic in what you can achieve in your given time frame. Overreaching your goal or underestimating how long a task will take might leave you challenging your abilities, furthering your desire to put them off in the future. It also doesn't hurt to try out a reward system for each task. By only doing your favourite things once you've carried out a task, you might be more likely to achieve your goals. You can also do some of these simultaneously: play your favourite TV show while you're doing household chores like ironing, or eat your favourite snack only while you do school work.

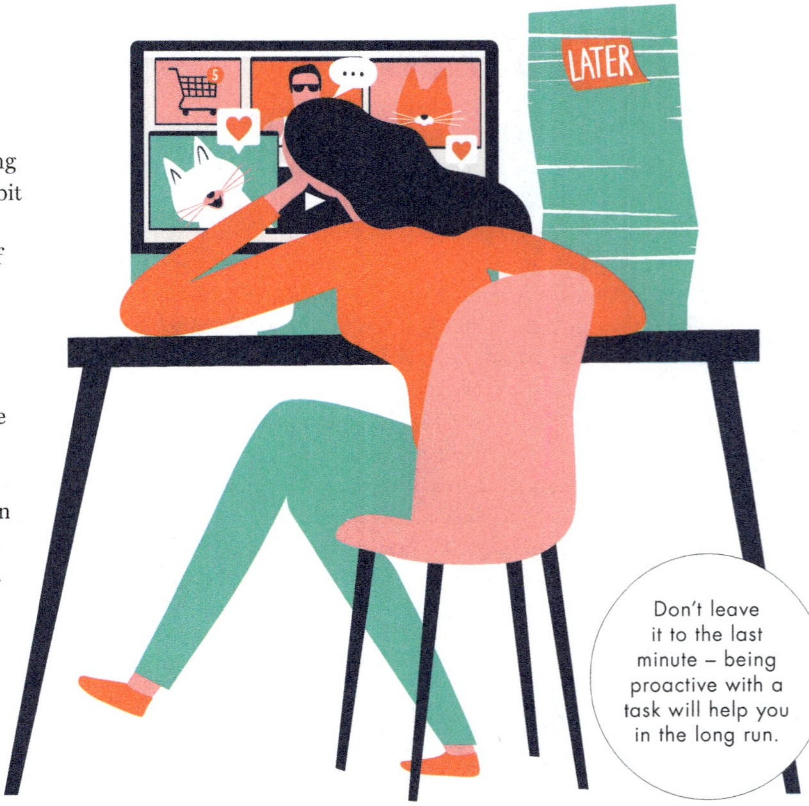

Don't leave it to the last minute – being proactive with a task will help you in the long run.

TO PREVENT PUTTING TASKS OFF UNTIL THE LAST MINUTE, SET YOURSELF A DAILY SCHEDULE, LISTING SIX OR SO OF THE MOST IMPORTANT THINGS YOU NEED TO ACHIEVE THAT DAY

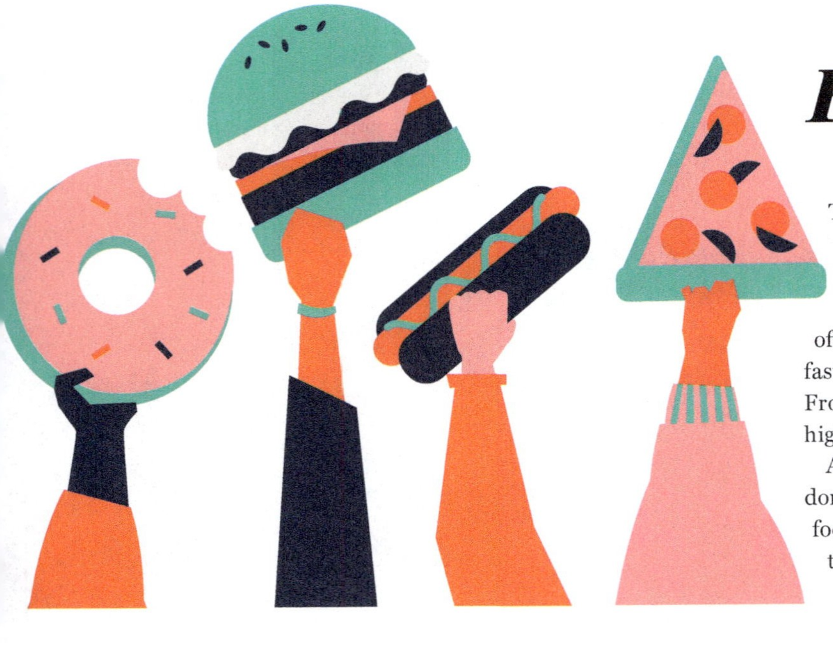

Eating fast food

The temptation to grab a juicy cheeseburger or a greasy bucket of chicken can be hard to fight. And while having a cheeky fast food meal every once in a while isn't necessarily a 'bad habit', when a server at your favourite burger joint knows your order off by heart, it's probably time for a change. It's no surprise that fast food can have negative effects on health when eaten regularly. From heart disease to obesity and diabetes, eating food filled with high levels of fat and sugar can wreak havoc on your body.

A good way to help ditch a fast-food habit is to make sure you don't reach the point of feeling overly hungry. When ravenous, junk food presents itself as a quick fix, meaning we are less likely to take the time to make a home-cooked meal. By creating a weekly plan you can stay on top of your hunger and out of a greasy spoon.

IMAGE SOURCE Getty Images

Wasting food

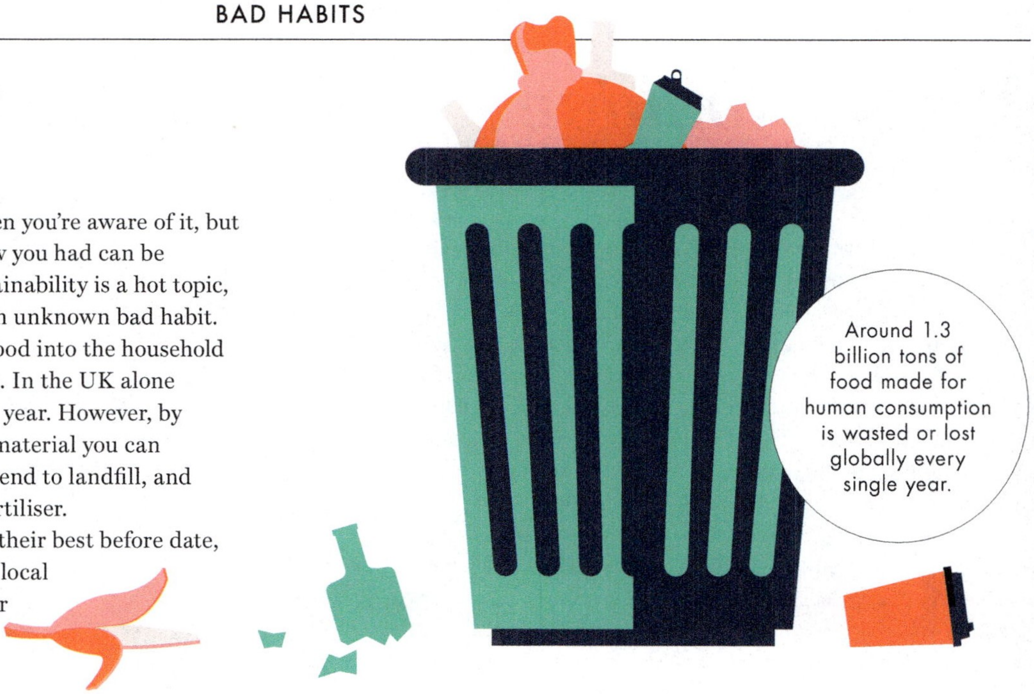

It's difficult enough to break a bad habit when you're aware of it, but trying to change a habit that you didn't know you had can be seriously challenging. In a world where sustainability is a hot topic, how we dispose of food waste could reveal an unknown bad habit.

It often comes naturally to simply throw food into the household waste bin without giving it a second thought. In the UK alone around 7 million tons of food is wasted each year. However, by purchasing a garden composter for organic material you can drastically reduce the amount of waste you send to landfill, and your garden will benefit from a nutritious fertiliser.

For those foodstuffs that are approaching their best before date, many community apps such as Olio connect local people to exchange and give away food rather than disposing of it.

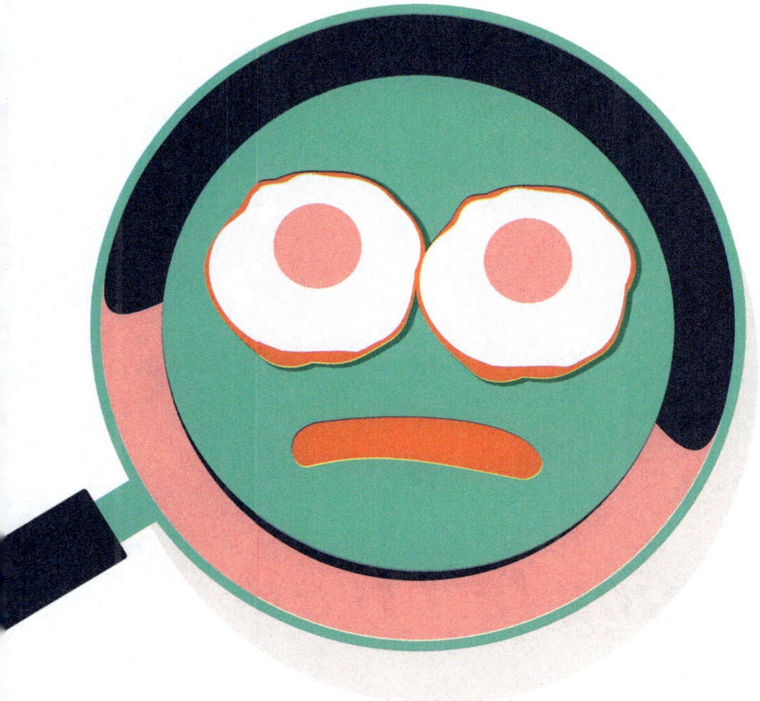

Skipping breakfast

It might not seem like a bad habit to ditch the morning toast and head straight to work, but repeatedly ignoring a critical meal of the day can be a routine with negative consequences. There's a reason why they call it the most important meal of the day, and that's because it kick-starts your metabolism. Leaving it until later in the day to chow down has been linked to health concerns such as weight gain and blood sugar fluctuations. To keep your metabolism in check, make sure you grab a bite bright and early.

Interrupting

Life is full of uncontrollable interruptions, whether it's an unexpected flat tyre or a nonsense marketing phone call. But there is something particularly annoying about being interrupted during a conversation. Cutting someone off mid-sentence is something many people have been guilty of, but being a repeat offender can be socially detrimental, particularly in the workplace. Verbal interruptions can suggest that you regard what you have to say as more important than what someone else is saying, leaving others to feel less so. In the workplace this behaviour may change; for example, people are less likely to stop their boss mid-sentence.

If you are guilty of this, try to take a second before you speak and let the other person finish. If what's on the tip of your tongue is a critical comment to the conversation and you're worried you might forget it, simply jot it down on a notepad and wait for the right moment to speak without cutting anyone off.

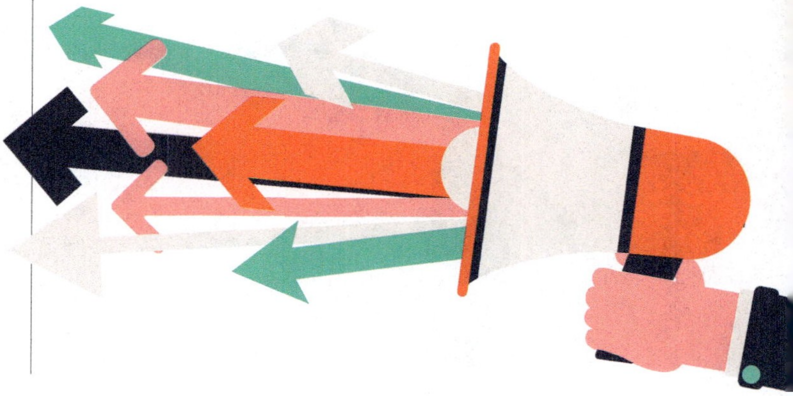

Not using sunscreen

If you love to bask in the sunlight during the summer months but neglect to apply sunscreen in the hopes of developing a golden tan, you may be unwittingly exposing your skin to a whole host of future problems. Exposing unprotected skin to ultraviolet (UV) radiation can increase the risk of developing skin cancer and promotes premature ageing. While sunbathing, UV rays weaken the fibres in the skin that keep it smooth and youthful, leaving skin wrinkled and leathery. The same can be said of visiting sunbed salons. The UV radiation from a tanning booth produces the same radiation found in the Sun, presenting the same risks.

To beat the burn and stay safe during summer, always carrying a travel-sized sunscreen in your bag is a great way to make sure you have protection against the Sun with you at all times. You can also harness the power of modern technology, which has taken away most of the guesswork when it comes to keeping an eye on the Sun. Downloading apps such as UVLens can notify you when the UV levels in your area are high and when to apply sunscreen to avoid getting a burn.

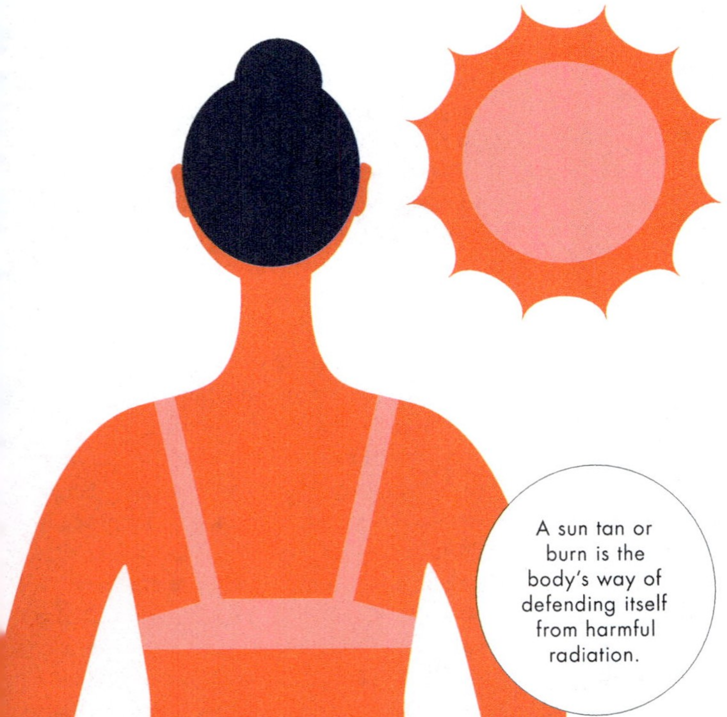

A sun tan or burn is the body's way of defending itself from harmful radiation.

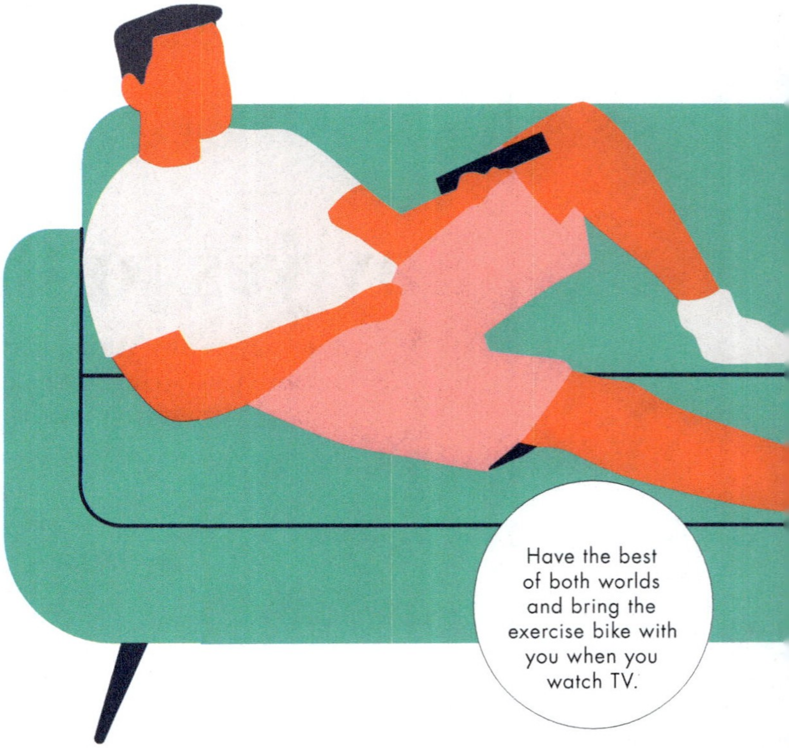

Have the best of both worlds and bring the exercise bike with you when you watch TV.

Being a couch potato

Slumping across the sofa in front of the TV after a long day at work or on a lazy Sunday afternoon might be considered by some as the perfect 'me time' – the ideal way to chill out and unwind. Perhaps for an hour or two a day that might be true, but what about for five hours or even an entire day? Getting into the bad habit of spending extended periods being sedentary increases the risk of depression, obesity and can even affect your personality, making you less agreeable and conscientious.

Keeping an active routine and rigid TV schedule is the best way to prevent becoming a couch potato. It's recommended that you only spend around two hours per day sitting watching TV and at least 30 minutes exercising. Channel surfing or binge-watching the latest Netflix show can be hard to resist, so only tune in to watch a specific show and try to limit how many episodes you watch in a day. If you just have to see how the series ends, take the treadmill or exercise bike from the spare room, put it in the living room and exercise while you watch.

"ALWAYS CARRYING A TRAVEL-SIZED SUNSCREEN IN YOUR BAG IS A GREAT WAY TO MAKE SURE YOU HAVE PROTECTION AGAINST THE SUN WITH YOU AT ALL TIMES"

IMAGE SOURCE Getty Images

Say yes to the power of no!

Agreeing to everything may keep others happy, but often at a personal cost. Here's why developing the habit of sometimes saying no means saying yes to self-worth

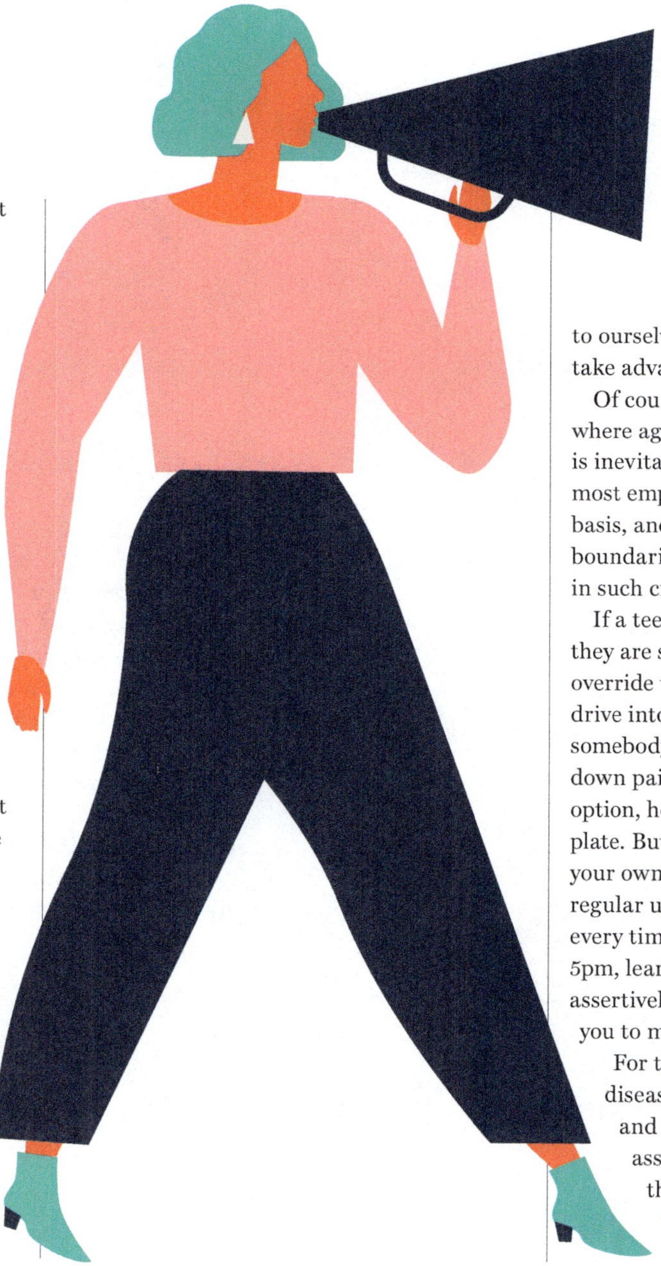

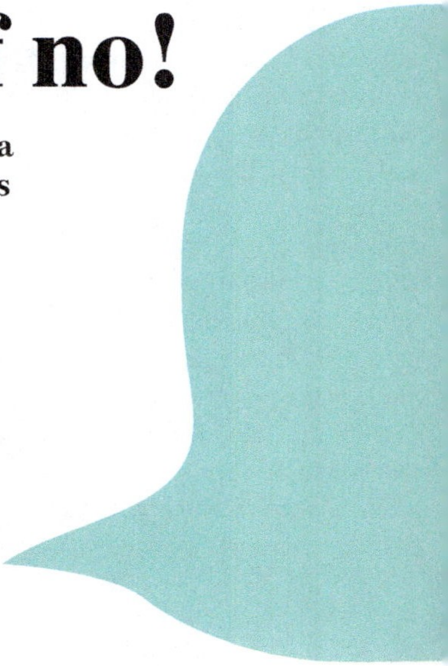

Growing up, we are generally taught that saying no all the time is considered impolite. And while young children have no problem using the word freely, sometimes as adults we need reminding of our right to it.

It's one thing to want to help others, but people who feel as though they simply can't say no suffer from an uncontrollable need for approval, and they may have deep-seated fears of anger and confrontation. As the late, acclaimed psychologist Dr Harriet Braiker pointed out in her *New York Times* bestseller, *The Disease to Please: Curing the People-Pleasing Syndrome*, "For many, the difficulty may start innocently enough with genuine and generous attempts to make others happy. But this seemingly harmless passion to always be 'nice', to put others first and to compulsively please them even at the expense of your own health and happiness rapidly spirals into a serious psychological syndrome with far-reaching physical and emotional consequences."

It's obvious that continually adding to a heavy workload because you can't say no to anything risks causing physical exhaustion. But we are less likely to consider how emotionally unhealthy it is too. Always shelving our own needs and desires to meet someone else's effectively sends out the message that we don't deserve to have our own needs met – both to ourselves, as well as others, who may then take advantage.

Of course, there are numerous situations where agreeing to things we don't want to do is inevitable or essential. Every parent and most employees will be used to this on a daily basis, and even people with healthy boundaries would find it impossible to say no in such circumstances.

If a teenage son or daughter calls to say they are stranded, safety concerns will override the fact that being woken at 3am to drive into town wasn't on our agenda. For somebody struggling financially, turning down paid overtime may not feel like an option, however much they have on their plate. But if there's the expectation you'll drop your own plans (or lose sleep) to provide a regular unpaid taxi service, or to work late every time a report is dropped on your desk at 5pm, learning how to say no gracefully, assertively and firmly is an essential skill for you to master.

For those suffering from the 'please disease', this may take some groundwork and self-examination. First, you need to assess why you continually agree to things you don't want to do. Examine what saying no represents. Is it rejection from social circles? A fear

No!

of being disliked, or not doing your job properly? Or perhaps it's concern for being seen as a 'bad' parent or partner? Did you grow up seeing it as essential to toe the line to avoid difficult situations? Remind yourself that self-care is not the same as being selfish, and it isn't your job to take on everyone else's problems or practicalities. If low self-esteem is the main issue, work on this with a qualified counsellor. Then follow our top tips for regaining the right to say no:

Start small. Like any habit, saying yes to everything can be something that is hard to stop doing. Some people will find it a lot easier to say no to things than others. Start with little things and build up from there.

–

Give yourself time. If your default response is to immediately agree, say that you need to check arrangements. Just be sure that you don't let this turn into a period of procrastination and guilt.

–

Focus on the positives of a negative and your desired outcome. Saying no to something that isn't a fit for you means being able to say yes to something that is.

–

> "REMEMBER THAT SELF-CARE IS NOT THE SAME AS BEING SELFISH"

Be prepared for some people to be taken aback or try to persuade you, particularly if they are used to you agreeing to everything. Stay polite but firm.

–

Try to avoid rambling explanations. "That sounds lovely but I have plans on Friday," is enough. As American etiquette expert and author Judith Martin once acknowledged, "Part of the skill of saying no is to shut up afterwards and not babble on, offering material for an argument."

–

Give an alternative suggestion if there's a compromise that works for you, as long as you don't end up agreeing to something else that doesn't. It's pointless saying no to manning a stand at a fête only to get lumbered with making umpteen batches of cupcakes when you don't have time for either.

Finally, if you regularly struggle with how to answer a request or demand, heed this simple line of advice from Brazilian novelist Paulo Coelho: "If you must say yes, say it with an open heart. If you must say no, say it without fear."

WORDS Sara Niven

IMAGE SOURCE Getty Images

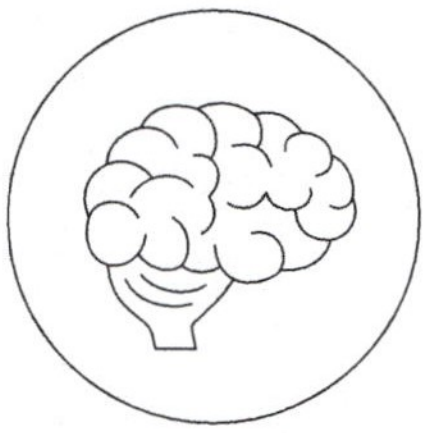

Stop worrying, start socialising

Are you more likely to get butterflies at a social event than be a social butterfly? Find out how to burst more confidently out of your cocoon

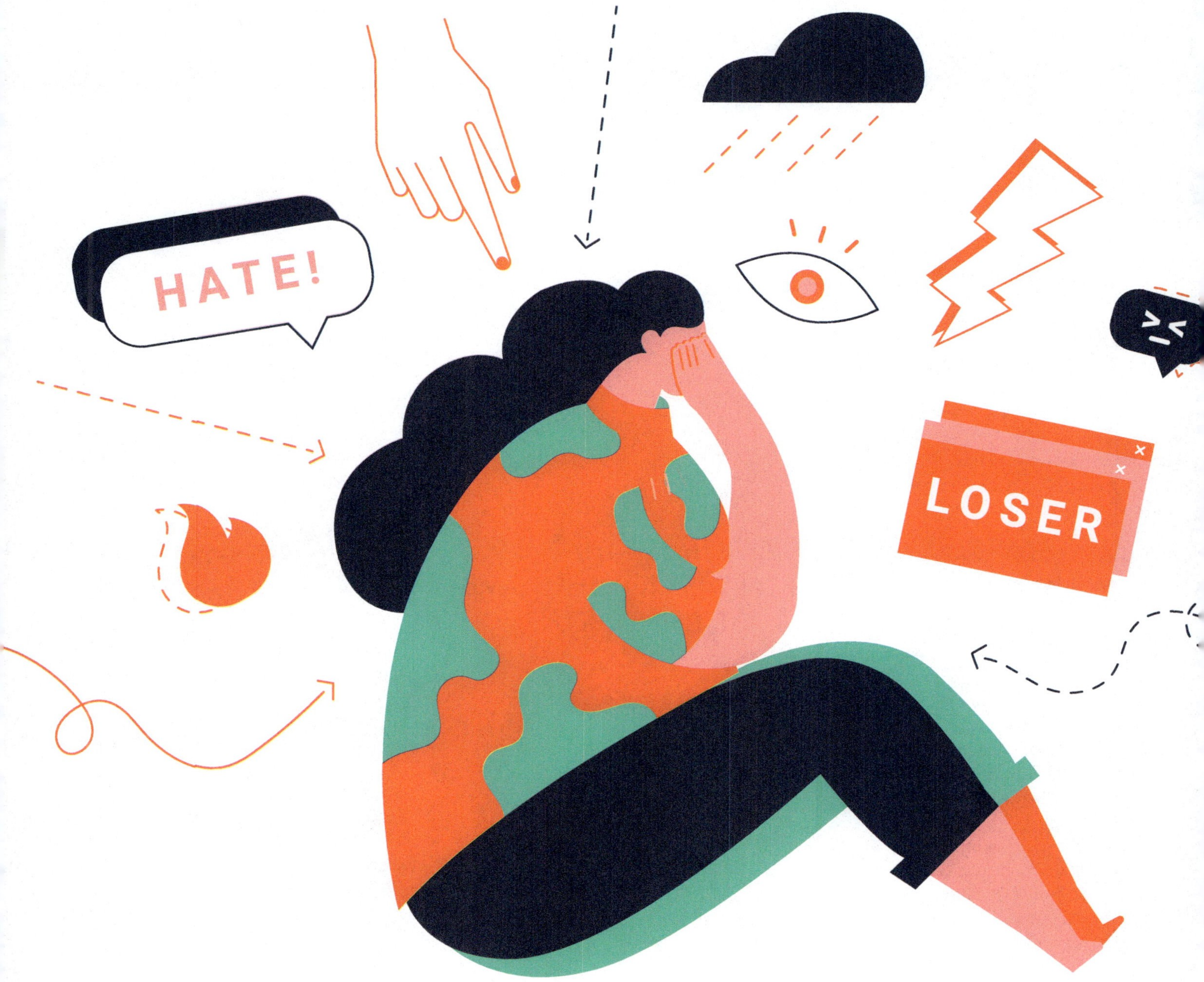

Getting an invitation to a party, wedding or night out is something we are generally expected to be pleased about. Choosing what to wear, meeting new people and the chance to be part of a special event or get together are all seen as positives.

Not everyone feels that way, however. Although a few nerves can be natural, people who experience physical stress-related symptoms, worry about events weeks in advance or avoid them altogether could have social anxiety disorder, or social phobia as it is otherwise known.

This recognised mental health condition is considered one of the most common anxiety-related issues and the third most prevalent psychiatric disorder after depression and alcohol dependence. Defined by mental health professionals as 'persistent fear and anxiety when it comes to social interaction', sufferers feel exposed to possible judgement or evaluation, especially by strangers.

According to Professor Nick Neave at the Psychology Department of Northumbria University, this actually makes some basic biological sense. "As human beings, we evolved from small kin-based groups, where individuals were surrounded by relatives and everyone knew their place in the social hierarchy. In modern times we are faced with anonymous, large, complex societies that may involve meeting strangers every day, particularly when it comes to social occasions. This causes anxiety because we constantly have to work out where we stand with them and never know if they mean us harm." In the past, anxiety might have helped us to stay aware of any potential danger, but it can cause daily distress for those struggling with it today.

So how can you deal with nerves ruining your enjoyment of occasions or preventing you from going altogether? It can be useful to consider any specific anxiety triggers. Most of us feel more comfortable in certain situations over others, and there's nothing wrong with gravitating towards those we see as a fit and turning down those we don't. Glastonbury may be out of the question if crowds and camping make you nervous, but perhaps you'd feel more at ease seeing a live band at a low-key event?

If it boils down to fears of being judged, it may be useful to explore any long-held beliefs or conditioning contributing to this.

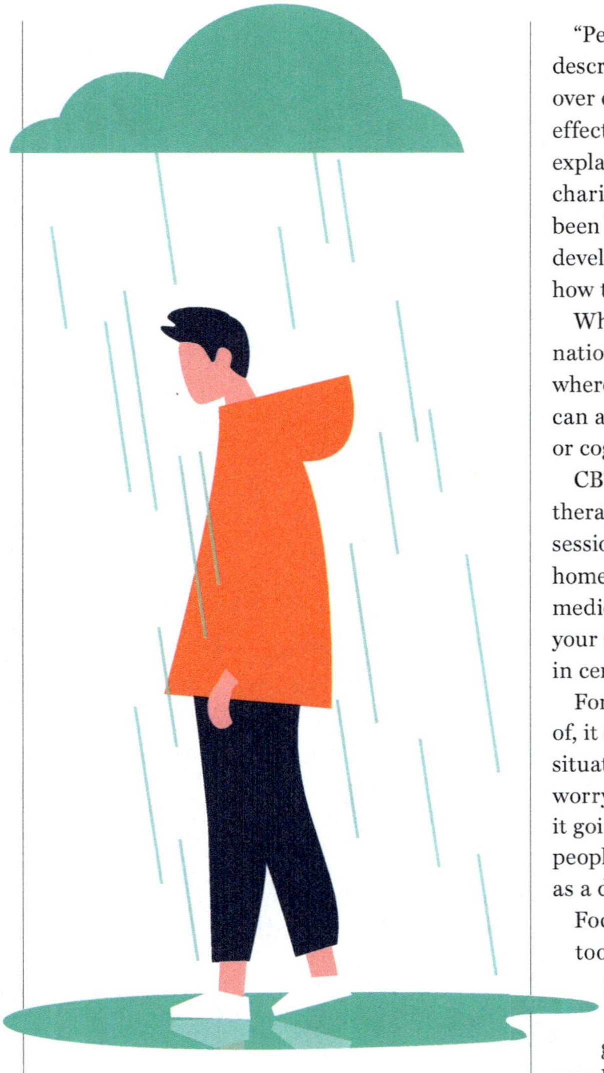

HOLD THAT THOUGHT

Challenge your thinking if you recognise the following:

AWFULISING
This is always imagining the most 'awful' outcome. It's one thing to be prepared for not knowing many people and another to decide that if no one immediately approaches you you're a total social failure.

PERSONALISING
This refers to thinking you are the focus of everyone's attention in a negative way. For example, if a group of people are laughing, you immediately decide they must be poking fun at you, when it is far more likely they are just having fun.

ALL OR NOTHING
There's a middle ground between feeling pressure to be the life and soul and not attending at all. You could decide to go and see how you feel after an hour and make a polite excuse if you're struggling. Over time, you may start to feel more at ease in similar situations.

"People who experience social anxiety often describe their parents as over protective and over critical, which can have a long-standing effect on their social interaction with others," explains a spokesperson for the national charity Anxiety UK. "Equally, some may have been bullied at school, which led them to develop a negative view of themselves and how they perceive others see them."

Whatever the cause, Anxiety UK has a national accredited talking therapy service where anyone struggling with social phobia can access counselling, clinical hypnotherapy or cognitive behaviour therapy (CBT).

CBT is seen as a particularly helpful therapy for dealing with anxiety, with sessions often including practical steps or homework. Not everyone is keen on taking medication, but it may be worth speaking to your GP to see if they feel it could be helpful in certain circumstances.

For big events you feel particularly fearful of, it can be useful to work through the situation in your head, but instead of worrying about what may go wrong, picture it going well. Visualising yourself greeting people, smiling and even enjoying it can act as a dress rehearsal for the real deal.

Focusing on others can also be a valuable tool. Have a few suitable questions prepared that invite people to talk about themselves. Good listening skills and genuine interest will be appreciated and may help you to start feeling less self-conscious and anxious.

If you find yourself completely overwhelmed in a social situation, the mental health charity Mind suggests a number of breathing exercises and relaxation techniques. Find out more on its website: **www.mind.org.uk.**

WORDS Sara Niven

For further details about the treatment of social anxiety see
NICE Clinical Guideline CG159
www.nice.org.uk/guidance/cg159

For information on the support services provided by Anxiety UK call
03444 775 774
or visit: **anxietyuk.org.uk**

IMAGE SOURCE Getty Images

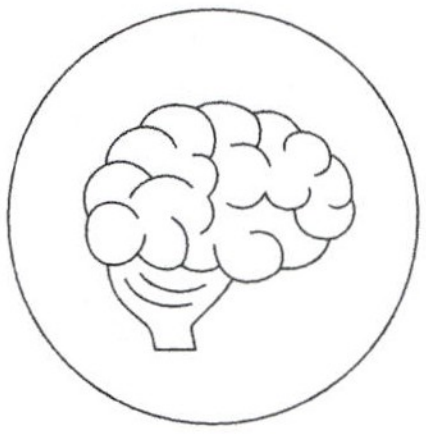

Group habits

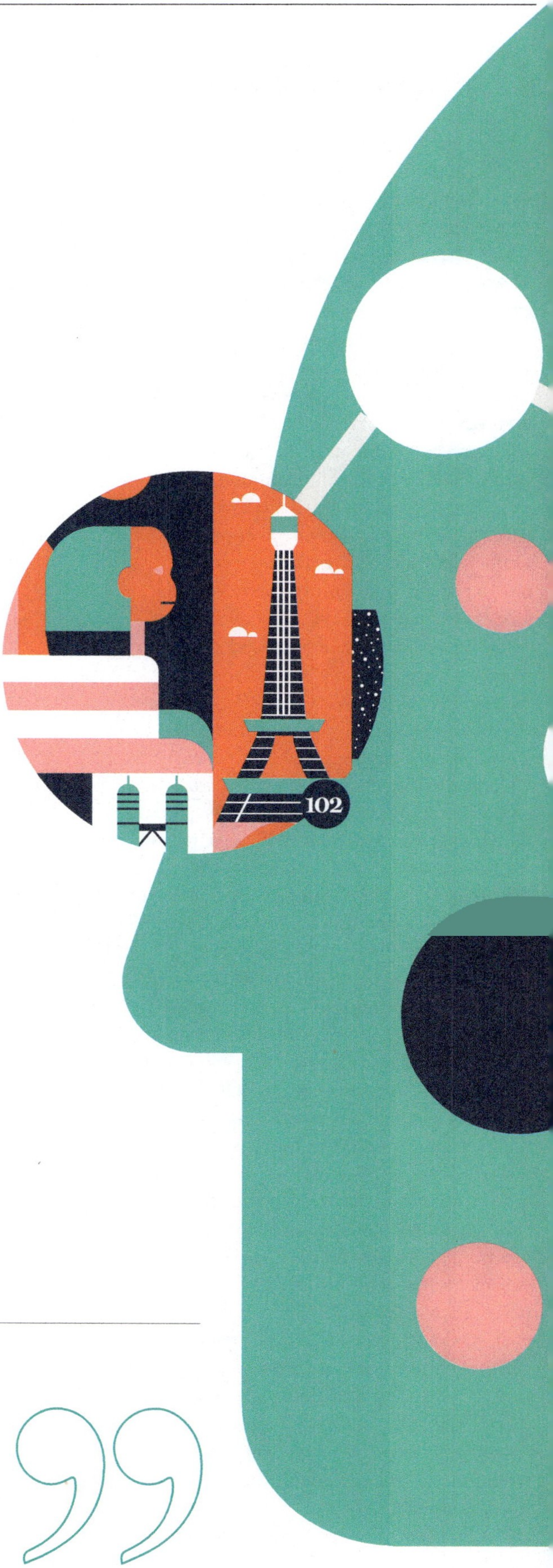

> SIMPLE DAILY HABITS CAN ALSO UNDERSCORE SUCCESS IN SUBTLE WAYS, SUCH AS GETTING A GOOD NIGHT'S SLEEP REGULARLY

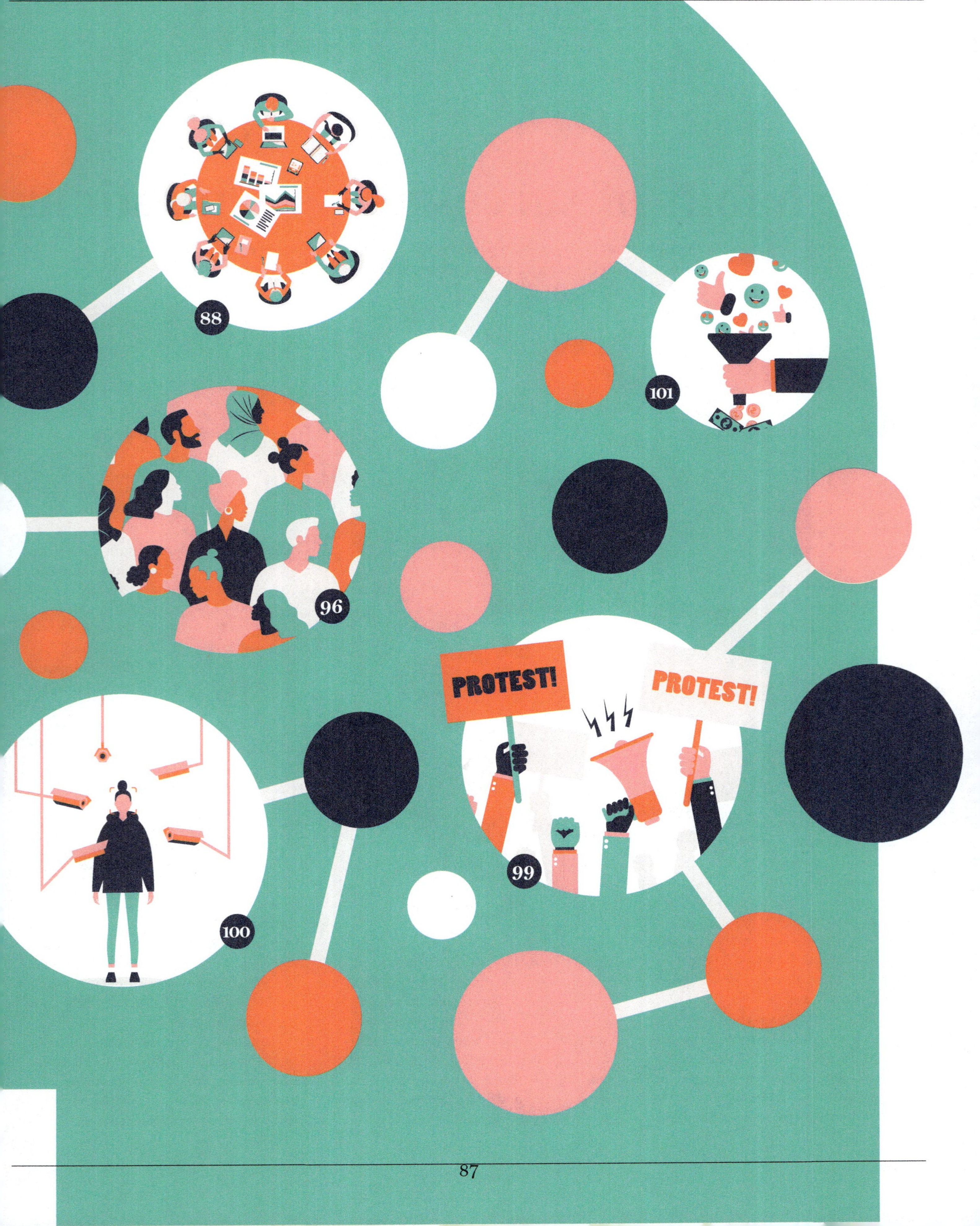
88
101
96
PROTEST!
PROTEST!
100
99

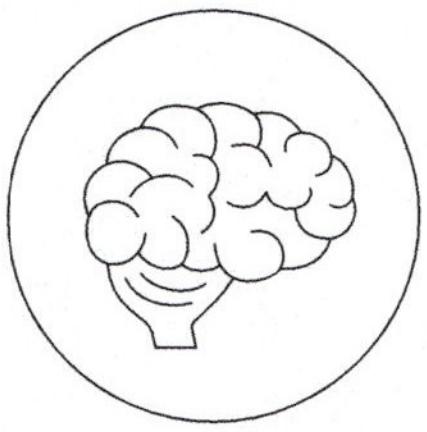

The habits of successful organisations

From a tenacious mentality to a good night's sleep, a decent combination of habits can propel teams to reach their goals

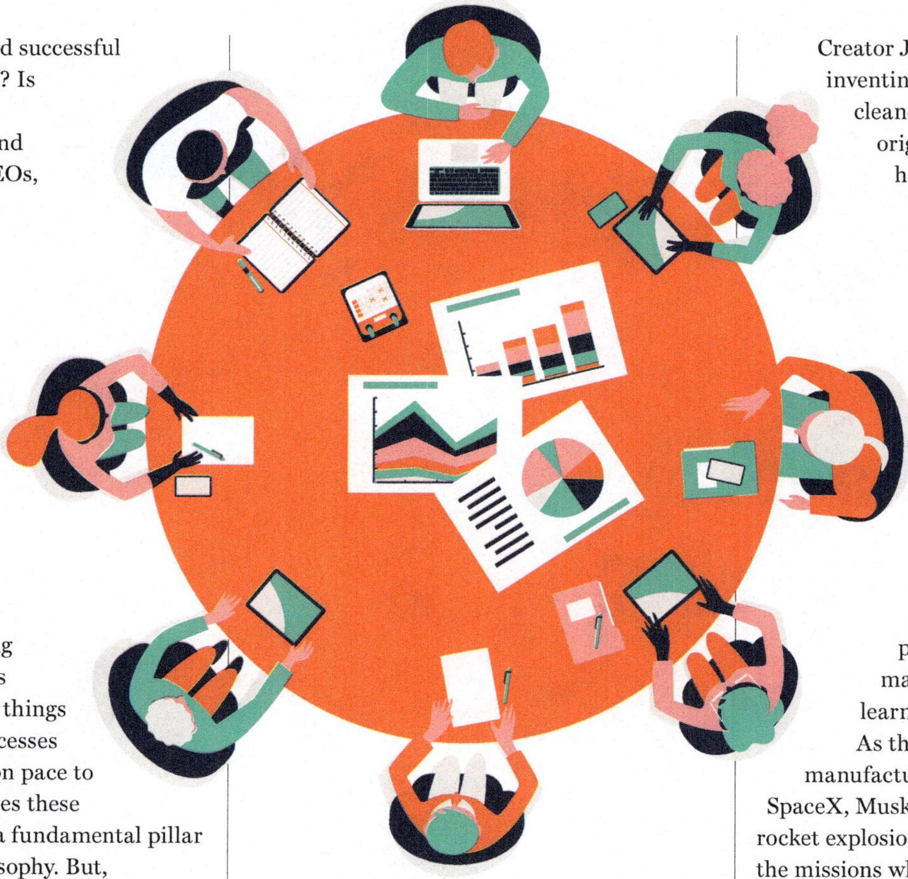

What lies behind successful organisations? Is success owed primarily to innovative and audacious leaders and CEOs, their hard-working and ingenious teams, or simply luck and inertia? It undoubtedly differs from organisation to organisation, but whether success comes from the top, the bottom or somewhere in between, all exceptional teams will have the same thing in their favour: a set of habits or behaviours that drives them towards being extraordinary. Sometimes these habits can be small things that help get thought processes whirling or keep a team on pace to reach its goals. Other times these habitual principles form a fundamental pillar of an organisation's philosophy. But, fascinatingly, despite the diversity in agendas and desires of organisations in different fields, we see these similar successful habits appearing time and again.

Let's begin with an often-cited but seemingly counterintuitive habit that garners success: learning how to fail. Failure is portrayed largely positively in business circles, with the often-touted mantra of 'fail fast, fail often' regularly used. Critics of such a course have warned that adopting a lackadaisical approach to failure can be a dangerous philosophy to instil in a huge company where a slew of individuals have sufficient freedom to make costly mistakes (banking springs to mind). But the benefit of this habit comes into its own in the hands of entrepreneurs and leaders steering their organisations to success.

Creator James Dyson rose to fame after inventing the Dual Cyclone vacuum cleaner and has since pioneered original hand driers, fans, heaters, purifiers and more. But before his meteoric rise he spent 15 years creating over 5,000 insufficient versions of his eventual landmark product. As Dyson has said, "You never learn from success, but you do learn from failure."

Coupling failure with positivity is a habit also championed by Tesla and SpaceX CEO Elon Musk. With a similar mindset to Dyson, Musk believes progress can only be made by making – and then crucially learning from – mistakes.

As the head of aerospace manufacturer and space travel company SpaceX, Musk has persevered through rocket explosions on the launch pad and, on the missions where the rocket successfully ascended into space, toppling and exploding upon landing. As the head of Tesla, he's had to contend with batteries spontaneously combusting and falling seriously behind with his production timetable.

The ability to learn from failure, then, is inevitably tied to the habit of positivity and perseverance. Speaking to Freakonomics Radio, James Dyson spoke of the importance and eventual rewards gleaned from

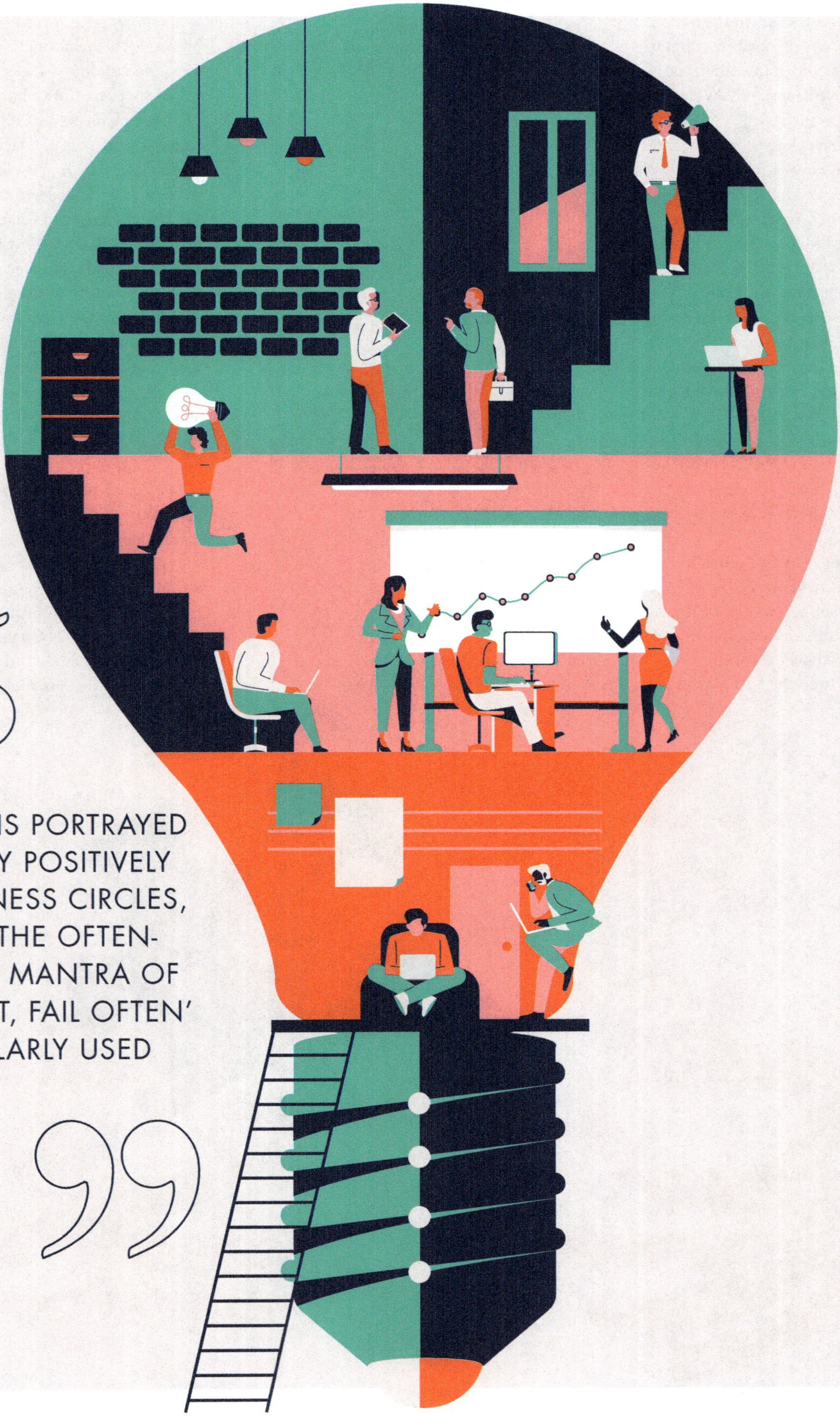

> FAILURE IS PORTRAYED LARGELY POSITIVELY IN BUSINESS CIRCLES, WITH THE OFTEN-TOUTED MANTRA OF 'FAIL FAST, FAIL OFTEN' REGULARLY USED

IMAGE SOURCE Getty Images

perseverance: "And just when you've had enough, and you think you're never going to get the answer, that's the point where you must try even harder. Because that's the point where everybody else gave up."

Persistence in the face of failure is a common theme that runs through the stories of many entrepreneurs, but perhaps none so famously as Steve Jobs, co-founder of Apple. Jobs' habit of perseverance manifested itself in a bizarre way, in that he often didn't acknowledge his failures as mistakes. Likewise, he could be notoriously impatient with the failures of others. And yet his journey stands as testament to the power of harnessing the lessons from failure and the benefits of a tenacious attitude.

In 1985 Jobs was forced out of Apple and subsequently failed to make a success of a new computer company he founded called NeXT. However, the determined entrepreneur went on to invest in a fledgling Pixar and, eventually, was welcomed back to lead Apple once again. With the knowledge of his failures tucked behind his ear, Jobs had become a more mature and developed leader. His second stint as Apple boss went significantly better than the first. Under Jobs' leadership the tech titan launched a range of hit products including the iPhone, one of the most revolutionary device in decades.

The sporting world, however, perhaps holds the most inspiring testament to courageousness in the face of failure. After the Wales football team defeated Belgium – which was ranked second in the world – in the UEFA European Championship quarter-finals in 2016, manager Chris Coleman delivered a rousing speech about failure. Finding humility in his elation, the manager said, "... four years ago I was as far away from this as you can imagine and look what's happened. If you work hard enough and you're not afraid to dream and you're not afraid to fail. Everybody fails. Don't be afraid to fail. I've had more failures than successes, but I'm not afraid to fail."

Those who persevere in the face of adversity typically engage in a complementary and equally powerful habit: they actively look towards and aspire to attain a better future. Sometimes this vision manifests as a long-term dream, other times it's a micro-goal to be achieved over the next day or working week. Indra Nooyi, the former CEO of PepsiCo, has spoken of imagining

IT'S ALL ABOUT MENTALITY

How football manager Pep Guardiola used social culture to take his team to the top

Success in sport is as much about mental preparedness as it is about physicality. When football club Manchester City hired one of the world leaders of the sport in Pep Guardiola, it was clear the team was bringing in a strategic genius of the game. What was perhaps less clear was the hire of Guardiola the leader, a man who would encourage and drive his players to new heights by transforming the mental fabric of the team.

Guardiola espouses the idea that the success of the team outstrips the desires of the individual, and he swiftly educated his players to feel the same way. Guardiola taught each player to be a servant to a cause greater than themselves; to want to be a piece of the winning team. By raising an individual's accountability from just themselves to their team, failure to invest the effort didn't just disappoint the player and their manager but all their team-mates. The social culture thus established, players would strive to be the player that their team-mates lifted into the air and showered with praise at full-time for striding the extra mile, instead of being the one denied to even join training because they arrived late. Together with his technical prowess, Guardiola has used his homogeneous unit to shatter records and establish a formidable football legacy.

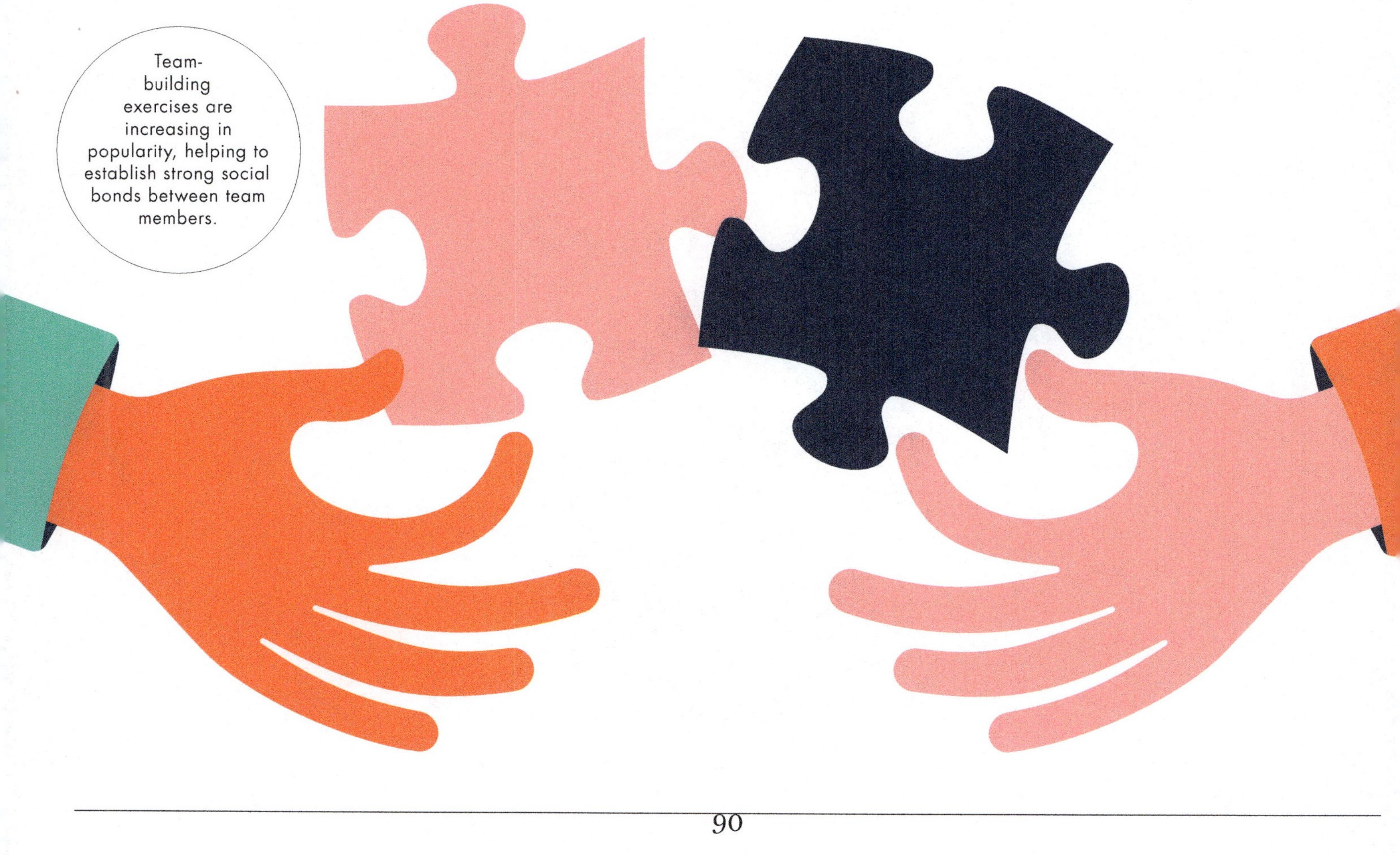

Team-building exercises are increasing in popularity, helping to establish strong social bonds between team members.

Adopting a habit of failure and learning, although disheartening, has led to fantastic innovation.

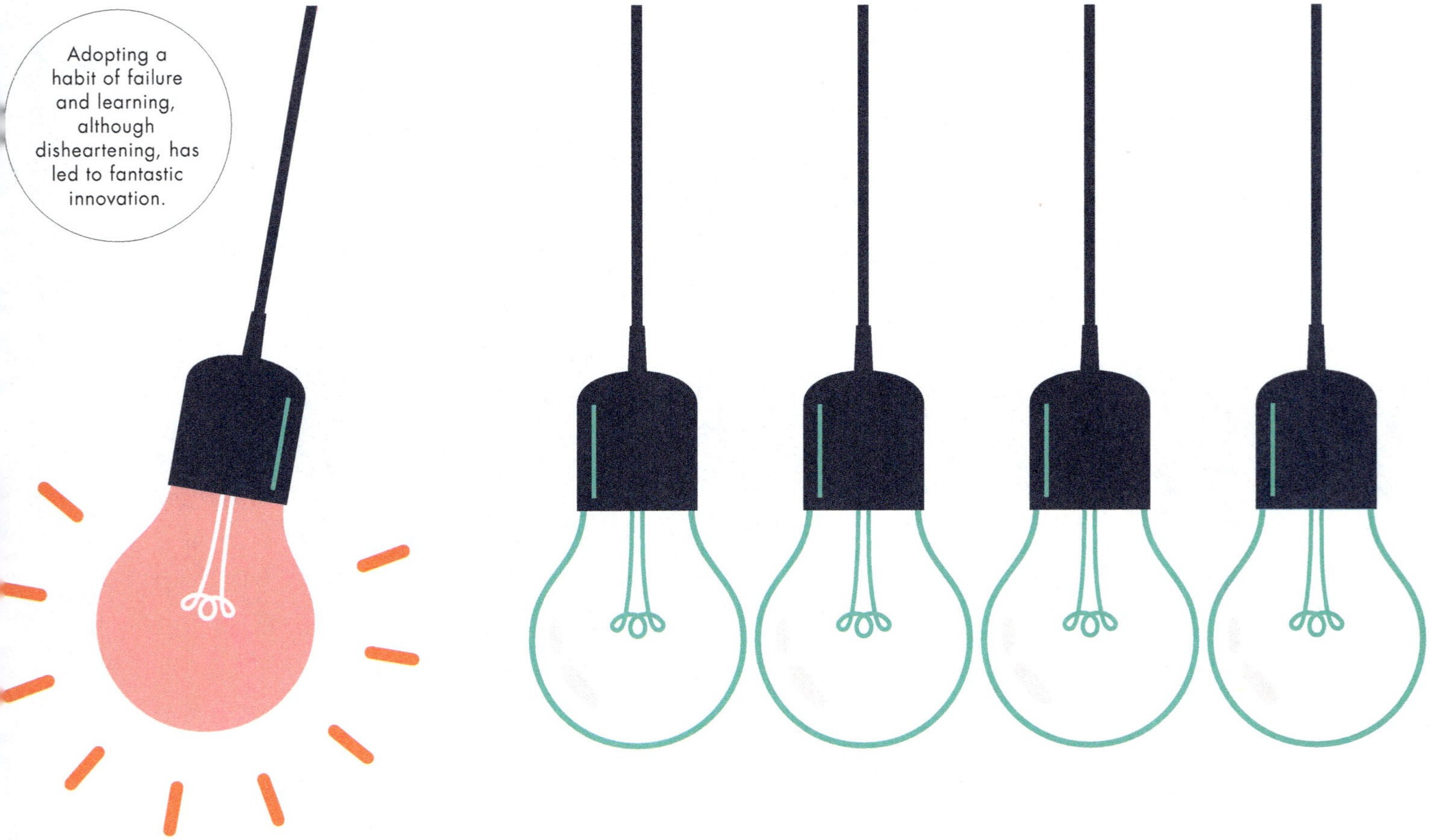

herself as a leader long before she took the reigns of the gargantuan food company. This was a belief instilled in her as a child, as she would take turns with her sister to play the part of president of India each night at dinner. Nooyi's mother would ask, "If you were inaugurated as president, what would you say?" This empowered a young Nooyi to dream of achieving great things from a young age. As adults within the workforce, however, we're often aided by smaller, more readily attainable goals.

Sheryl Sandberg, chief operational officer at Facebook, has advised harbouring a long-term dream but coupling it with habitually creating an 18-month plan that helps people stay on course and realise their personal ambitions. Facebook's chief executive officer Mark Zuckerberg also sets himself regular yearly goals.

Powerful state-of-mind habits rightly earn a significant place in the story of successful organisations, but simple daily habits can also underscore success in subtle ways. Getting a good night's sleep regularly is a prime example. In 2016, Yoshinori Ohsumi received the Nobel Prize in Physiology or Medicine for his work on autophagy – a key process of cellular recycling that happens in our brain as we sleep. Autophagy clears out useless cellular debris and toxins and, put simply, rejuvenates our cells. These lessons from biology regarding the benefits of a good night's sleep on productivity are reinforced by the successes of leading business figures. Facebook's Sheryl Sandberg, Amazon's Jeff Bezos and PepsiCo's Indra Nooyi have all testified to the importance of sleep in their busy working lives.

> "SIMPLE DAILY HABITS CAN ALSO UNDERSCORE SUCCESS IN SUBTLE WAYS, SUCH AS GETTING A GOOD NIGHT'S SLEEP REGULARLY"

It should be noted that some studies suggest adopting the opposite approach, reporting that length of sleep is often inversely correlated with earnings. This means that the more you earn, the less you typically sleep. Elon Musk, for his part, has been reported to make do with as little as six hours sleep a night due to his congested schedule. But what happens when we expand our viewpoint from leaders and take a look at the productivity of a sleep-deprived workforce? A 2015 study focusing on the Kansas State Employee Wellness Program discovered that sleeping difficulties caused, rather predictably, increased absence and

IMAGE SOURCE Getty Images

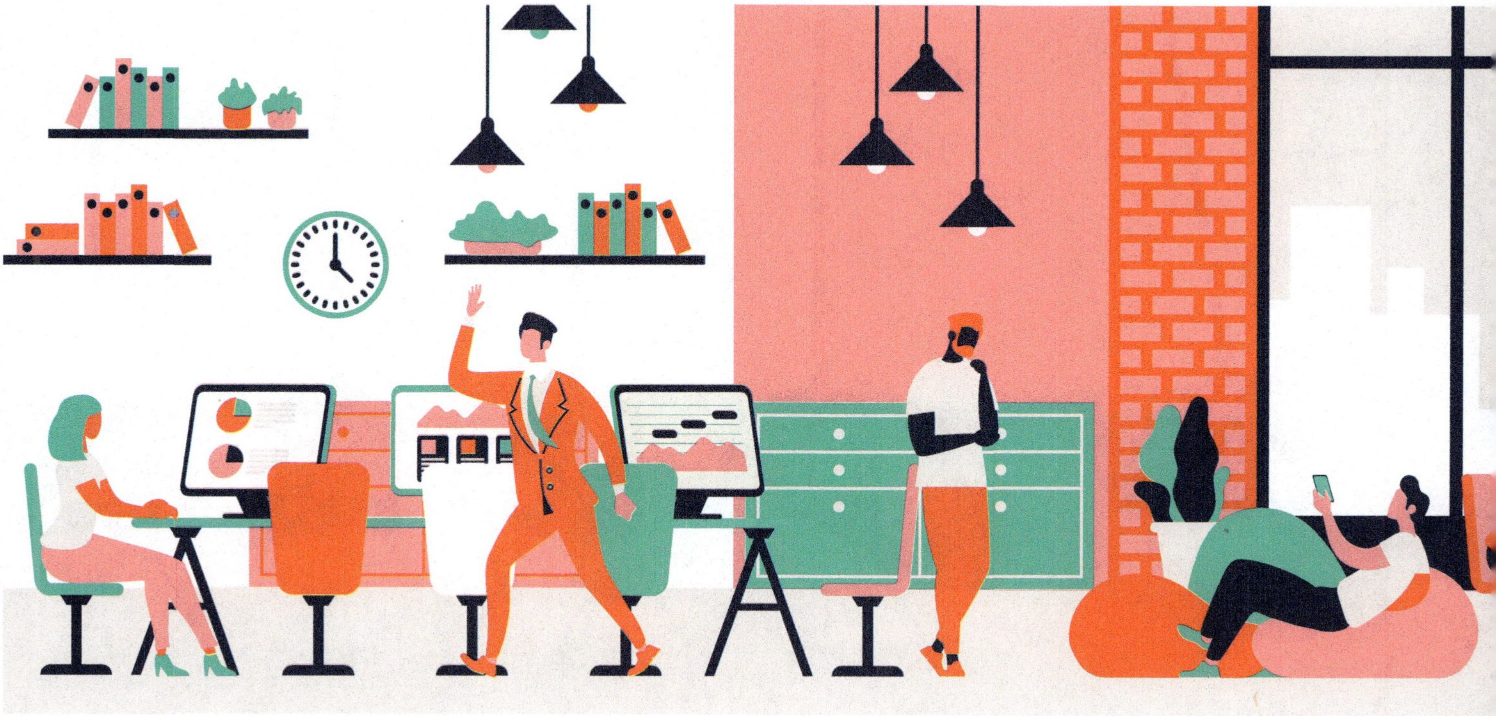

lower productivity in the workplace. Another piece of research tracked the sleeping habits of night-shift workers and found that successive nights with little sleep inevitably took its toll on worker output. Of course, the amount of sleep an individual requires for optimal activity varies significantly from person to person, but a habit of regular, uninterrupted sleep of sufficient length appears to be a routine we could all do with adopting. Failing that, some companies have turned to implementing 'nap rooms' to cater for their employees.

Google has equipped its headquarters in Mountain View, California, with EnergyPods that are specifically designed to accommodate a hard-working employee and grant them a soothing power nap. The EnergyPod reclines its occupant in the optimal relaxing position for blood flow and after an allotted time gently brings them out of their slumber using light and vibration. Space agency NASA and car company Mercedes-Benz are also fans of the innovative EnergyPods. New York City's *Huffington Post*, meanwhile, has also embraced nap rooms after its co-founder Arianna Huffington collapsed from exhaustion brought on by sleep deprivation.

The simple activity of sleeping may seem like an underrated habit behind successful companies, but it's not unique in its simplicity. Mark Zuckerberg, the founder and CEO of Facebook, is an advocate of walking to improve productivity. He has been noted to take his meetings outside so that he and his team can think as they walk. Steve Jobs, too, was known to host meetings on the move and go for regular walks in search of inspiration. This habit is another that's reinforced by scientific research.

> "MARK ZUCKERBERG, THE FOUNDER AND CEO OF FACEBOOK, HAS BEEN NOTED TO TAKE HIS MEETINGS OUTSIDE SO THAT HE AND HIS TEAM CAN THINK AS THEY WALK"

Marily Oppezzo and Daniel Schwartz of Stanford University found that creativity was bolstered when walking and continued for a short time after an individual returned to a sitting position. Amazingly, they observed that even simply walking on a treadmill while staring at a blank wall doubled creativity over being sat down and was comparable to walking outside. If that's the case, then why not bring the benefits of walking into the meeting room itself? That's exactly what Duke University's School of Nursing did when they replaced their office chairs with raised desks and treadmills, allowing the staff to type and walk as they spoke.

In addition to increasing creativity, the treadmills had the added advantage of encouraging the staff members to exercise. This is another organisational habit that's growing in popularity, with internal gymnasiums springing up in all manner of office spaces. Naturally, Google is also at the forefront of this strategy and has already

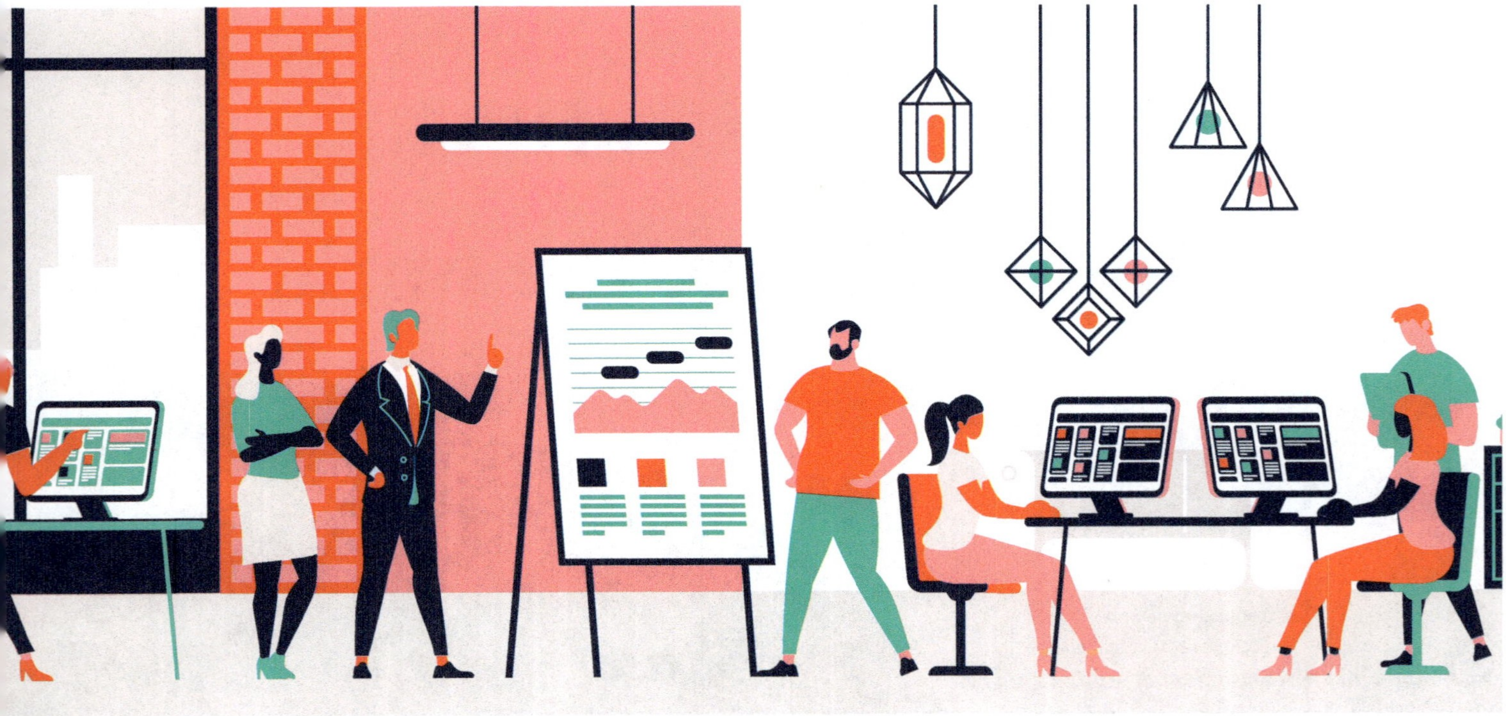

incorporated free gymnasiums and gym classes at its headquarters. More broadly, forerunner companies are beginning to pay more attention to employee happiness.

Hilton, which runs some of the world's most beautiful hotels, has a stellar reputation for plush decor in its lobbies and customer spaces, but it has recently begun upgrading the staff-only sections of its buildings so that its workers can share in a degree of luxury. Hilton also teamed up with clothing company Under Armour to design more lightweight and comfortable workwear for its staff. These efforts helped Hilton to recently top *Fortune*'s list of best companies to work for. Following close behind in second place was the company Salesforce, which has also turned its attention to improving staff welfare. Alongside traditional career goals targets, the company now includes well-being objectives for employees to strive towards.

As well as caring and catering for their staff, another critical element organisations are adopting is a customer-first focus. Indra Nooyi, during her time as CEO of PepsiCo, would often imagine herself as a customer when judging how her companies' products looked on the shelves. Likewise, the California-based grocery chain Trader Joe's encourages its staff to go the extra mile in finding the exact product their customer is after, whether or not they're needed elsewhere. In a similar vein, the popular brand Kimpton Hotels & Restaurants rewards staff members for making a client's visit especially memorable.

Habits can be difficult things to change. Once we've adopted them, they sink their claws in and we can find it hard to shake them off. This is as true for the individual as it is for organisations of people, as the familiar is always easier than the unknown. That being said, perhaps the most important habit employed by successful organisations is that of innovation. Those who habitually challenge the status quo, try new things, push boundaries and set pioneering examples for others to follow set the stage for their habits to become standard practice in many companies. Individuals who sleep well, exercise regularly, learn from their mistakes, keep pushing and set themselves goals and exceed them may have all the ingredients for establishing a successful company. Yet perhaps the biggest challenge is having the courage to swap out office chairs for treadmills and exchange meeting room spaces for nap pods once the organisation has grown. The most successful organisations are always adapting, evolving and moving away from archaic norms, thereby finding new habits along the way.

WORDS James Horton

UNDERSTANDING HABITS

How organisations improve by appreciating their employees' most effective styles

Instilling habits within an organisation can be a critical component of building success. Yet a good organisation is served well by also appreciating the habits that are already present in its workforce. As the simple-but-effective maxim goes, play to your strengths. Organisations that recognise the habits and personalities of its individual team members and adjust to accommodate them may soon reap the rewards of increased productivity. This can be achieved by helping individuals to work in their optimal environment and aiding their team-mates in understanding their personal drives.

Some companies have used insights from psychology to build tools that help team members and their managers down this path. One such company, Insights Discovery, boasts partnerships with England football player Jamie Vardy, the UK's National Health Service and food company Danone, among others. Insights have used research from Swiss psychologist Carl Jung and his student Jolande Jacobi to build a 'four-colour energy' wheel that assigns personality types to employees after completion of a questionnaire. This simple colour spectrum system can help leaders place their staff in roles that suit their skill set and equip team members with a new appreciation of their colleagues' behavioural traits.

IMAGE SOURCE Getty Images

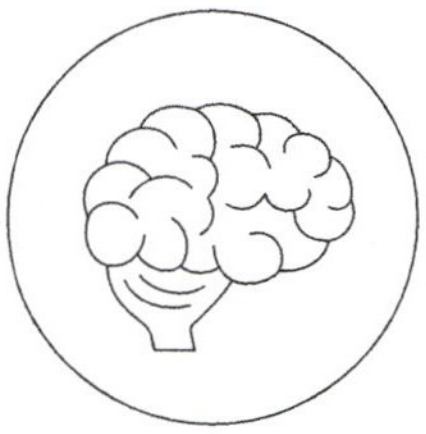

How to change the world

The study of social change and how to bring it about

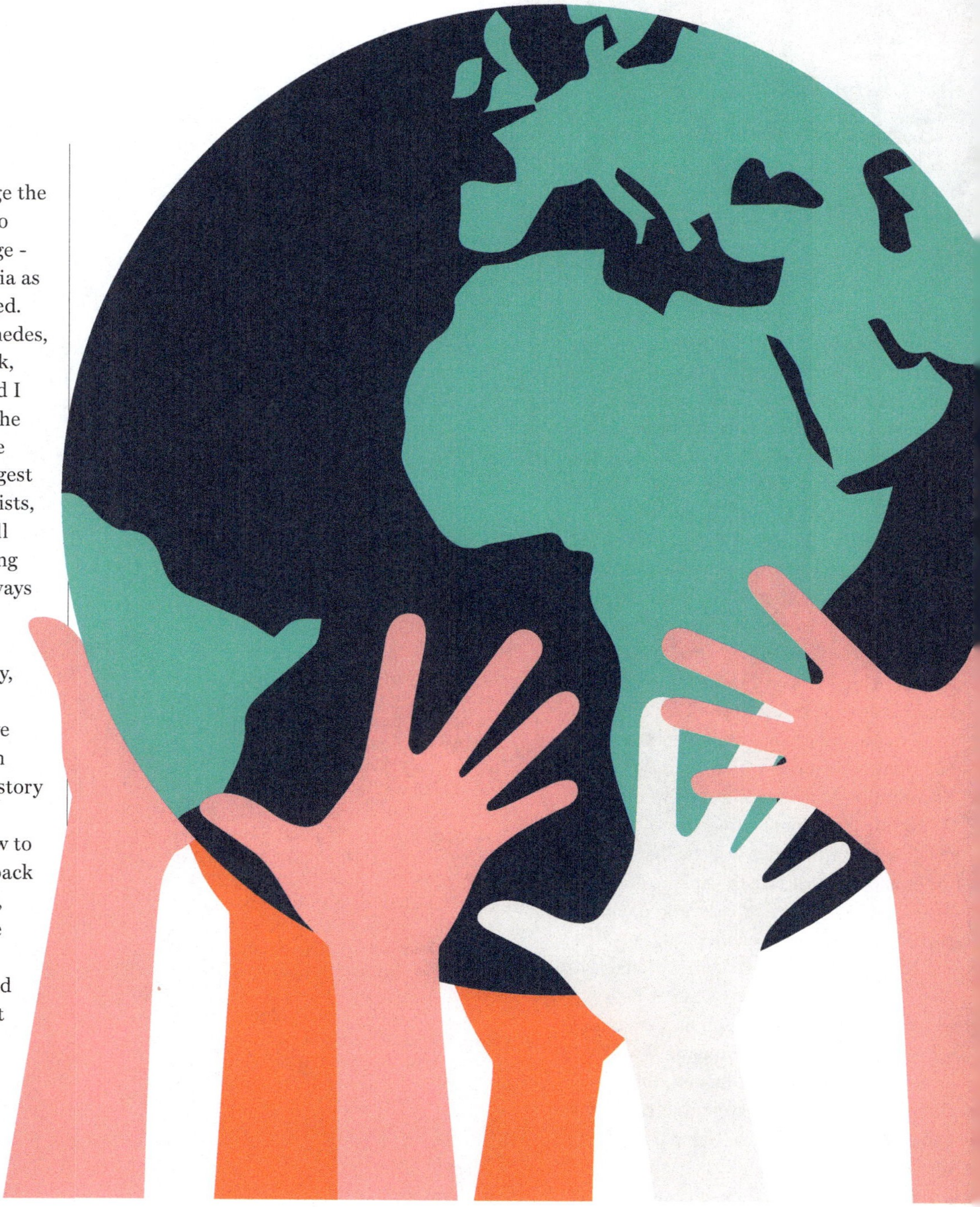

So you're young, impassioned and empowered. You're going to change the world. But how are you going to do that? Worlds aren't exactly easy to change - indeed, societies have just as much inertia as massive objects: they resist being changed. But as the Greek mathematician Archimedes, flush with his analysis of how levers work, asserted, "Give me the place to stand and I shall move the earth." If that applies in the realm of physics, can the same insight be applied to human societies, from the largest to the smallest? Philosophers, psychologists, sociologists and systems analysts have all looked to answer this question, developing answers deriving from their particular ways of looking at the problem.

Once upon a time, though, the bigger question was can societies change? Today, living in a time of considerable social development, that question seems to have been answered, but it is worth bearing in mind that throughout most of human history advancement has been slow and often imperceptible. And before we look at how to bring about change, it's worth stepping back and asking, are you sure, absolutely sure, that the change you're advocating will be for the better? In 19th-century Russia, people chafed against Tsarist tyranny and the Okhrana, the Tsar's secret police. But at worst, the Okhrana executed a few thousand (probably fewer) opponents of the regime. Following the Bolshevik Revolution and the overthrow of the Tsars, the communist regime was responsible for the death of

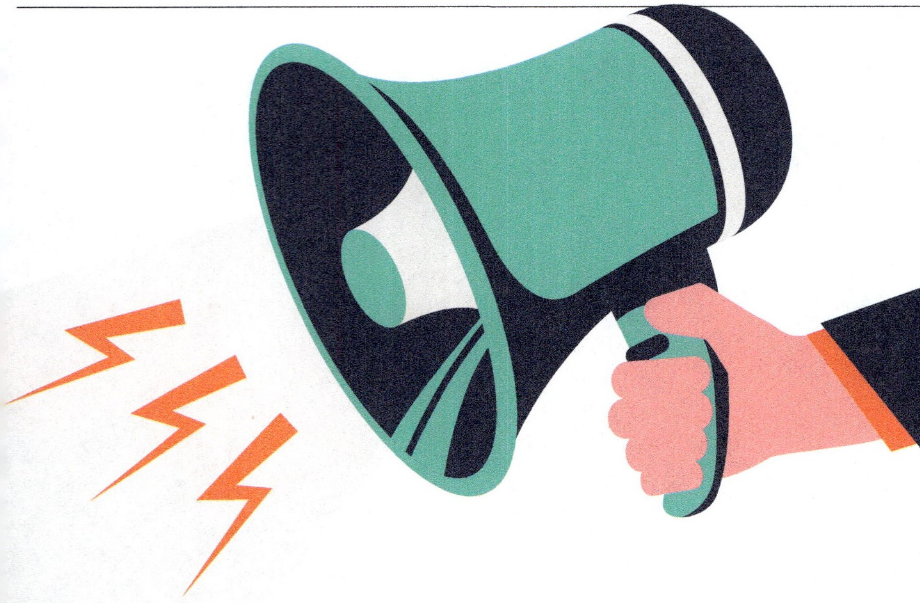

approaching 20 million Russians. Sometimes, change is not for the better.

This idea was once fundamental to human thought about change. The two oldest concepts of change are decline and fall, where humanity plummets from a previous state of Edenic grace and plenitude to its present condition of moral and physical deprivation, and cyclical change, where the world and societies go through a repeating pattern of growth, decay, death and then rebirth.

Added to these two fundamental ideas, the fusion of Christian and Jewish notions of linear time moving towards a culmination with Enlightenment ideas of the gradual freeing of humanity from the superstitions that encumbered it produced the third great view of change: progress.

What goes around comes around

The oldest of the ideas of change, that all is a cycle, is based on the clearly visible rhythms of the natural world: winter, spring, summer, autumn and then winter again before a new spring; day and night; the phases of the Moon; the rise and fall of tides; and in Egypt, the regular, life-giving flooding of the Nile. In the calendar ancient civilisations developed based on these natural phenomena, we have similar cycles. The seven days of the week, however, was adopted from the Jewish calendar, with its divinely mandated day of rest. Many other cultures had no days of rest, at least not for the poor or slaves. Modern-day theorists have advanced ideas of cyclical change, from the business cycles of boom and bust proposed by Nikolay Kondratyev to theories of the birth, growth, decadence and death of civilisations put forward by Arnold Toynbee and Oswald Spengler.

Everything is going to pot

The belief that humanity has fallen from a previous golden age to its present parlous state is present in many ancient cultures, from the Classical idea of the four ages – Gold, Silver, Bronze and Iron – to the idea of original sin developed by Saint Augustine of Hippo in the 5th century.

The idea recurs under different cultural colours but its universality suggests its importance in human cultural development: for most of history societies have been deeply conservative (with a small 'c') and resistant to change. Under this view, change is necessarily for the worse, a belief that was adopted by nomads, pastoralists and early farmers. Change, in their cases, normally wasn't a good thing.

One-way tracks

The other pole of Judeo-Christian thought, that of history having a narrative, with a beginning, middle and an end, also became thoroughly embedded in thinking about change, leading to the rise of ideas of social

OFF THE BUSES

The bus boycott in Montgomery, Alabama, was the first step towards desegregation

On 1 December 1955, Rosa Parks was sitting on a bus when the driver told her to get up from her seat to make room for a white man. The law in Montgomery required strict segregation on buses, with the front ten seats reserved for white and the ten rear seats reserved for blacks. That left 16 seats in the middle that filled from the respective reserved sections. However, if the white seats were all full and a white person got on, then all the black people in the foremost row of unreserved seats had to get up and stand so that the white person would not have to sit next to a black person.

On that December day, the bus driver told Rosa Parks to get up and stand so that a white man could sit down. Parks refused. She was arrested, found guilty and fined. But Parks, with support from the Montgomery Improvement Association, appealed against the decision, while the Association, which included Martin Luther King among its leaders, organised a boycott of all Montgomery bus services. The movement was hugely successful, and despite boycotters, black churches and dwellings – including King's – being attacked, the boycott held, attracting support from across the country.

On 13 November 1956, the United States Supreme Court found that the laws mandating segregation aboard Montgomery buses were unconstitutional, and on 20 December the city changed its laws, allowing black passengers to sit anywhere on its buses. Against the odds, the boycott had succeeded.

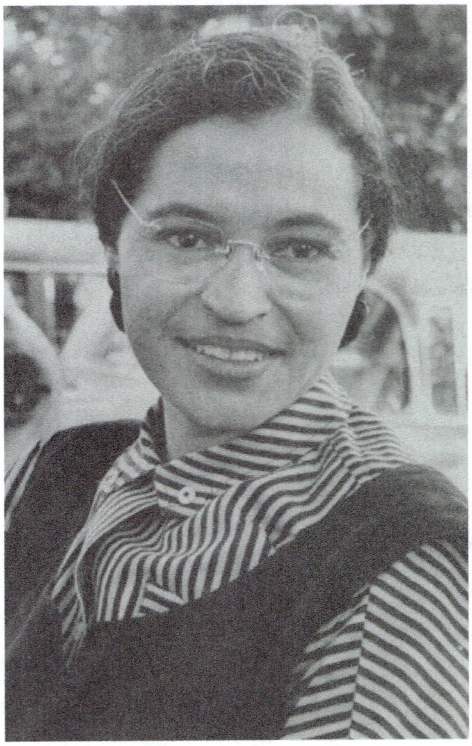

IMAGE SOURCE Getty Images

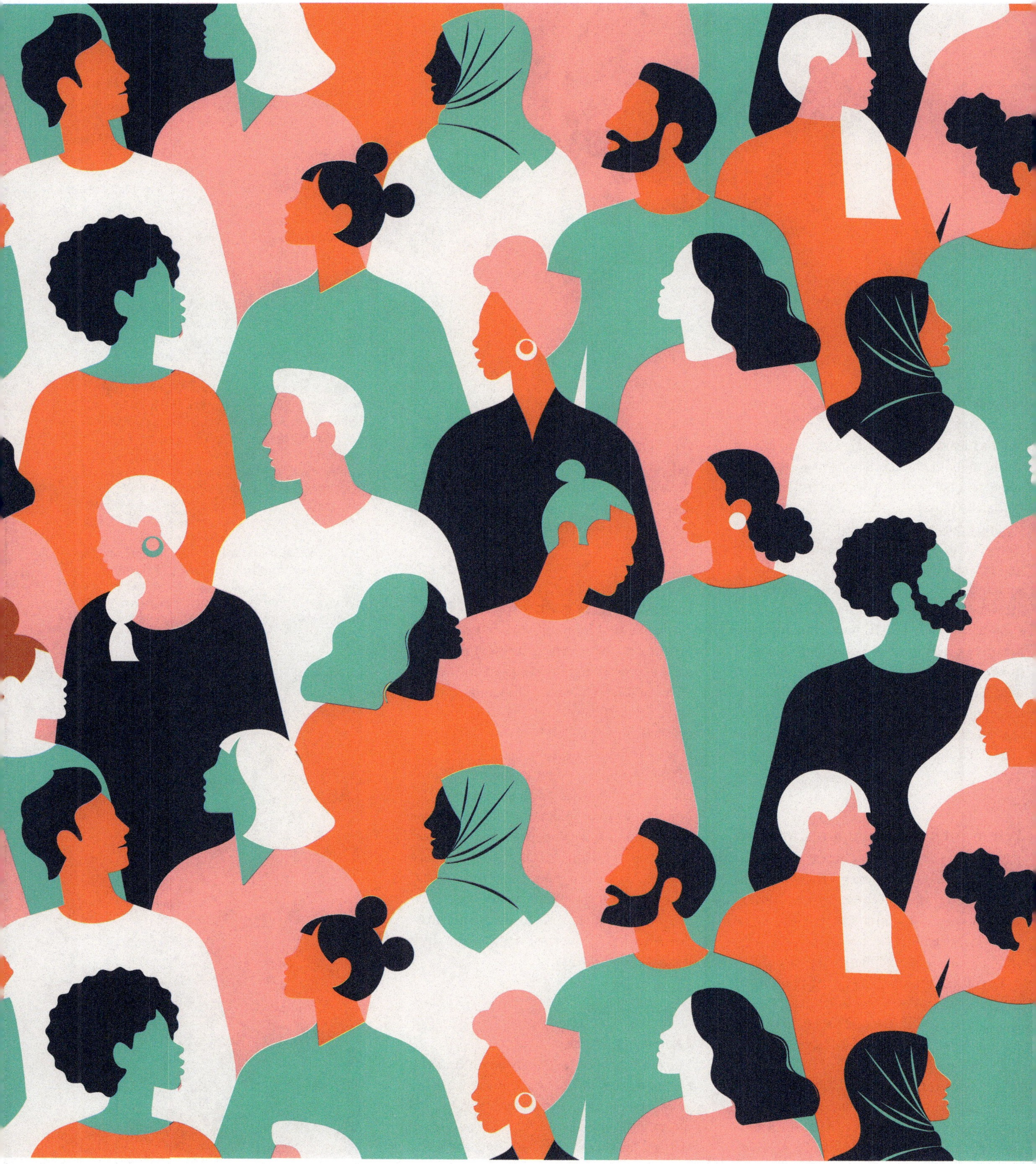

and cultural progress, these ideas usually being disguised to conceal their inheritance from Christian thought. So Auguste Comte's theory of the three stages of social evolution, from theological to metaphysical to positivist (empirical) and Herbert Spencer's linking of cultural to biological evolution all follow from the overarching idea of history having a narrative that was inherited from Christianity. In the 19th century it led to the work of Karl Marx and his dialectical theory of historical progress leading, inevitably, to a final communist paradise. The efforts of 20th-century communists to bring about this paradise led to literal hells on earth, in the Soviet Union, communist China, Cambodia and too many other places to mention here.

But leaving aside the theorists of the ineluctable march of history, it's clear that there are one-way developments in societies, from the adoption of agriculture through to population growth and resource depletion.

Mix and match

With systems as complex as human cultures, change is inevitably a result of the interplay between one-way and cyclical transitions. However, the transformation of medieval, largely agrarian cultures into the modern technological world is a process where a number of one-way interactions have multiplied each other, including urbanisation, population growth, commercialisation, division of labour, the growth of science and the spread of the nation state. Such a complex change is not necessary – there is no natural law rendering it inevitable – but once achieved, the power attendant to modern civilisation tends to make it both dominant and infectious.

The best example of this is 19th-century Japan, which had sealed itself off from the rest of the world for centuries. When the rest of the world came knocking in the ironclad shape of the warships of Commodore Matthew Perry of the US navy in 1853, the Japanese realised that if they did not wish to be dominated by these technologically superior visitors they had no choice but to modernise themselves, which they did, to such effect that 60 years later Japan defeated Russia in a war, the first Asian country to defeat a European power in the modern era.

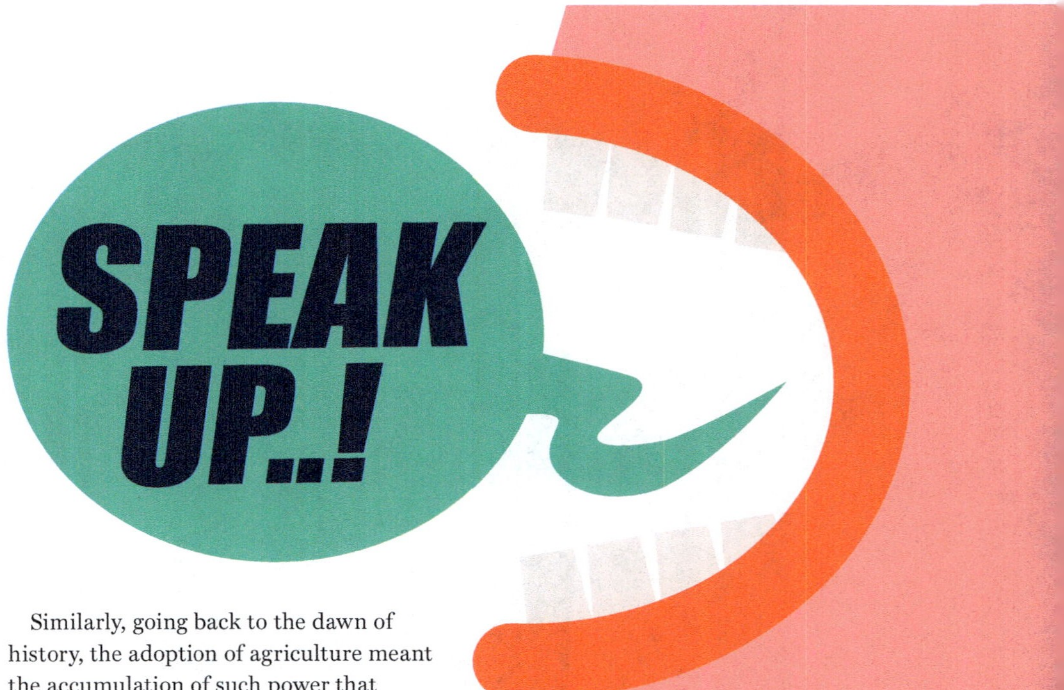

Similarly, going back to the dawn of history, the adoption of agriculture meant the accumulation of such power that nomads and pastoralists had no option but to retreat to less-productive, marginal land that was not coveted by farmers and the societies they underpinned.

Where to stand and how to push

The Greek scientist Archimedes quantified the laws of levers. With sufficient leverage it is possible to move any object. But societies are far less definite than objects. How can you change them? This was a question that preoccupied environmental scientist Donella Meadows (1941–2001). As lead author on the book *The Limits of Growth*, she proposed that there are physical limits to human economic growth because of the Earth's carrying capacity.

While still contested, Meadows' conviction that economic growth had to be restrained in order to save the planet led to her thinking hard about the ways to change complex systems, from companies through to cultures, and the result of this was her groundbreaking essay *Leverage Points: Places to Intervene in a System*.

In this work, Meadows sectioned systems into lower, intermediate and higher levels and suggested where pressure had to be applied in order to bring about change in the system. These 12 leverage points are the most systematic approach on how to modify societies so far developed.

> “MEADOWS SECTIONED SYSTEMS INTO LOWER, INTERMEDIATE AND HIGHER LEVELS AND SUGGESTED WHERE PRESSURE HAD TO BE APPLIED IN ORDER TO BRING ABOUT CHANGE”

IMAGE SOURCE Getty Images

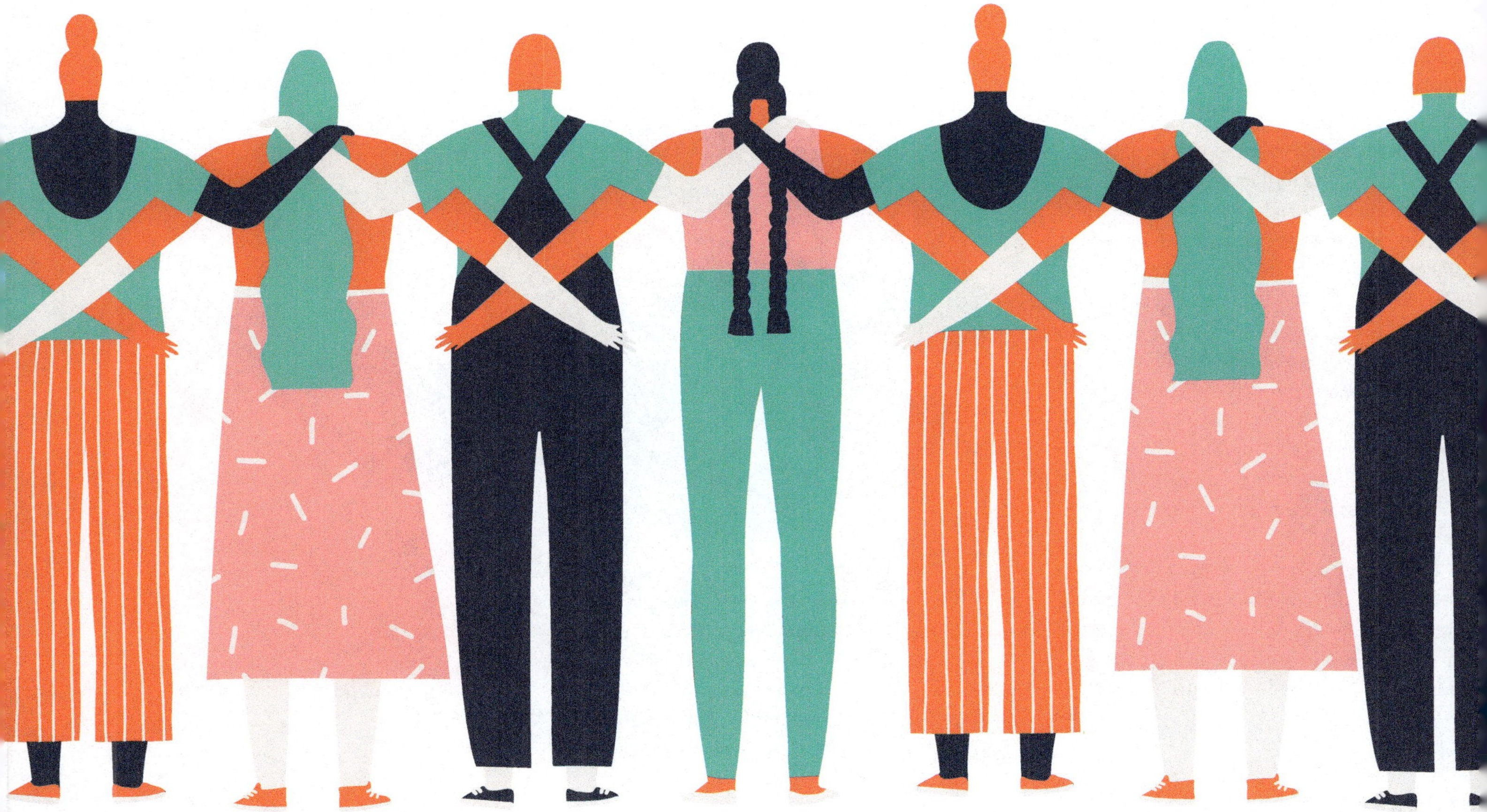

Where not to push

The researchers who inspired Meadows had found that people often have an intuitive idea of where a system might be altered by applying pressure – that is, making changes – but, paradoxically, often apply exactly the wrong pressure to bring about the change they seek and instead make the situation worse. A classic example is subsidised housing for people with low income. In a city such as London, which has very high costs of living, policymakers have typically sought to help people with low incomes by providing subsidised housing. But subsidising housing actually reduces the well-being of the city, even for the poor. The point is that applying this model without commensurate efforts to create jobs and opportunities creates unemployment, worsens the ratio between employment and housing and increases the cost of welfare far beyond that of subsidising the housing in the first place. So, yes, housing costs are key, but putting pressure solely on this one point actually has the effect of pushing the system in the opposite direction to the one intended.

> “ATTEMPTS TO MAKE SOCIETY MORE EQUAL ARE ALSO HAMPERED BY THE POSITIVE FEEDBACK LOOPS INHERENT TO BEING RICH”

The 12 points

At number 12, and thus the least effective point of leverage, are the parameters, the numbers of the system, such as taxes and subsidies. An example would be the chancellor of the exchequer increasing tax on petrol and diesel vehicles to encourage drivers to switch to hybrid and electric cars.

Number 11 are the system's buffers, the reservoirs within it that enable it to resist disruption, which are a good thing but also make it harder to change. Businesses might keep a large stock of goods in their warehouses to guard against disruptions in supply or sudden surges in demand.

Number ten is the physical structure of the system. Think of a railway network. Where the tracks and station are placed profoundly influence their surroundings, but because these structures are difficult and time-consuming to alter, it is difficult to influence a system by changing them. In social terms, think of the changes produced by the Baby Boomer generation born in the decade after World War II: the societal changes effected during the 1960s were in

part down to simply having a lot of people being young together.

Number nine refers to how quickly the system can respond to feedback and its propensity to over- or undercompensate because of this feedback. Imagine you're standing in a shower and it gets too hot. You turn the water colder, but it's still too hot. You turn it colder. Still too hot. You turn it colder again, and then suddenly it comes through like ice and you whack it back up, only for the water to scald you. Poor feedback produces wild oscillations in systems that can spiral out of control.

Negative feedback loops are at number eight, guarding against the runaway destruction of the system. In democratic societies this is provided for by the franchise. A topical recent example is Brexit, where part of the explanation for the referendum result was that a significant proportion of the population of the UK felt itself sufficiently divorced from one of the key agents of globalisation, the EU, and opted to leave it.

Positive feedback loops are at number seven, providing means of reinforcing changes to a system, with sometimes catastrophic results in the case of an epidemic. Attempts to make society more equal are also hampered by the positive feedback loops inherent to being rich: the best educations and opportunities usually go to the wealthy, meaning that the children of rich people tend to accumulate even more wealth at the expense of those without their income.

At six are information flows or, to be a bit more precise, new information flows. Suppose a company emptying effluent into a river has to publish an annual report of how much lead and mercury it pumps into the river. Soon enough this public report, even without any legislation, will cause it to start treating its waste.

Number five are the rules, the laws of the system. Change the law and you change society. Look at the extraordinary changes that have occurred following the decriminalisation of homosexuality. Until 1969 it was against the law; in 2014 gay marriage became legal in the UK.

Number four brings us to the key feature of living things and societies: the ability to organise and change themselves. In creatures this involves things such as the immune system responding to new pathogens; in societies it's anything from the adoption of new technology to social revolutions. New structures are extremely effective ways of bringing about social change. Think of the Anti-Slavery Society that succeeded in bringing about a ban on a practice that was as old as humanity.

At number three are the goals, the aims of the system, whether it be a company, a club or a culture. Change these and everything else will shift to accommodate that.

Number two are the unwritten but accepted rules, the paradigm of a society. Today we take equality as a given and strive for it. But change this unspoken acceptance of equality as a good thing and society will be transformed.

At number one is the power to change the societal paradigm entirely. To do this, establish a religion. Religions create cultures, and the founders of religions – Jesus Christ, the Buddha, Muhammad – have been the most influential figures in human history. To change everything, change the paradigm.

WORDS Edoardo Albert

HOW THINGS CHANGE

The underlying mechanisms that transform societies

A number of competing theories exist to explain the deep social changes that have occurred throughout human history. The idea of the accumulation of knowledge becoming embedded within societies and leading to growth in populations and new knowledge is the obvious underpinning to all the other theories. But there can be no doubt that we know more collectively today than people did 5,000 years ago.

However, set against this are theories on the limits of growth, often imposed by ecological and environmental constraints, that suggest that growth cannot continue in a straightforward linear path. Among the constraints faced are other, competing cultures, and theories of cultural competition suggest that it is precisely this struggle that drives social change: few events bring about quicker and more profound societal changes than warfare.

Yet social change need not necessarily be a result of conflict: in particular, new ideas can diffuse into a society, either arising from within or coming from another culture. In today's world these are the early adopters, the young people driving information technology and its concomitant cultural changes. What is clear is that the rate of social change is showing no sign of slowing down.

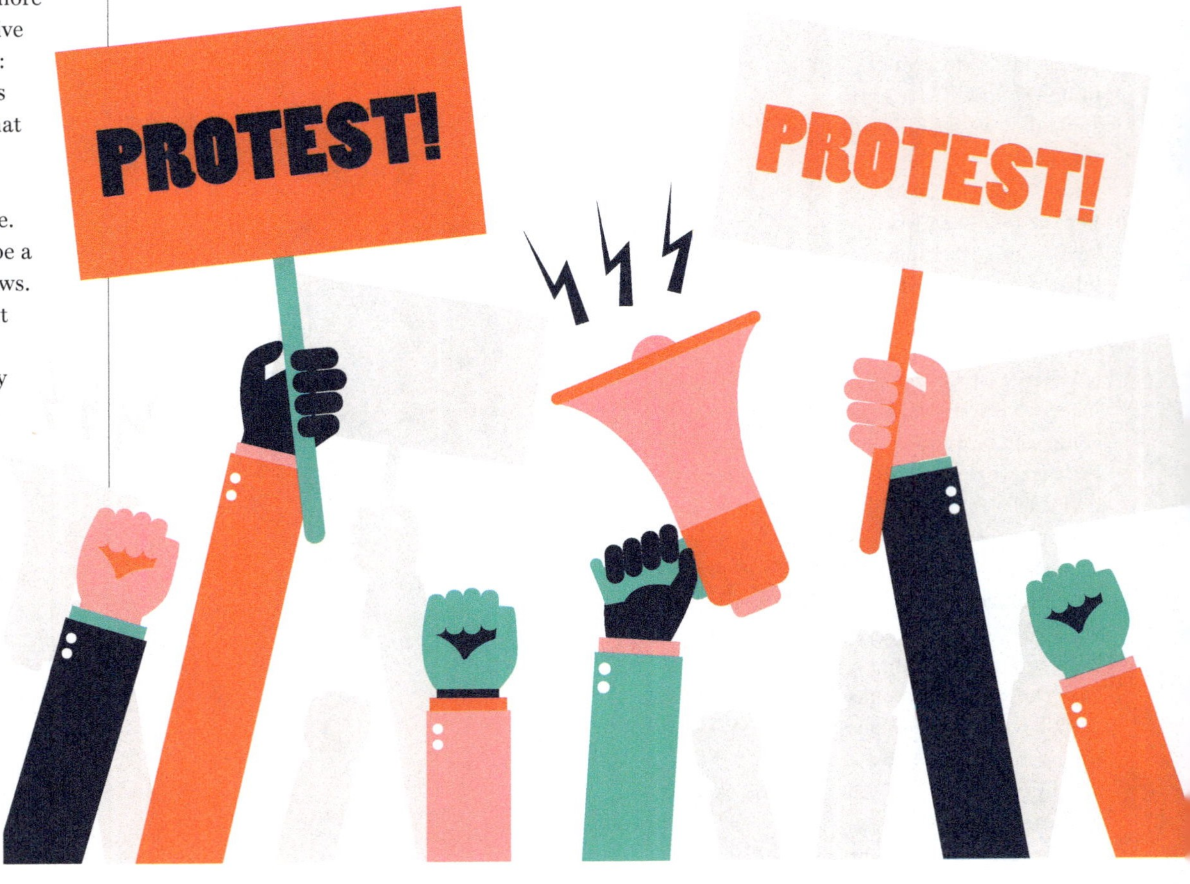

IMAGE SOURCE Getty Images

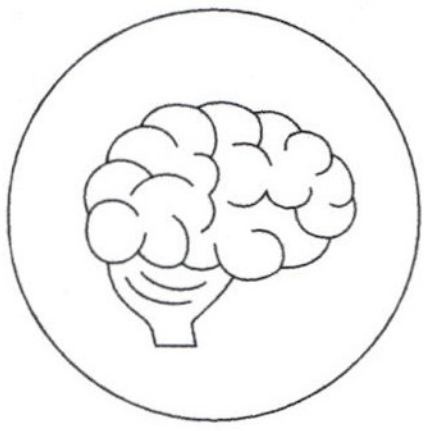

Tracking our habits

How companies track you on the web and monetise your habits

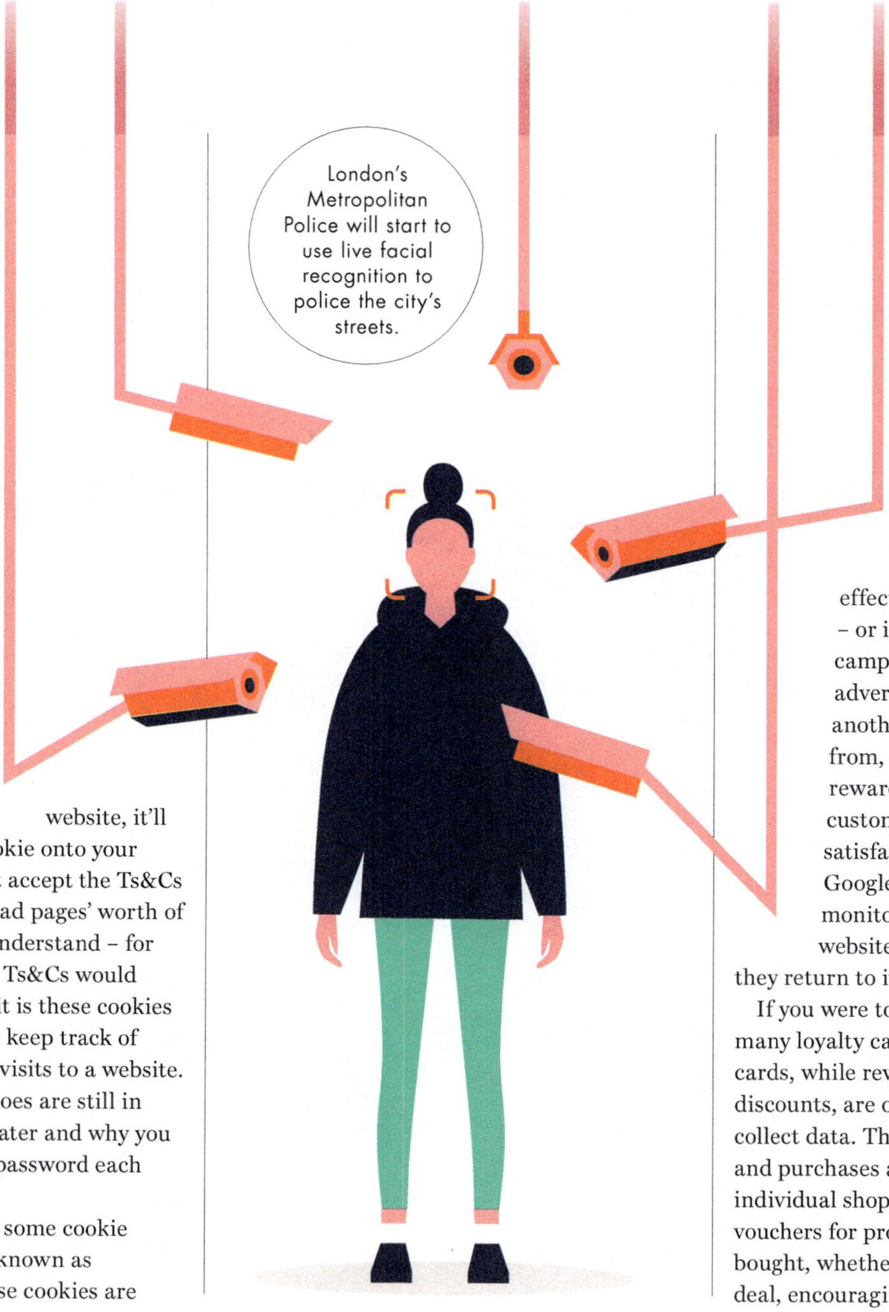

We wake up and check our emails and messages. On the way to work we scroll through Facebook. Before we head into the office, we grab a coffee and croissant and post a picture on Instagram. During our lunch break, we decide to do a bit of online shopping. Later the same day, we see adverts for the coat and shoes that we were looking at earlier. For the following week we keep seeing the same adverts pop up, and we start to wonder if the internet is spying on us.

When we first visit a website, it'll place what's known as a cookie onto your computer. Normally we just accept the Ts&Cs because we don't want to read pages' worth of text that we're unlikely to understand – for example, reading Amazon's Ts&Cs would take about nine hours. But it is these cookies that identify you, helping to keep track of what you're doing and your visits to a website. They're why the coat and shoes are still in your shopping basket days later and why you don't have to re-enter your password each time you use that website.

While this is useful to us, some cookie trails are less so. These are known as third-party cookies and these cookies are placed by web pages that you're not surfing but by the adverts that have been linked to that webpage. They let advertisers and analytics companies track your browsing history on websites that have their adverts. So they know that you've been searching for shoes using a number of different websites. Cookies can be an effective way of seeing how effective – or ineffective – an advertising campaign is. When you click on an advert, it may use a cookie to tell another website where a user came from, allowing the company to reward another for referring a customer. In the name of customer satisfaction, analytical tools like Google Analytics allow companies to monitor how many people use a website, for how long and whether they return to it.

If you were to look in your wallet, how many loyalty cards would you find? Loyalty cards, while rewarding customers with discounts, are one easy way for companies to collect data. They track our shopping habits and purchases and target promotions to each individual shopper. They are why we get vouchers for products that we've previously bought, whether that's toothpaste or a meal deal, encouraging us to spend more money.

Most of us use Google's services each day, and this activity enables Google to build a picture of who you are, where you go and your interests simply by examining your web searches, location history and the apps that you use. Google can figure out that you're a cyclist if you were to search for 'cycling routes' on Google Maps and 'cycling gear' using Chrome. They may then show an advert for cycling gear on YouTube. As they collect more data about you they can build up a more accurate picture of who you are to create more personalised adverts. Perhaps you've noticed that Google Maps has made a coffee shop recommendation – it would have made one based on similar coffee shops that you've been to before.

Have you ever wondered how Netflix knows what films and TV shows you'll enjoy? The reason for Netflix's success is that it knows what the customer wants. With approximately 160 million subscribers around the world, this large number of people generates a lot of data.

Netflix's interaction with its audience using the simple thumbs up/thumbs down system means more people are likely to respond, which results in greater personalisation for the user. Netflix can also track what new series you're watching, how much of it you finish and what genres you like. It can then make recommendations so that you don't have to spend three hours trying to decide what to watch.

Netflix also uses data to commission and licence content in different parts of the world and decide whether they should keep a programme or cancel it. And, as a paid-for service, they are not harvesting your data.

We all realise that Facebook and Google know too much about us, but every company that collects or uses our personal data has a responsibility to keep their customers' data secure. If they don't, they can expect severe repercussions when things go wrong.

In 2019 the Information Commissioner's Office fined British Airways nearly £184 million (approximately $240.4 million) after the personal details of around 500,000 customers were stolen. This was the first case of its kind under the UK's new privacy laws, the General Data Protection Regulation (GDPR), which came into force in May 2018.

WORDS Baljeet Panesar

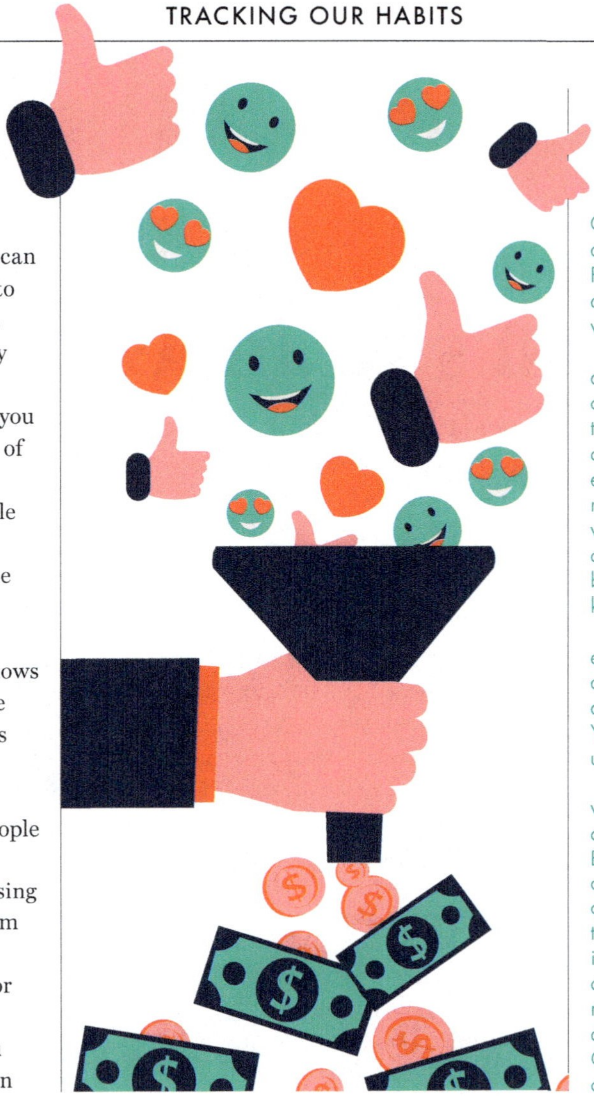

SURVEILLANCE CAPITALISM

Can something ever just be free?

Have you ever wondered why Facebook and Google keep advertising camping equipment and sleeping bags after you buy a tent? Perhaps it was headphones the time before that, after you bought a new phone? Welcome to the world of surveillance capitalism.

A term popularised in 2014 by American academic Shoshana Zuboff, surveillance capitalism refers to your personal data being treated as a commodity. Often completed by online services that are free, such as search engines and social media platforms, companies monitor our online behaviour – what we search, what we buy, what we like – to collect data that can later be sold, usually without us knowing, to businesses who want to know us better than we know ourselves.

Given we make 40,000 Google searches each second, 3.5 billion searches every day and 1.2 trillion per year, this creates huge amounts of data – and profits for companies. Yet we don't fully know where the data will end up or the extent of the surveillance.

After the Cambridge Analytica scandal, the way in which companies and organisations use our data has rightly caused concern. This 'Big Brother'-like surveillance threatens our privacy in a world where we always remain connected to our devices, and with the rise of smart devices, the amount of data that we produce has increased more quickly than ever before. Such companies can influence our decisions, manipulating our behaviour and maybe, one day, even taking away our free will. Could Orwell's famous novel *1984* be a glimpse into our future?

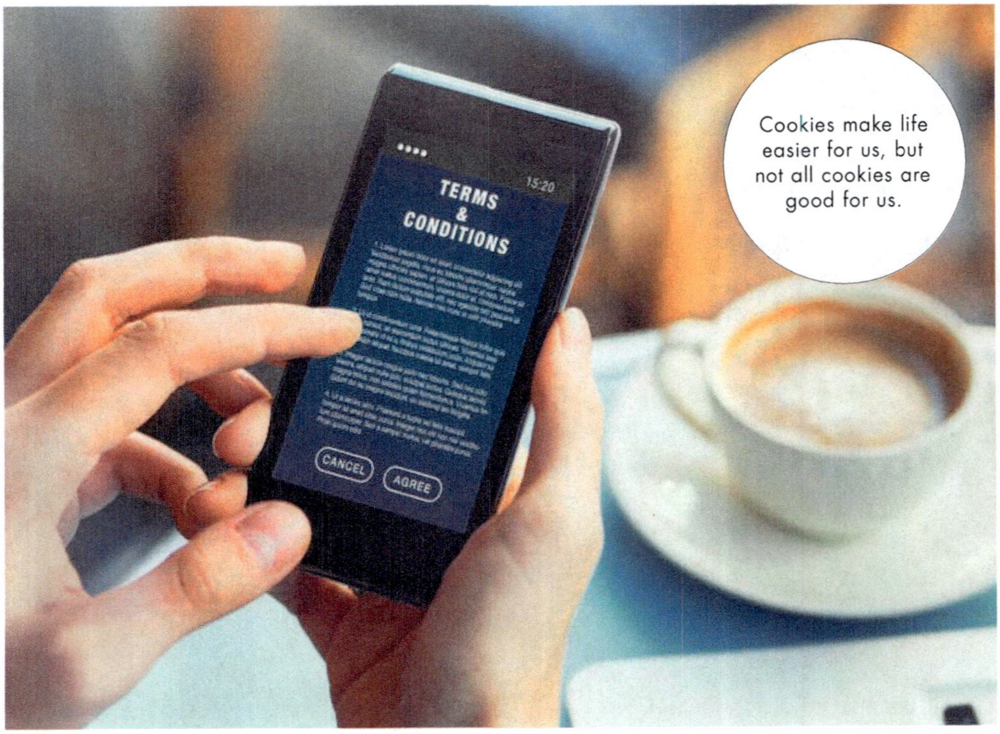

Cookies make life easier for us, but not all cookies are good for us.

IMAGE SOURCE Getty Images

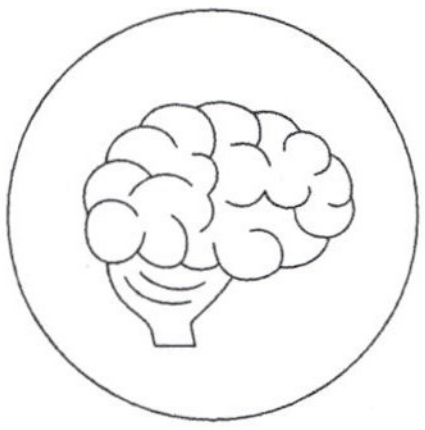

The world's strangest customs

Discover some of the weird, quirky and terrifying customs from around the globe

From cheese rolling and bog snorkelling in the UK to the Monkey Buffet Festival in Thailand, these customs and habits may appear strange to us, but they are an important part of the culture from which they originate. Each custom is passed down from generation to generation, connecting us to our ancestors and reminding us of our history.

We have come a long way since the beginnings of civilisation, and we now live in a world that is a beautiful, culturally diverse place. There are more than 7.5 billion of us living on this planet, made up of thousands of peoples; from those who live in cities to those who are part of a tribe, people from all around the world have developed complex customs and unique habits that express their heritage, which they have been taught since they were born.

Even the way we celebrate our birthdays is unique – it depends on where you live and where you were born. In the UK we're gifted our favourite cake and presents, but in Norway you typically get a chocolate cake and you have to choose someone to dance with you. In Vietnam all birthdays are celebrated on one day of the year, known as Tet, and not the day you were born.

Depending on where you are in the world, this list may seem strange, and some of these customs might appear bizarre, but each of them are an important part of a culture's heritage and preserving its way of life.

WORDS Baljeet Panesar

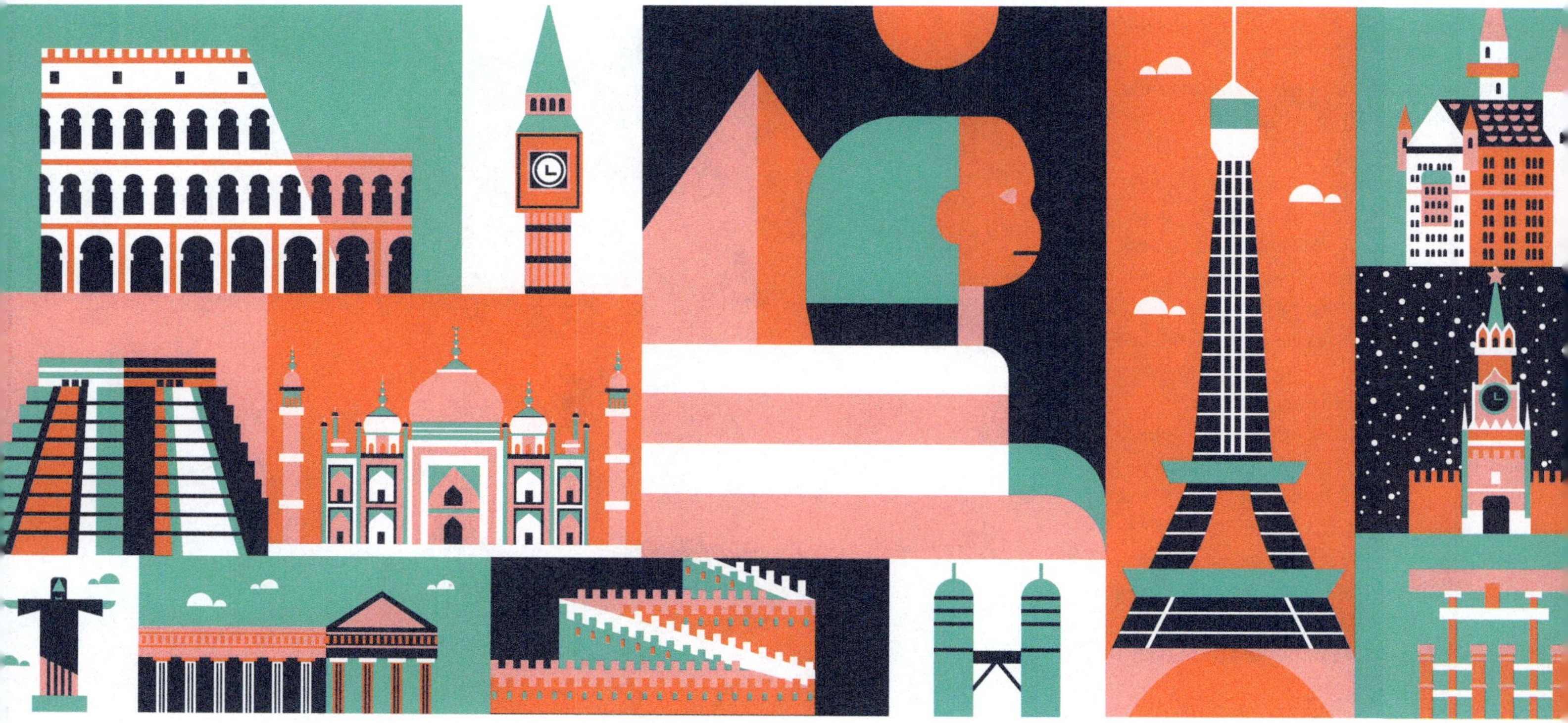

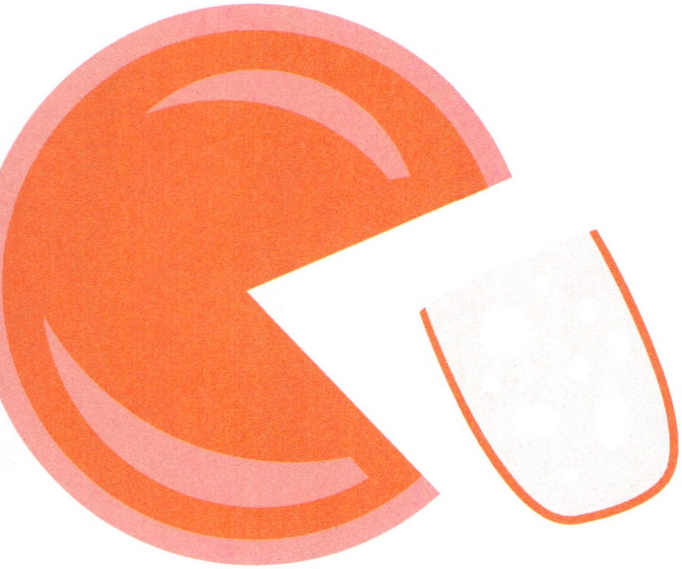

Cheese rolling

COUNTRY OBSERVED: UK
ORIGIN DATE: 1826

Every spring bank holiday thousands of people from all over the world gather on Cooper's Hill near Gloucester, England, for an annual cheese-rolling festival.

The rules are simple. A three-to-four-kilogram, round Double Gloucester cheese is sent rolling down a steep hill, and the participants have to catch it. This may sound easy, but the cheese gets a second head start and can reach speeds of up to 110 kilometres per hour. The first person to reach the bottom of the hill and cross the finish line is crowned the winner. For their efforts they get to take home the cheese. Technically, it's the first person to catch the cheese, but this is near impossible given how quickly it gains speed. This might sound like fun to some, but it is also dangerous – spectators have been injured by the rolling cheese, and some people have tumbled their way to broken bones.

Although cheese rolling was first reported in the 1800s, it's thought that its origins lie centuries earlier, but the exact beginnings of this eccentric British tradition remain a mystery. Some believe it started as a way to claim grazing rights around the common. Others think it dates back to the pagan custom of rolling bundles of burning brushwood down a hill to welcome a new year. This belief means that sweets, buns and biscuits are still scattered over the hill, which is said to encourage a fruitful harvest.

Krampus

COUNTRY OBSERVED: AUSTRIA
ORIGIN DATE: PRE-CHRISTIAN

On the night of 5 December a creature that's half-goat, half-demon visits children to see if they've been naughty. The creature's name is Krampus and he is the 'Christmas Devil' – a beast with a long red tongue, fangs and horns that belongs in your nightmares.

Since the 17th century Krampus has been keeping Saint Nicholas company, who rewards good children with sweets. But according to legend, on Krampus Night, or Krampusnacht, the creature swats misbehaved children, stuffs them into a sack and hauls them off to his lair to be eaten or tortured. Today, adults may dress up in fur suits, wooden masks and carry cowbells to scare children, or they can partake in a Krampuslauf, a ritual that is supposed to get rid of ghosts. Those who survive Krampusnacht are rewarded with presents on Nikolaustag (Saint Nicholas' Day) on 6 December.

This mythical figure has been a part of Christmas tradition in Austria and southern Germany for centuries. Like Krampus, other countries have their version of Saint Nicholas' helpers – Knecht Ruprecht in Germanic folklore and Hans Trapp in French legend.

But Krampus has had his difficulties. In the 12th century the Catholic Church tried to ban Krampus celebrations because of his resemblance to the devil, and a further attempt by Austria's Christian Social Party followed in 1934. Both were unsuccessful, though, and Krampus is becoming even more popular.

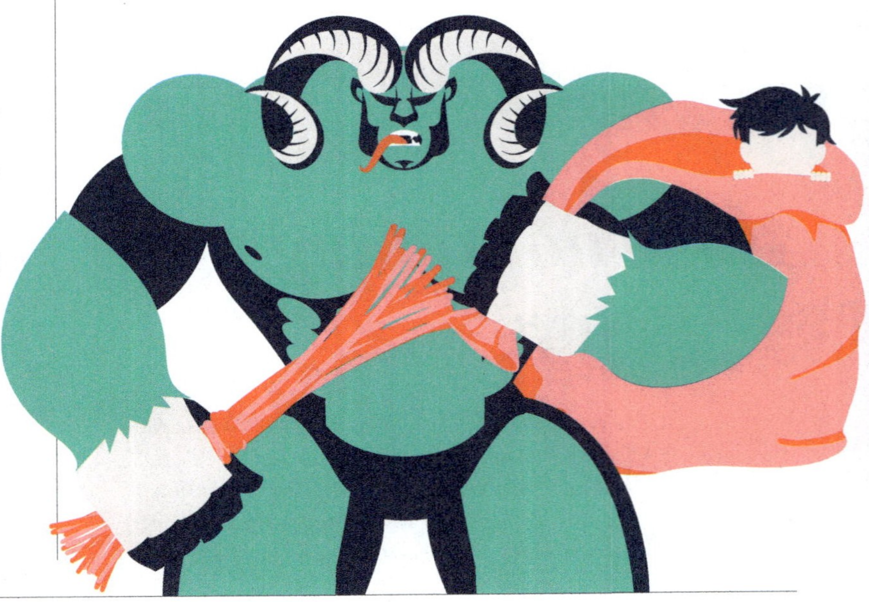

"THE FIRST PERSON TO REACH THE BOTTOM OF THE HILL AND CROSS THE FINISH LINE IS CROWNED THE WINNER. FOR THEIR EFFORTS THEY GET TO TAKE HOME THE CHEESE"

IMAGE SOURCE Getty Images

Bull jumping

COUNTRY OBSERVED: ETHIOPIA
ORIGIN DATE: UNKNOWN

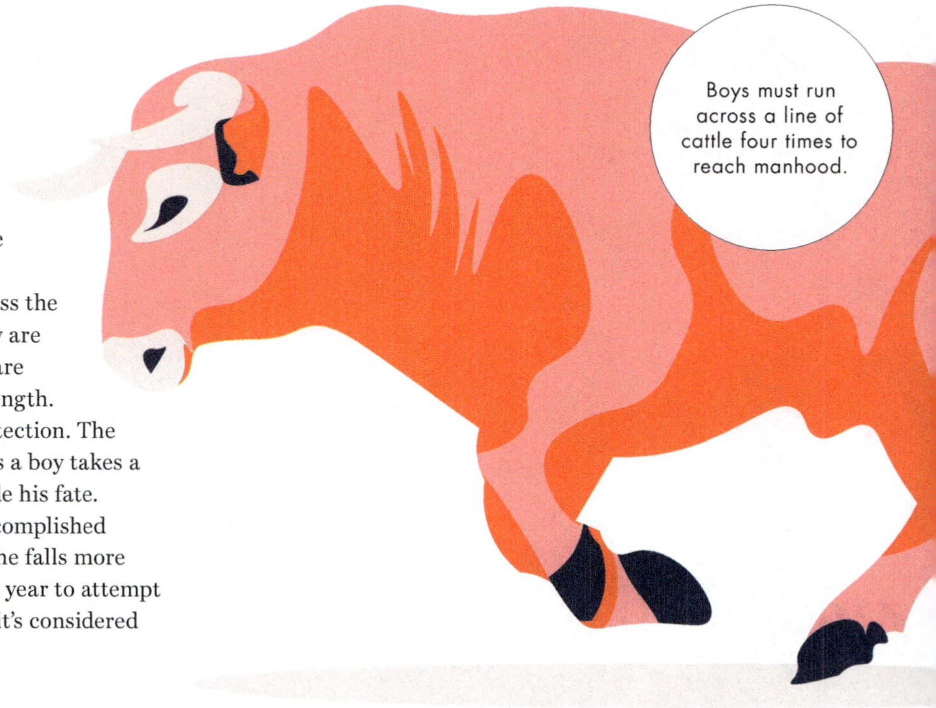

For a boy in the Hamer community, this is one coming-of-age ceremony that decides whether or not he can be called a man and marry.

During this rite of passage, the boys have to run across the backs of cattle. The boys that take part in the ceremony are rubbed with sand to wash away their sins, their heads are partially shaven and they're smeared with dung for strength. Each boy is stripped naked, with only tree bark for protection. The bulls, too, are coated in dung to make them slippery. As a boy takes a leap of faith, his strength, bravery and agility will decide his fate.

If he succeeds he becomes known as a Maza – an 'accomplished one' – and can take the first of up to four brides. But if he falls more than four times, he will have to wait until the following year to attempt the feat again. Failure really isn't an option, however – it's considered the most important day of a boy's life.

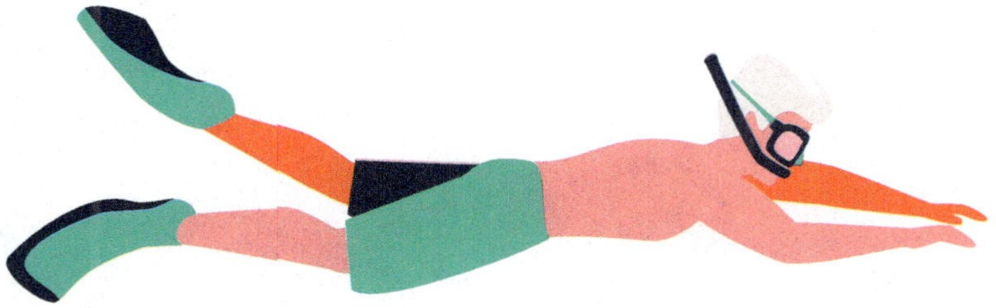

Bog snorkelling

COUNTRY OBSERVED: UK
ORIGIN DATE: 1976

Every August, the Waen Rhydd peat bog in Llanwrtyd Wells, Wales, draws over 150 people to a sporting event that tests competitors' endurance and skill. But this isn't a marathon of the conventional sort. Instead, the challengers have to swim through a muddy bog. This eccentric sport is said to have been created as part of a bar bet in 1976, and it attracts people from all over the world.

During the event, the brave participants have to swim two lengths of the bog, which is 55 metres long. Equipped only with a snorkel and flippers – a wetsuit is highly recommended too – competitors rely on the power of their kicking to secure the fastest time. To make things even more difficult, you can't use traditional swimming strokes. But if you think that's still too easy, there's also a bog triathlon where participants complete a 13-kilometre run, a length of the peat bog and a 19-kilometre mountain cycle.

Cockroach racing

COUNTRY OBSERVED: AUSTRALIA
ORIGIN DATE: 1982

Each year, on Australia Day (26 January), a clutch of cockroaches are given the chance to race to victory – and their freedom. These speedy insects can reach 50 body lengths per second; that's the equivalent of us reaching 320 kilometres per hour.

The race takes place in a six-metre-wide ring, with about 14 races throughout the day, each lasting just a few seconds. The winning cockroach joins a coveted position in a hall of fame, and the winning owner wins roughly £100 (about $135) to spend at the pub.

The race, the story goes, was born from an argument between two people at a bar about who had the biggest and fastest cockroaches in their suburb. The argument was settled with the insects the following day and since then a cockroach race has taken place each year at the Story Bridge Hotel in Brisbane, Queensland, attracting guests from Australia, New Zealand and further afield.

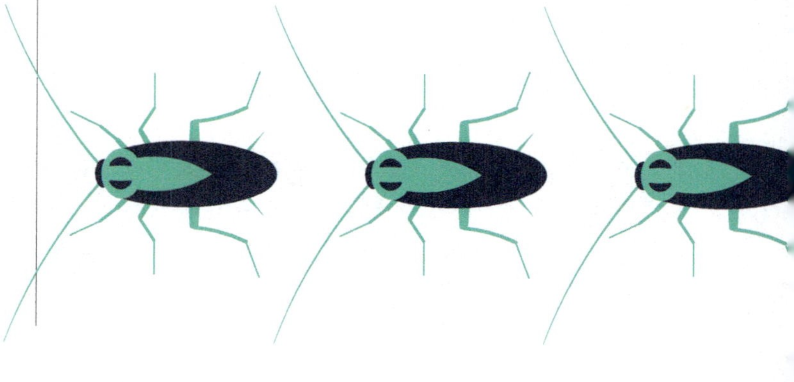

A WEEK OF FESTIVITIES CULMINATES IN 100 TONS OF TOMATOES TRANSFORMING THE STREETS INTO RIVERS OF TOMATO SAUCE IN AN HOUR

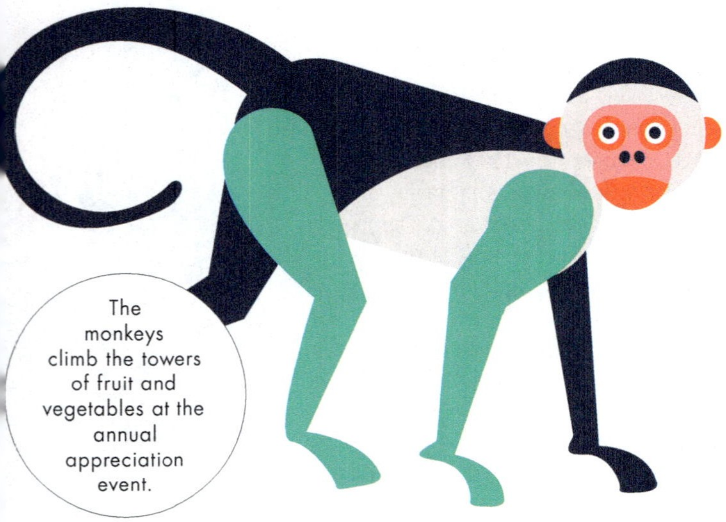

Monkey Buffet Festival

COUNTRY OBSERVED: THAILAND
ORIGIN DATE: 1980S

On the last Sunday of November in the city of Lopburi, thousands of long-tailed macaque monkeys gather at the ruins of the 13th century Phra Prang Sam Yot temple. Here, a banquet of fruit, vegetables and sweet treats await the guests of honour, who are thought to bring good luck to the community and promote tourism in the surrounding area.

A week before the event the macaques receive invites to the feast, attached to which are cashew nuts. The festivities begin with performances from locals dressed in monkey costumes, attracting the primates to the temple. Once they have arrived, locals indulge their guests with 2,000 kilograms of fruit, vegetables and other treats that include durians, grapes, pineapples, watermelons, rice and even cans of cola.

Historians trace Thailand's appreciation of the monkeys to the 2,000-year-old tale of Rama. In the epic, the monkey king Hanuman and his army help the divine prince Rama rescue his wife Sita from the clutches of an evil demon lord. Some of the locals regard the monkeys as descendants of Hanuman, and the Monkey Buffet Festival is one way to show their respect.

La Tomatina

COUNTRY OBSERVED: SPAIN
ORIGIN DATE: 1945

Every August, 20,000 people make their way to the Valencian town of Buñol to take part in the world's biggest food fight, just for fun.

In a town of only 9,000 people, a week of festivities that involves music, parades, dancing and fireworks culminates in this tomato-throwing event where more than 100 tons of over-ripe tomatoes transform the streets into a river of tomato sauce in an hour.

Although the origins of the festival are largely unknown, a popular story tells of a group of teenagers who were at a street parade where a fight broke out and people started to throw tomatoes at each other. The following year, the teenagers brought their own tomatoes from home and instigated a pre-planned fruit fight, starting the annual event.

In 1957, when the festivities were cancelled, a tomato burial was held in protest. The ban was lifted in 1959, and nearly 25 years later it was televised for the first time. Since then, La Tomatina's popularity has continued to grow, with people coming from all over the world to witness it first-hand. In 2002 the event was added to Spain's Fiesta of International Tourist Interest.

La Tomatina has also inspired similar celebrations in other parts of the world including Chile, the US and South Korea.

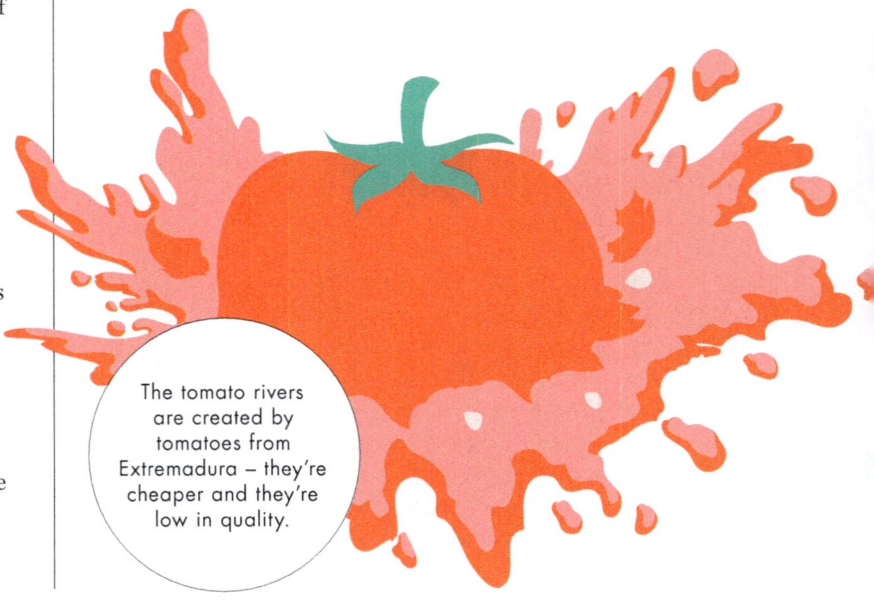

IMAGE SOURCE Getty Images

Bullet ant initiation

COUNTRY OBSERVED: BRAZIL
ORIGIN DATE: UNKNOWN

In a remote village in the Brazilian Amazon, the Sateré-Mawé people believe that to become a man you have to experience the bite of *Paraponera clavata*, the bullet ant, whose sting is said to be 30 times more painful than that of a bee.

To complete the coming-of-age ceremony, boys as young as 12 must first find the ants in the forest. The ants are then sedated and woven into gloves, with their stingers pointing inwards. The gloves are then placed on the boy's hand, and the angry insects continuously sting the skin. During the ritual the boy performs a dance to distract himself from the pain. After ten minutes, the boy can finally remove the glove but will continue to experience discomfort and possibly even muscle paralysis that will subside after 24 hours. To become a warrior, the boys have to wear the gloves 20 times, without crying or showing any weakness.

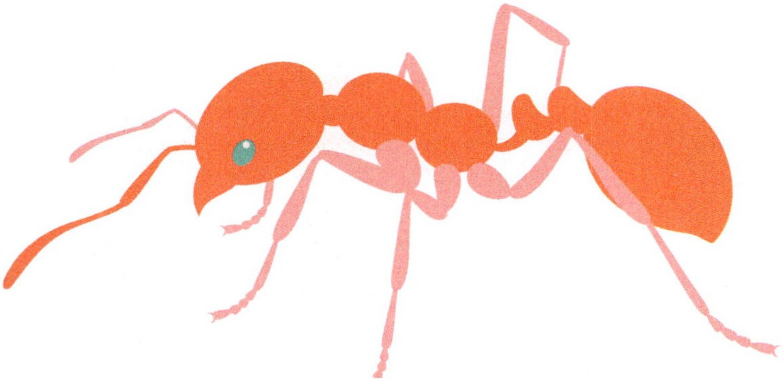

Wife carrying

COUNTRY OBSERVED: FINLAND
ORIGIN DATE: LATE 1800S

Every year thousands of visitors flock to the small Finnish town of Sonkajärvi – which normally has a population of 4,000 – to experience the wife-carrying contest, known as eukonkanto to the locals.

Competitors have to carry their wives using a fireman's lift, a piggyback or in the so-called Estonian style, completing a 253.5-metre sand track obstacle course that includes a one-metre deep- water pool. The fastest couple are crowned the champions, winning the wife's weight in beer.

Wife carrying was inspired by the tale of robber Herkko Rosvo-Ronkainen from the 1800s. Legend says that to be part of his gang, you'd have to carry grain sacks through an obstacle course that was chosen by the ringleader himself. Another theory is based on the practice of wife stealing. Other wife-carrying events take place in the UK, the US, Australia and Germany.

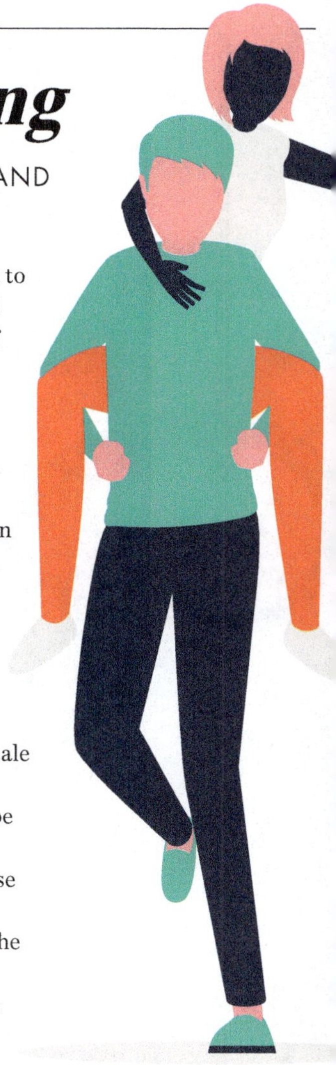

Battle of the Oranges

COUNTRY OBSERVED: ITALY
ORIGIN DATE: 12TH CENTURY

Every February in the northern Italian town of Ivrea thousands gather to celebrate a tradition that dates back to medieval times.

Wearing protective helmets and body armour, the villagers are ready for a three-day battle. But in this fight their choice of weapon are of the citrus variety – they are, in fact, oranges. It's an event that's happened every year since 1808.

Honoured with the title of the 'largest food fight in Italy', over 256,000 kilograms of the fruit are hurled among the villagers, with one of the nine teams declared the winners. If you fancy watching the event, make sure that you wear a red hat so that you don't become a part of this orange-tinged civil war.

Legend says that after the city's tyrant was decapitated by Violetta, a miller's daughter, the young woman led a revolt, storming through the streets and burning the tyrant's house with the people of Ivrea to celebrate their new freedom.

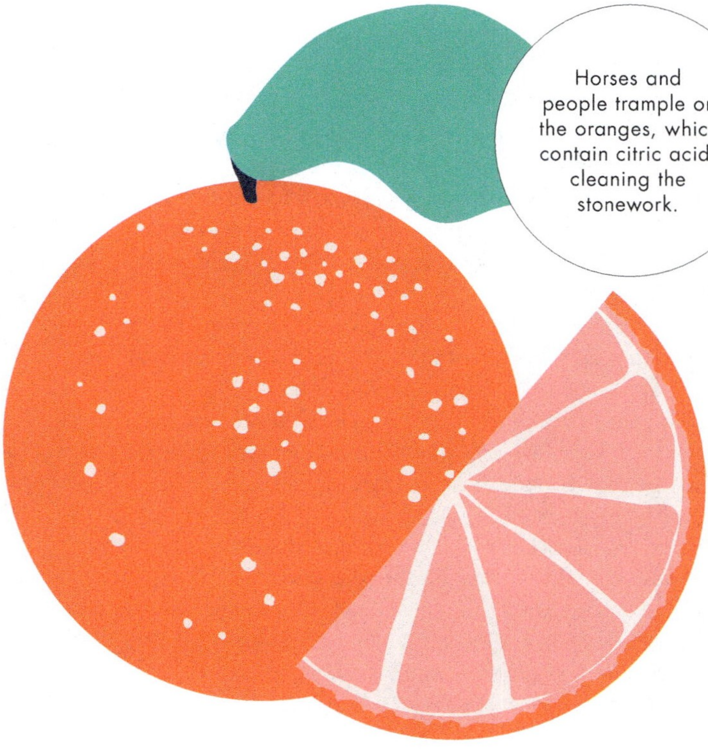

Horses and people trample on the oranges, which contain citric acid, cleaning the stonework.

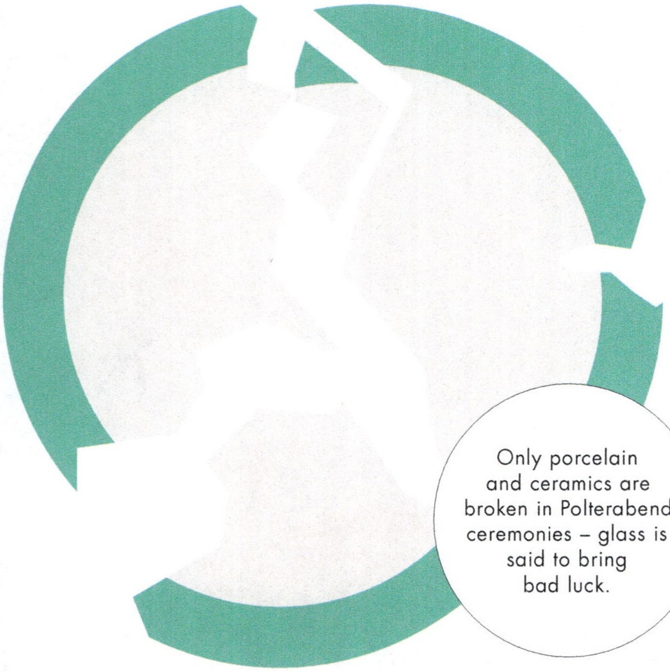

Only porcelain and ceramics are broken in Polterabend ceremonies – glass is said to bring bad luck.

Polterabend

COUNTRY OBSERVED: GERMANY
ORIGIN DATE: UNKNOWN

Around the globe, wedding traditions are an important affair. In Germany it's no different, and its people have a custom called Polterabend, which roughly translates to 'noisy evening'.

The night before the wedding, friends and family of the bride and groom gather at the house of the bride, bringing old crockery that will later be smashed. According to an old German saying, 'scherben bringen glück'– shards bring luck. The couple then have to clear the debris, symbolising that by working together they can overcome any difficulties they will face during their married lives.

Although the origins of this custom are not well known, it's thought to date to ancient Germanic tribes who broke shards to ward off evil spirits. A similar tradition is that of Baumstamm sägen, where the newlywed couple have to saw a log in half in front of their wedding guests, symbolising strength and endurance.

> THE COUPLE THEN HAVE TO CLEAR THE SHARDS, SYMBOLISING THAT BY WORKING TOGETHER THEY CAN OVERCOME ANY DIFFICULTIES THEY WILL FACE DURING THEIR MARRIED LIVES

Baby jumping

COUNTRY OBSERVED: SPAIN
ORIGIN DATE: 1620S

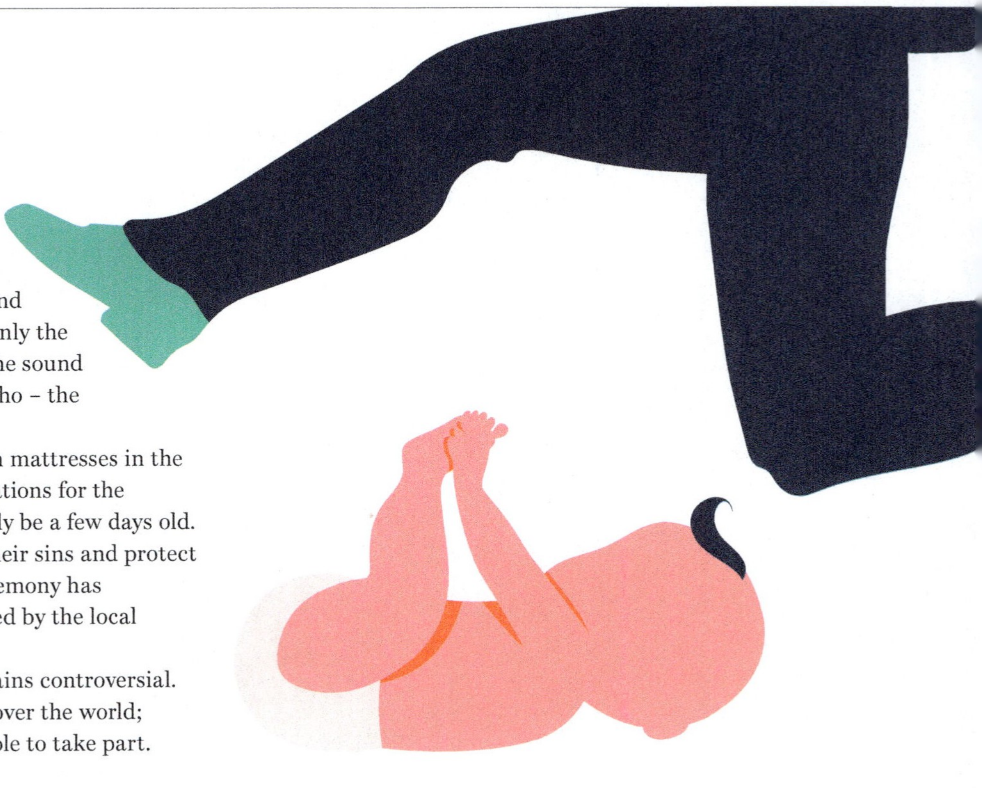

Every year, in the village of Castrillo de Murcia, red and yellow masked 'devils' run through the streets, insulting and whipping villagers with a horsetail on a stick. But this is only the beginning. Pious men, known as el Atabalero, appear at the sound of drums, driving out evil and starting the Salto del Colacho – the Flight of the Devil.

Babies that were born in the previous year are placed on mattresses in the street while the 'devils' jump over them. It's part of celebrations for the Catholic Feast of Corpus Christi, and some babies may only be a few days old.

This orthodox baptism is said to cleanse the babies of their sins and protect them from disease and misfortune. After the jumping ceremony has concluded the babies are showered with rose petals, blessed by the local priest and then collected by their parents.

To date, no babies have been hurt, but the practice remains controversial. In recent years, the festival has attracted people from all over the world; conventionally, only babies born in the village would be able to take part.

IMAGE SOURCE Getty Images

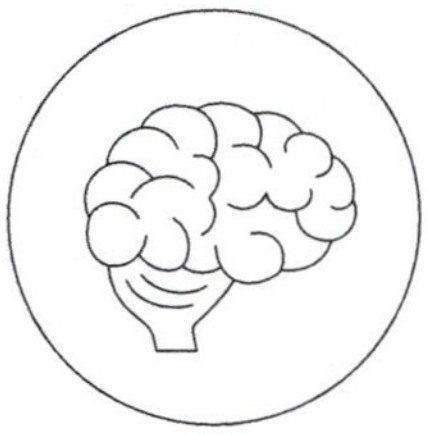

Animal habits

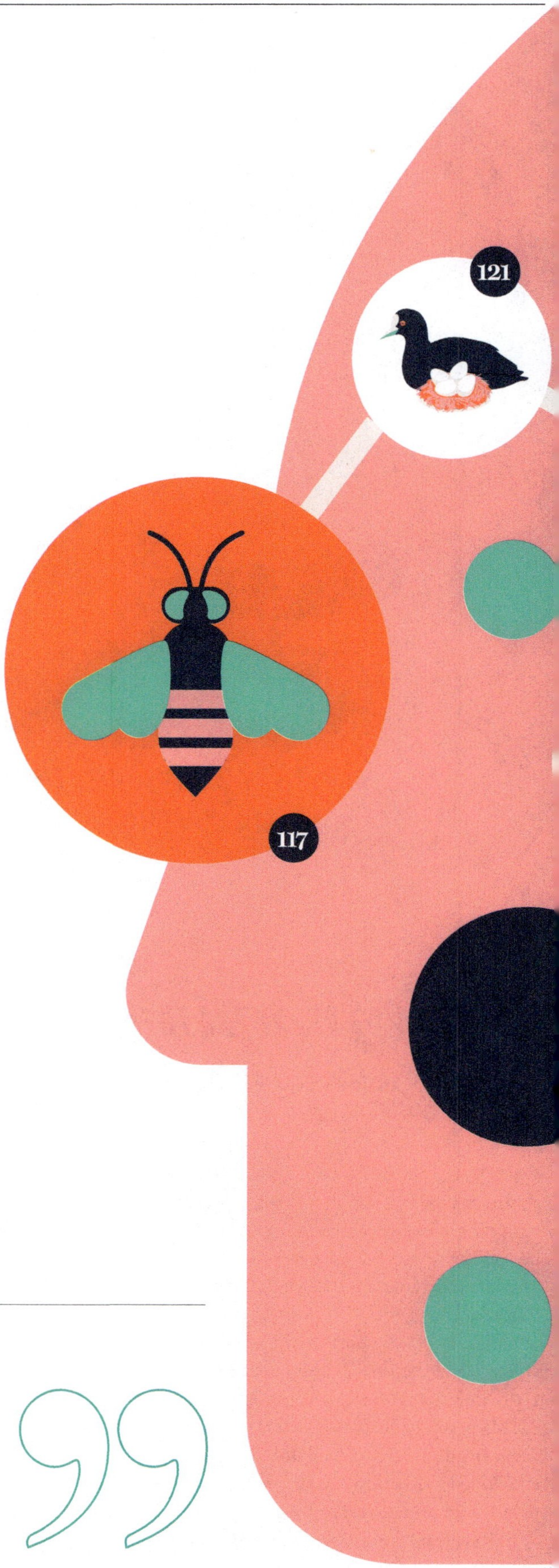

> "A LARGER HERD IS MORE LIKELY TO CONTAIN WEAK, OLD OR YOUNG ANIMALS, SO BEING ABLE TO JUDGE THE SIZE OF A HERD IS VERY BENEFICIAL"

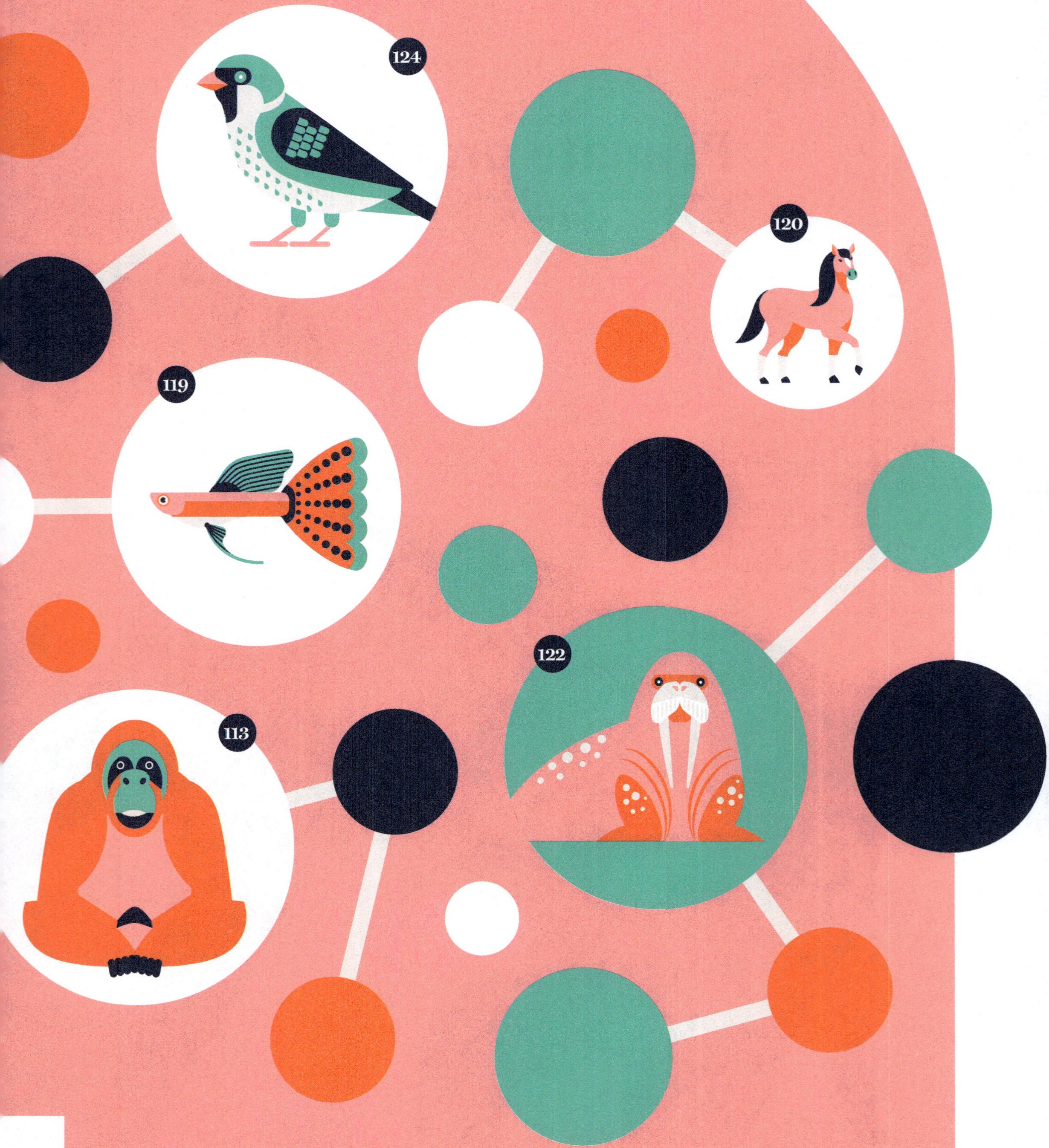
124
120
119
122
113

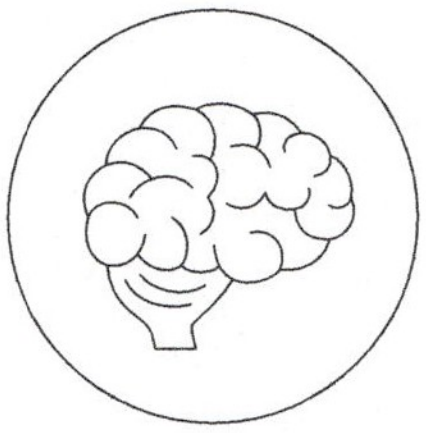

Primate practices

We look at the day-to-day habits of our closest relatives – the great apes

As our closest living ancestors, we have always been fascinated by the other members of the primate species. From the way they walk and interact to how they eat and sleep, it's easy to spot some of ourselves in them, despite the stark differences in our respective habitats. To an extent they can be viewed as a funhouse mirror of how we once were – almost a portal into the distant past.

Our focus in this article will be on the habits and routines of the 'great' apes: chimpanzees, orangutans, gorillas and bonobos, taking into account factors such as what they eat, how and where they sleep, the hierarchical structures of their groups and other facets of their day-to-day lives, as well as the kind of challenges they face. It will perhaps become clear that we are not quite so different after all...

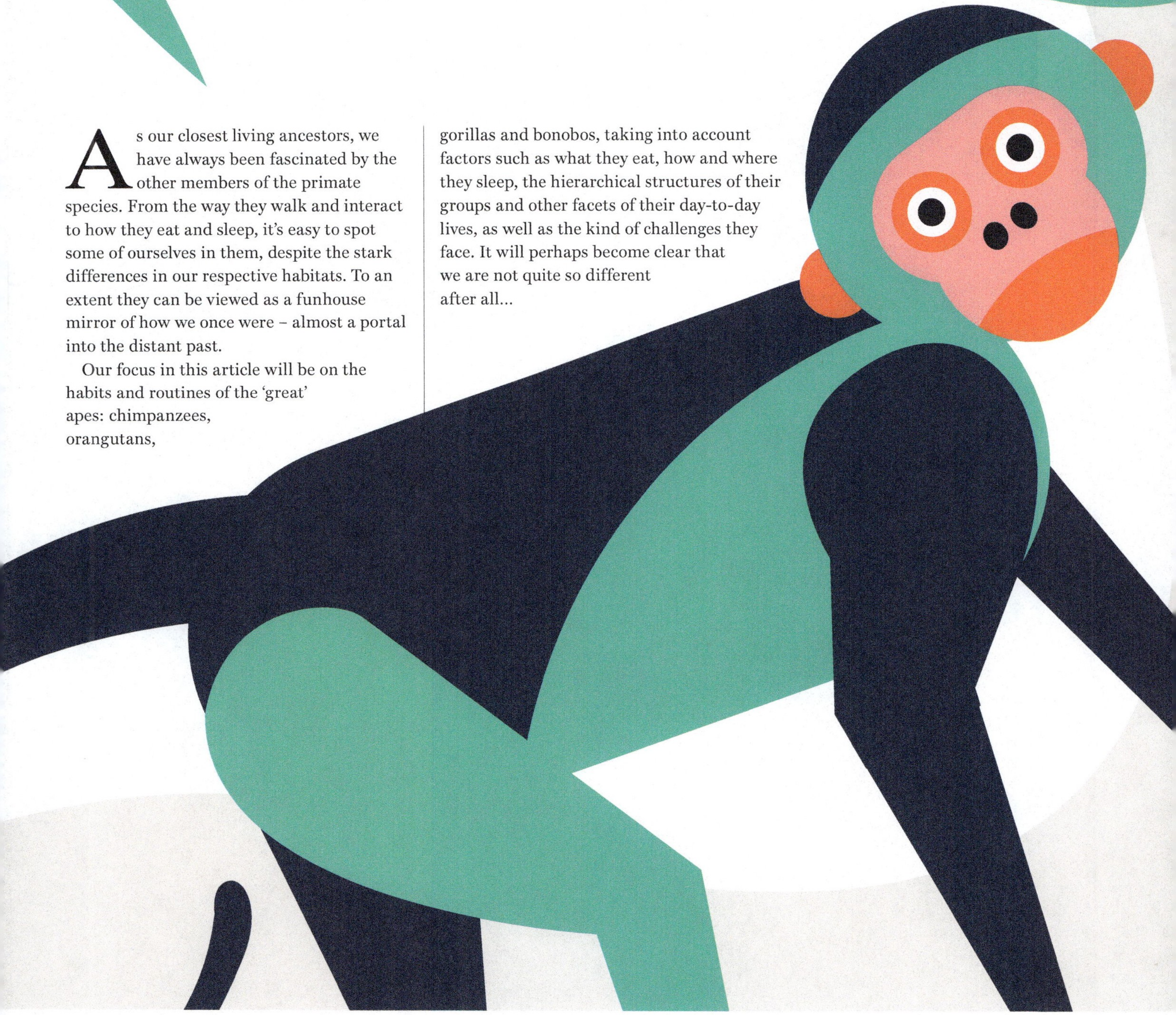

Chimpanzees

Our closest cousins (they share around 98 per cent of our genes), chimpanzees are arguably the most sociable of the great ape subspecies. Fiercely protective of their young, mothers pay close attention to their offspring, and they live in large groups of a few dozen for the duration of their roughly 50-year lifespan.

Female chimpanzees are able to give birth from about the age of 13 years old, with the infant staying as close to their mother as possible (clinging to her early on and later riding on her back) until the age of two. Males take longer to mature, not being considered to have reached adult status until they're 16 years of age.

Hierarchies are fairly strict in chimpanzee groups. There is usually an alpha male, aged between 25 and 30 years, who is responsible for maintaining order in the group, such as forming alliances and protecting the group from attack. The alpha will regularly display affection to assert his authority, although at the same time he has to retain support from other males to maintain dominance. Conversely, the female role in the group revolves more around rearing young, and they are rarely found in positions of power.

Chimpanzees have no trouble getting about; although they generally walk on all fours, they can stand upright and are partial to travelling by swinging through the rainforests that they call their home. Additionally, they are known to dwell in assorted woodlands and grasslands.

Varied eaters, they will often subsist on fruit and plants, but they are known to hunt live prey too. Using tools, they are capable of digging up insects like grubs from their nests, and if they happen upon it, carrion can also make for a meal. Another example of their human-like behaviour is their use of leaves to soak up drinking water and stones for smashing open nuts.

While chimpanzees have been known to display extreme levels of violence against different groups (see 'Fight Club'), at the same time they have a more affectionate side. They are often seen grooming each other – picking bits of dirt, dry skin and various parasites from one another's skin – for a variety of purposes. This cleaning ritual could be interpreted as a show of affection or simply to help keep their companions clean, but it's also used to reduce the stress of infants during weaning. Beyond this, grooming can play a genuine role in influencing the hierarchy in a group, helping individual chimpanzees form alliances with one another.

When it comes to sleep, chimpanzees display particular ingenuity. They'll nestle high up in the trees on branches, with nests constructed from notably sturdy tree species like ironwood, giving them both a vantage point and a place of safety from ground-based predators. Here, they'll sleep for around eight to nine hours a night.

FIGHT CLUB

Inside the bloody gang wars of chimps

In an instance of the apple not falling too far from the tree, different primate factions have been known to fight each other, often with bloody results.

In recent years chimpanzees and bonobos have been the primary focus of studies into primate violence. A study conducted by the University of Minnesota, Twin Cities, observed 18 chimpanzee and four bonobo communities in Africa during a period covering over 500 researcher years. All in all, 152 primate deaths related directly to fighting were observed.

While the exact reasons for these disputes are unknown, a number of hypotheses have been posited. For instance, in light of greater human activity reducing the amount of land primates have, disputes between different chimpanzee factions (bonobos were observed to be relatively peaceful) have increased, resulting in violent encounters. These don't seem to be pitched stand-offs, however; more often than not encounters tend to consist of groups ambushing solo males.

Other theories include the desire to expand territory and acquire new mates (males tend to be the majority of the perpetrators). During one ten-year study in Uganda, ecologists observed a group of 28 chimpanzees cornering and attacking a small group of females and their offspring for a prolonged period of time.

"GROOMING CAN PLAY A GENUINE ROLE IN INFLUENCING THE HIERARCHY IN A GROUP"

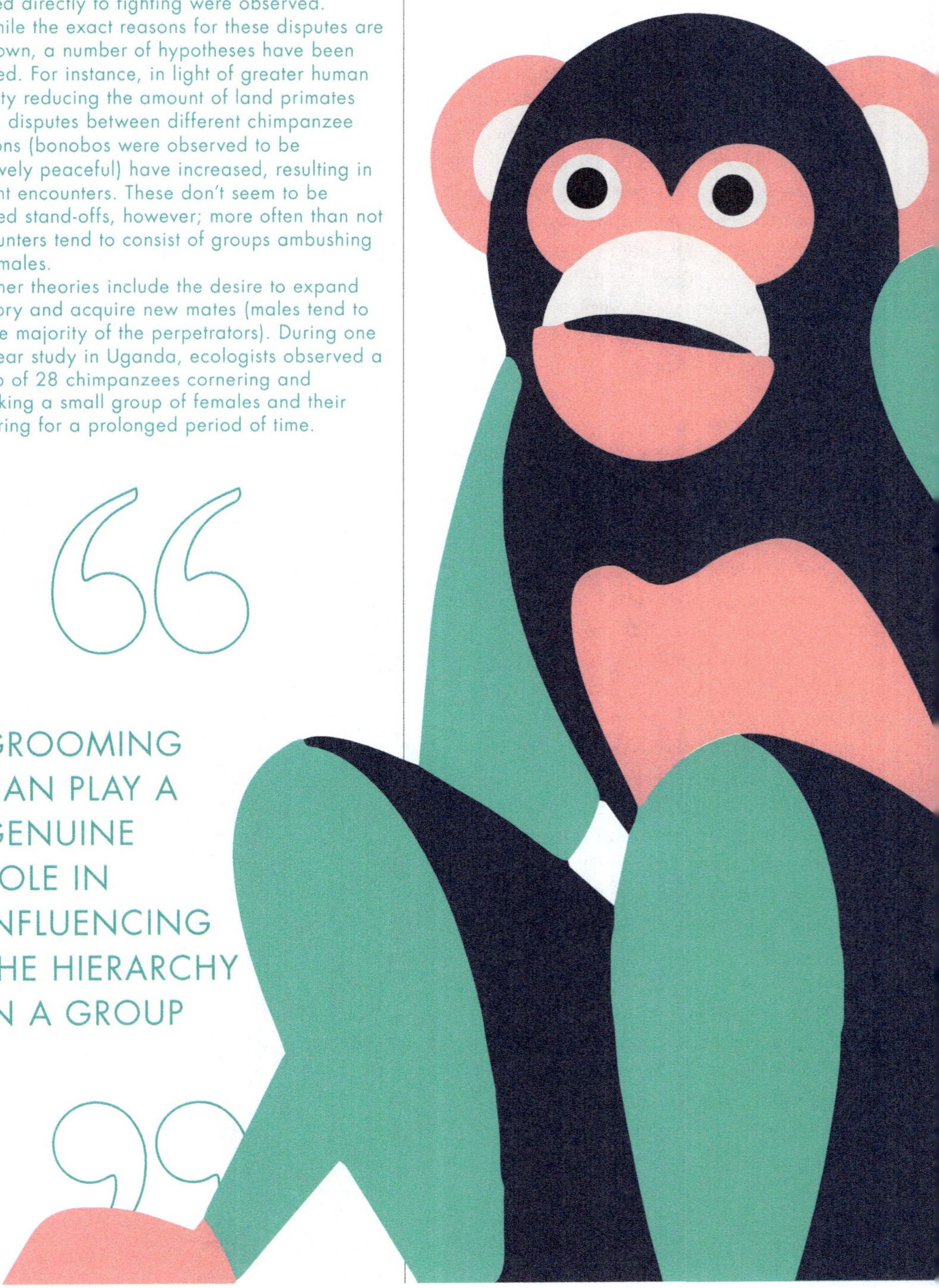

IMAGE SOURCE Getty Images

Gorillas

Native to sub-Saharan Africa, the gorilla can be divided into four sub-species: the eastern lowland gorilla (based around the Democratic Republic of Congo, near the border with Rwanda); the mountain gorilla (the Albertine Rift rainforests in Rwanda and Burundi); the western lowland gorilla (central Africa) and the lesser-known Cross River gorilla (on the border between Cameroon and Nigeria).

Like chimpanzees, gorillas have a rigidly defined social structure (numbers range from just a few to over 40 members), although their alpha is a far more imposing figure. Generally the oldest member of the group, the hue of his fur denotes his 'silverback' moniker. Accompanied by a 'troop' of younger gorillas, he asserts his authority with displays of dominance like pounding his chest and loudly shrieking. Despite this, gorillas are generally among the more mild-mannered of the primate species, only provoked into displays of violence when disturbed or threatened, and disputes between gorilla factions are much rarer than they are in other primate species.

Similarly to us, female gorillas give birth after a pregnancy period of around nine months, having reached sexual maturity at ten to 12 years (males do so at 11 to 13). Infants are entirely dependent on their mothers for the first year or so of their lives, clinging onto them while they move around until around the age of three. While males play little active part in bringing up their children, they – particularly the silverback of the troop – will protect them if needed.

Gorillas have a primarily vegetarian diet, sticking to things like plant stems, bamboo shoots and different types of fruit. They'll also go for various insects should the opportunity strike, with western lowland gorillas having a particular penchant for raiding termite nests.

Depending on the location, gorillas will sleep either on the ground or in trees in specially constructed nests (females tend to sleep in trees, whereas the males usually prefer to stay on the ground). They'll relocate every night, with each gorilla having to construct their own resting place all over again (save for the young, who share sleeping space with their mothers for the first few years of their lives).

While gorillas display the third-highest DNA similarities to human beings after chimpanzees and bonobos, there are other notably shared behavioural traits. Gorillas have been observed to partake in displays of happiness and sadness, and the way their young behave (constantly playing and swinging through trees) is evidently childlike. Moreover, some gorillas in captivity have displayed the capacity to learn sign language taught to them by their human captors, a clear indication of intelligence.

Gorillas are generally relatively placid unless they feel threatened.

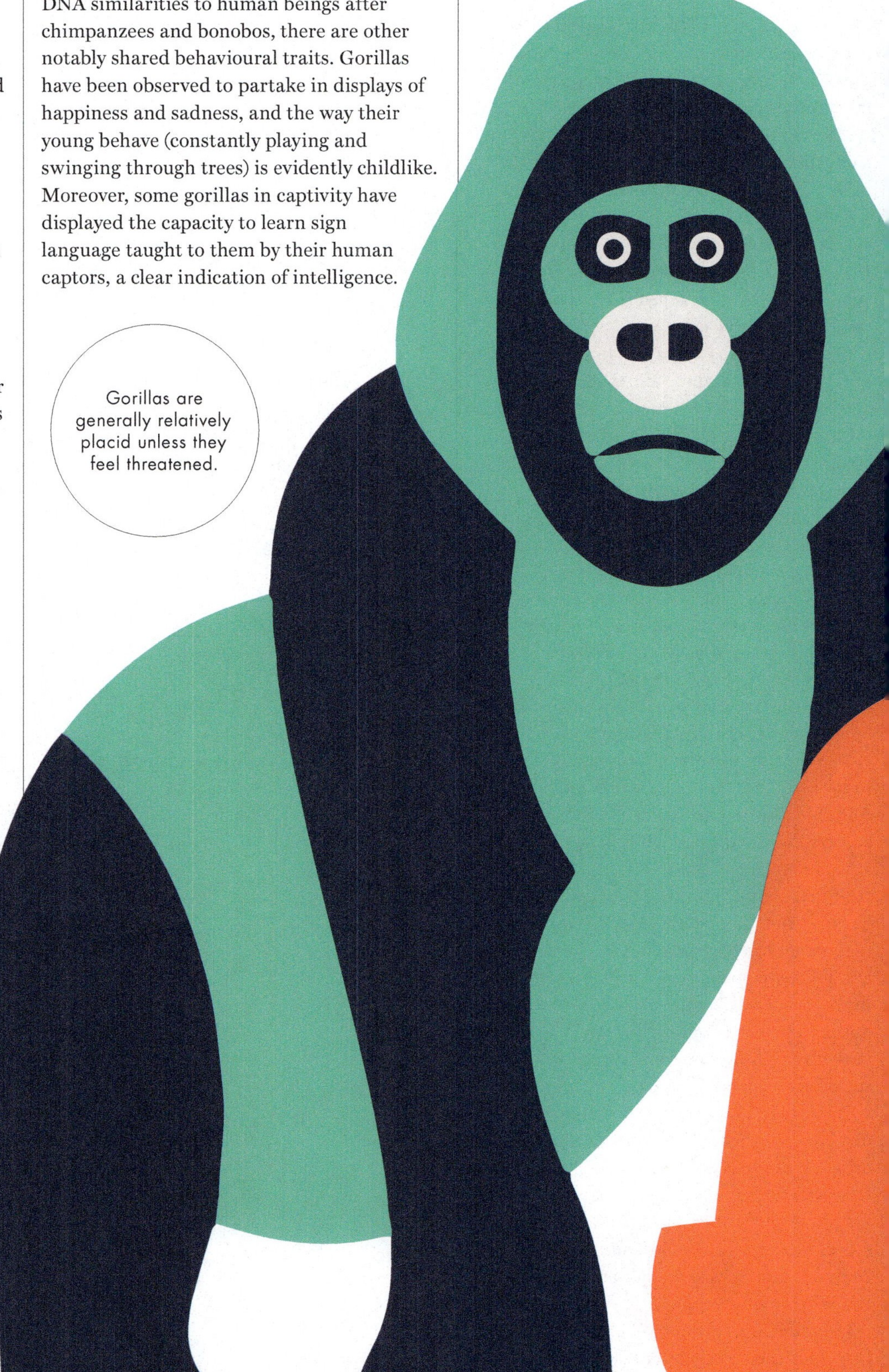

> ORANGUTANS ARE LESS VIOLENT THAN OTHER APE SPECIES; FIGHTS BETWEEN MALES ARE RARE

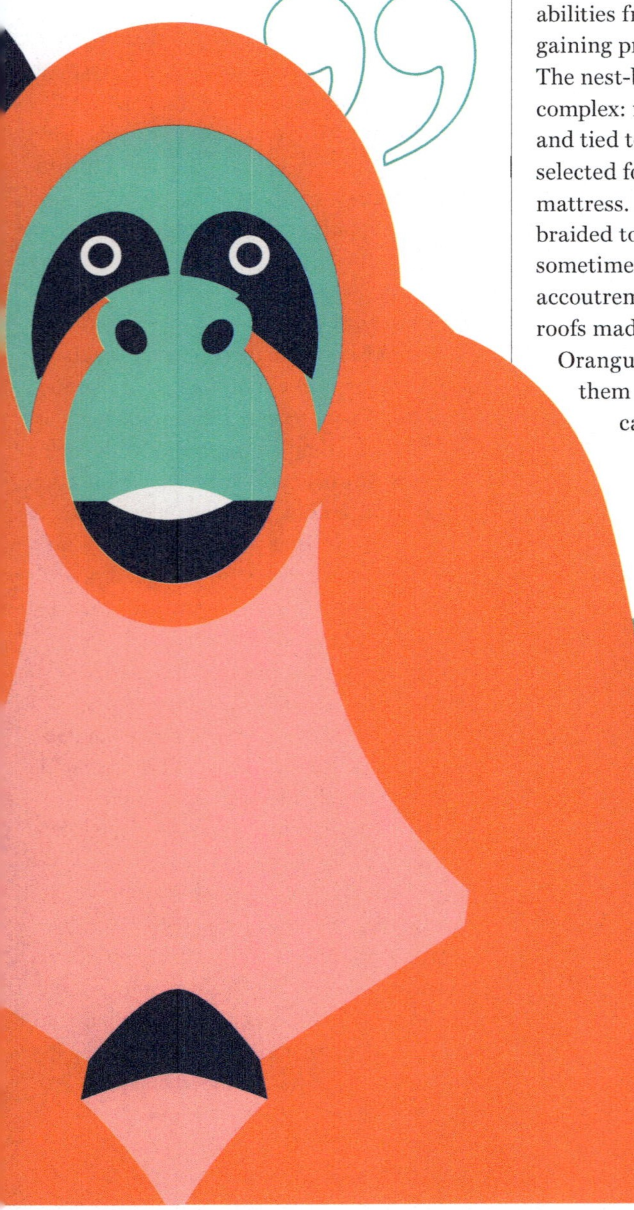

Orangutans

Found in the rainforests of Borneo and Sumatra, the orangutan's name literally translates as 'person of the forest' in Malay, and it's an apt description considering just how much of their time they spend in the trees. With their long arms stretching as far as 2.1 metres from fingertip to fingertip (which make them perfect for swinging), they are the most distant of the great ape species from us in terms of shared DNA, yet, as we shall see, one of the most intelligent in terms of adapting to their habitat.

With their body structure ideally suited for life in the trees, it is no surprise that they spend so much time there. Nest building is an important skill among orangutans, with the young learning to replicate their mother's abilities from about six months before gaining proficiency after around three years. The nest-building process is surprisingly complex: first, branches are pulled together and tied to a point, then leafier branches are selected for the foundation to serve as a mattress. Finally, the tips of the branches are braided to form a mattress of sorts, sometimes accompanied by additional accoutrements like pillows, blankets and roofs made of leaves.

Orangutans' reproduction habits mark them out from other primates. Females can only give birth once every eight years – the longest duration for any animal. Both males and females reach sexual maturity at about 14 to 15 years, and they are one of the few primate species not to practice infanticide. For the first two years of their lives orangutan offspring are almost entirely dependent on their mothers (the fathers rarely play a role in their upbringing), being in physical contact with them at all times. From there they gradually gain independence, although they stay in contact with their mothers until the age of around six or seven.

Also unlike other primates, orangutans are far more likely to live alone. While mothers live with their children and adolescents may band together in small groups, adult males live a far more solitary lifestyle. This style of living lends itself to their foraging habits: fruit is the most popular choice, with tree bark, insects and bird eggs also considered acceptable alternatives. In some cases, Sumatran orangutans have been partial to living prey, notably the small loris. Moreover, orangutans are less violent than other ape species; fights between males are rare, with one of the most common causes of encounters being over the attention of a female.

Sadly, perhaps in part due to the inflexible nature of its lifestyle, the orangutan's existence is under threat. Due to the increasing threat of deforestation to their habitat, orangutans are in severe danger of becoming extinct.

Estimates place the current wild population at around 50,000-65,000, a stark figure indeed given that a century ago approximately 230,000 lived in the jungles of Borneo and Sumatra.

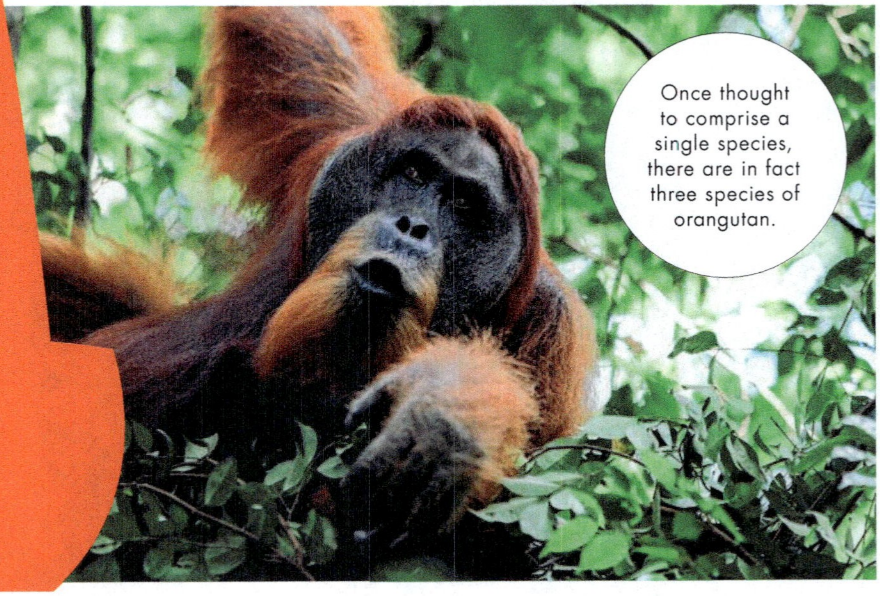

Once thought to comprise a single species, there are in fact three species of orangutan.

IMAGE SOURCE Getty Images

Bonobos

Arguably the most enigmatic of the great apes (thanks to the political instability in the Democratic Republic of the Congo, where the species are almost entirely located, relatively little study has been conducted in their natural habitat), bonobos are a bit of an oxymoron. While generally shy and wary of outsiders, in their own habitats they are seen to display a range of emotions while sharing little of the aggression seen in chimpanzees, their closest primate counterparts.

Unlike that of chimpanzees, however, bonobo society doesn't appear to be a patriarchal one. Rather, status among males and females appears to have some form of parity, with females even coming out on top in some respects. A lot of this is down to the high levels of sexual activity taking place among bonobos, with members of a particular group copulating with each other on a regular basis, both as a social nicety and as a means of reproduction – the rate at which they do so is the highest of any primate species. They are also one of the few species who will have sex facing each other, and homosexuality has also been recorded.

Additionally, males are also rarely able to assert physical dominance due to females teaming up with one another to combat them. The same dynamic applies during activities such as hunting: bonobos have been known to take down small forest antelopes, with females banding together to chase them out of the long grass. While, like other primates, they'll subsist on foods like berries, plants and eggs, they seem increasingly willing to take on small mammals like flying squirrels and anomalures.

Another area in which bonobos appear more flexible than chimpanzees (interestingly, until further study in the 1990s, bonobos were assumed to be a smaller variety of chimp) is in their daily habits. Usually found in groups of 100 or so, rather than staying together they will split up into smaller hunting parties throughout the day, only regrouping at night in order to sleep. For this, they'll construct nests in trees much like other primates.

As the second most similar species to humans after chimpanzees (again sharing around 98 per cent of human DNA), bonobos have been seen to share other traits with us. For instance, they communicate with each other vocally using consistent noises for the same thing, and they have even been seen to shake their heads as a means of saying 'no'. They also seem more keen to walk on two feet than chimpanzees do and generally appear to have more placid personalities.

Ultimately, what is most striking about the habits and routines of the greater ape primates is how distinct they are from one another, despite their undeniable similarities in lineage. Each has adapted to their environment in different ways – one of the few universally shared traits, however, is the negative impact that human activities have had on their environments, with all of the greater apes having their status jeopardised in one way or another. We live in hope that one day humankind as a whole can learn to live in such a way that reverses the potentially dark future ahead for these fascinating and beautiful species.

WORDS Steve Wright

IT'S GOOD TO TALK

How captive apes have been taught to communicate

While apes in the wild have their own methods of communicating with one another, their hosts in zoos have taken things one step further by attempting to teach them sign language.

In the 1960s, Allen and Beatrix Gardner at the University of Nevada – later succeeded by fellow academics Roger and Deborah Fouts – started working with a chimpanzee called Washoe. By the time of Washoe's death in 2007 she knew about 250 signs, putting them together to form word combinations like 'Gimmie Sweet' and 'You Me Go Out Hurry'. In turn, her daughter Loulis learned signs from her – the first instance of a chimpanzee learning from the same species rather than a human.

Although attempts have been made to teach apes how to speak – in the 1940s, a chimp called Viki in Florida was raised with a family, and taught (with someone moving her lips for her) how to say 'mama' – actual speech is impossible for apes. This is because apes' larynx (or speech box) is higher than humans', which, coupled with a thinner tongue, means they can't pronounce the sounds needed to produce what is recognisable to us as speech.

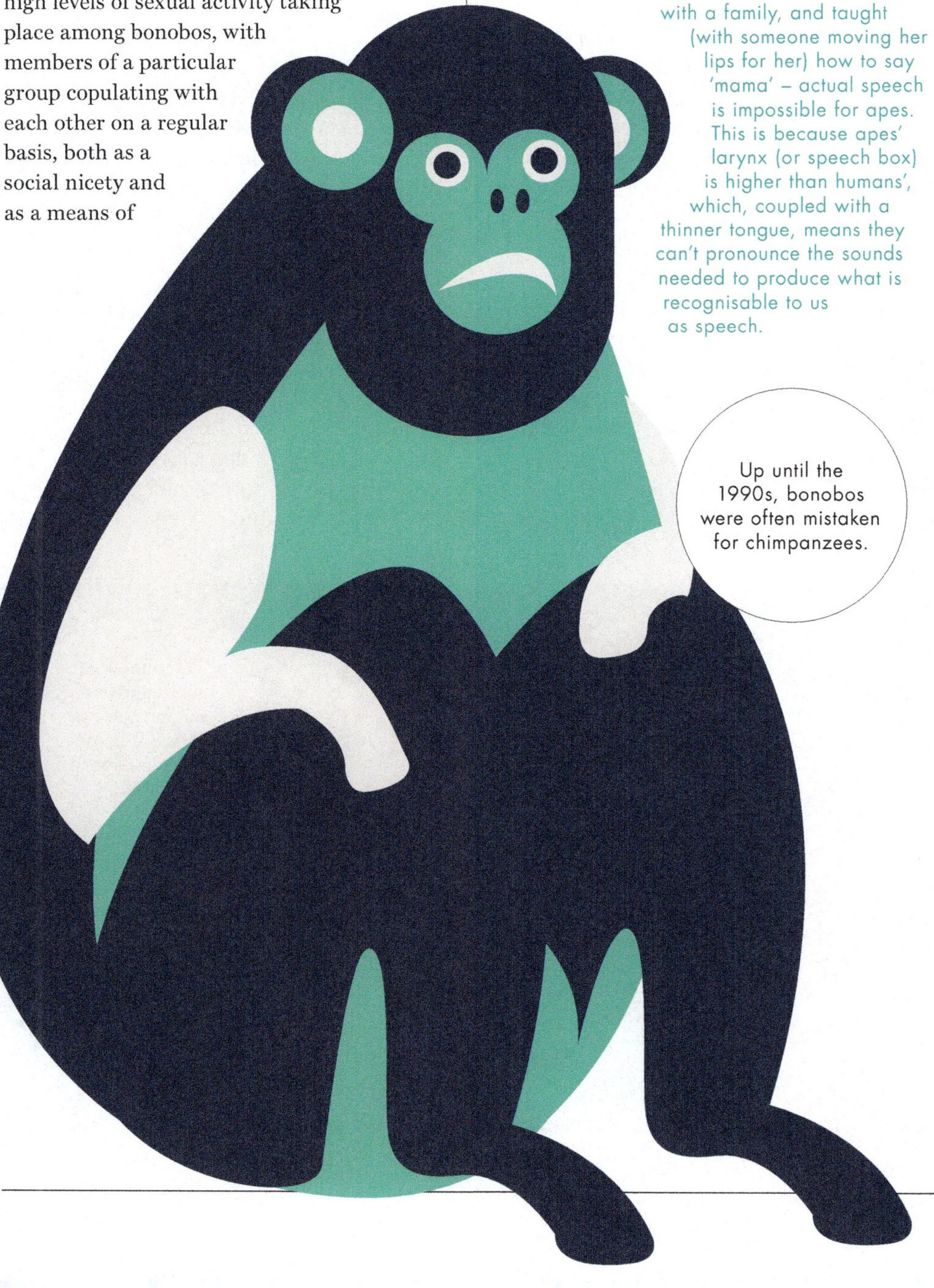

Up until the 1990s, bonobos were often mistaken for chimpanzees.

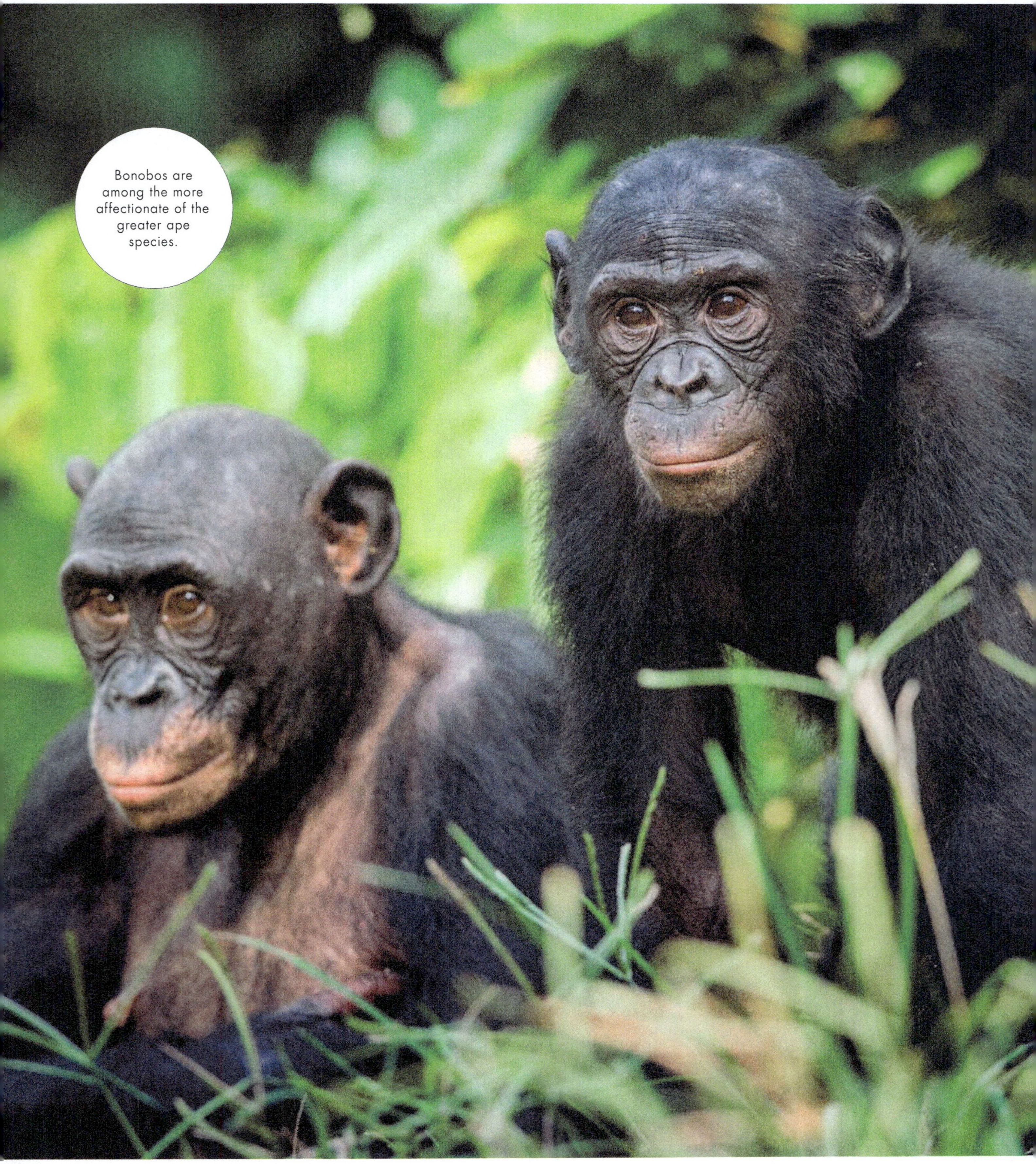

Bonobos are among the more affectionate of the greater ape species.

IMAGE SOURCE Getty Images

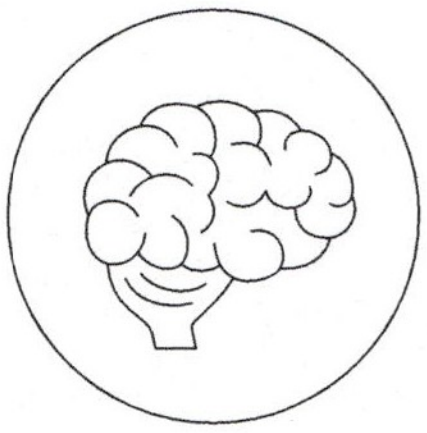

The skill that counts

Being able to count is an incredibly useful skill, and it turns out it's a far more common talent among animals than we realised

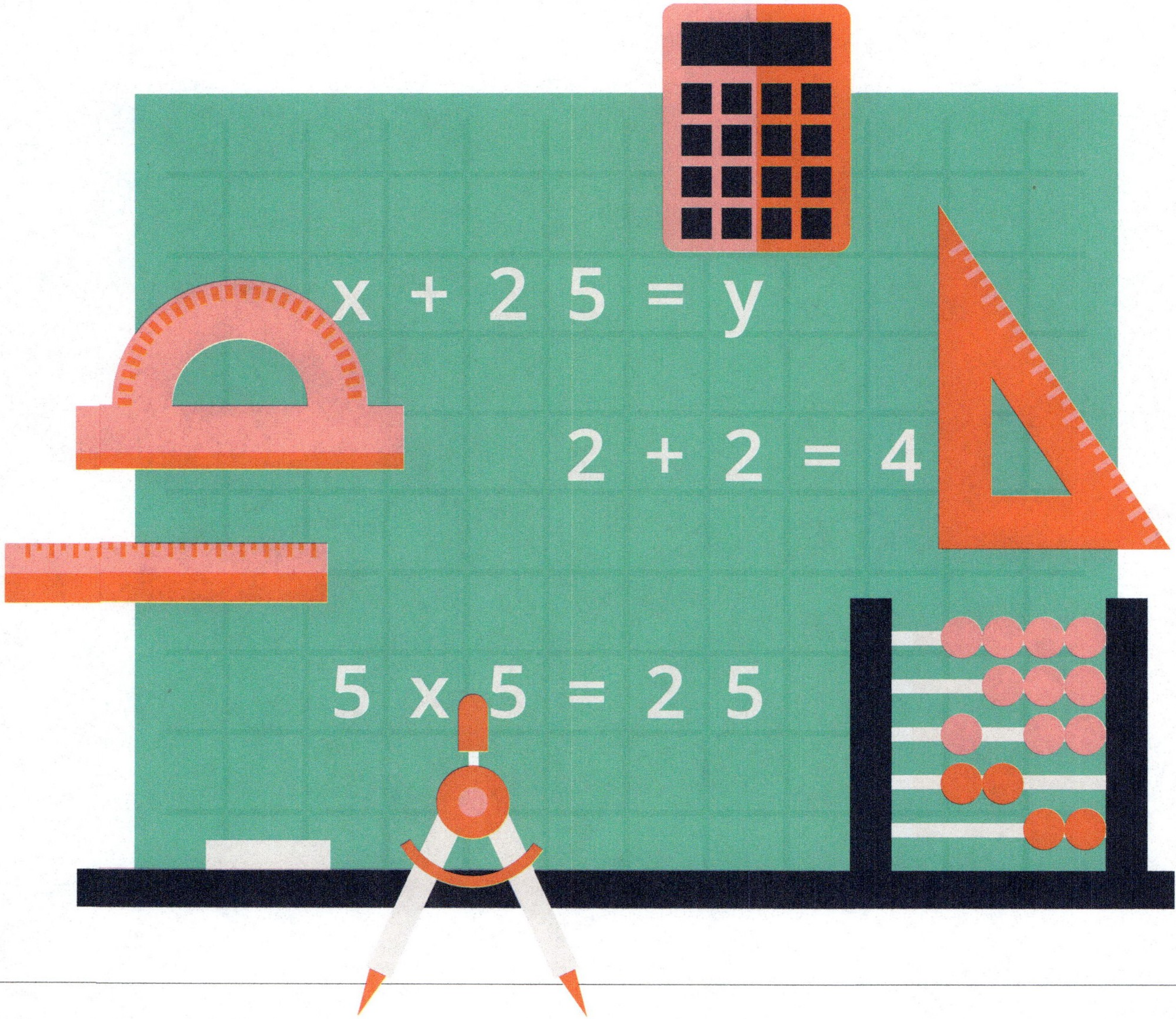

IF A PRIDE OF LIONS COMES ACROSS ANOTHER GROUP THAT IS SMALLER THAN THEIR OWN THEY ARE MUCH MORE LIKELY TO ATTACK IT

Lions avoid prides with more members

Judging another group's size is a useful strategy

For lions, living in groups (prides) allows individuals to join together to rear cubs communally and hunt larger prey. Another advantage is the ability to defend territory from other lions. One single lion group can roam an area of over 259 square kilometres, although boundaries often change over time.

As lions are well known for aggressive behaviour, such as infanticide, the size of a group can be very important. It's therefore not too surprising that lions are able to count the number of members in other groups they encounter. If a pride comes across another group that is smaller than their own they are much more likely to attack it.

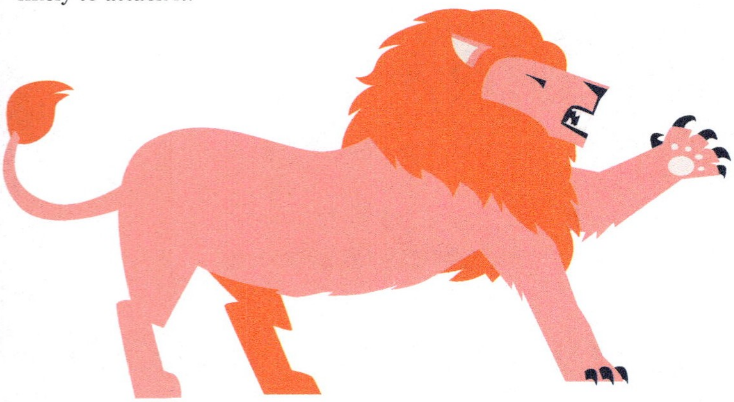

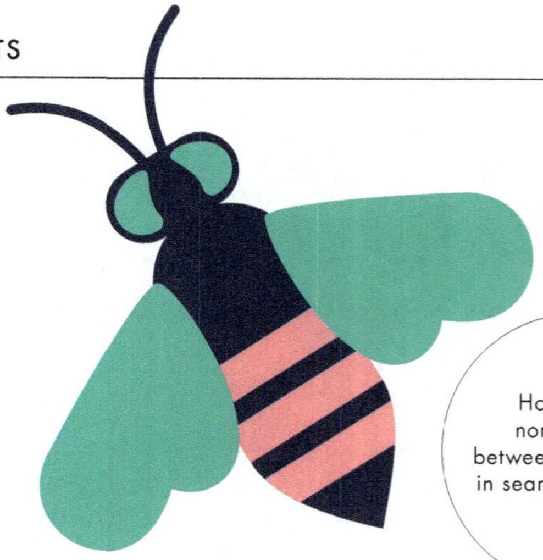

Honeybees normally fly between 0.8–6.4km in search of nectar.

Bees can judge distance

Knowing where to get the best nectar saves time

Honeybees live in large hives containing one queen bee, a few hundred fertile male drones and tens of thousands of sterile female worker bees. The entire colony needs to work together in order to ensure its survival, and so communication between individuals is very important.

All species of honeybees have been found to use abstract language, such as waggle dancing, to direct other bees to fly in a particular direction. The length of dance directly correlates with the distance at which the flowers can be found. Other bees are then able to accurately pinpoint how far to travel.

Chicks can count better than toddlers

Even newborn chicks can count up to five

Chickens are often thought to be rather lacking in intelligence, but it seems they might actually be a lot smarter than we give them credit for. Several studies have found that even tiny chicks are able to count up to five. One experiment even discovered that they are able to add and subtract small numbers of objects hidden behind screens and reliably pick the larger number.

Overall, newborn chicks are actually able to outperform human toddlers in many intelligence tests. Given that chicks leave the nest after only a couple of days and are independent within a few weeks, they need to be able to learn and adapt very quickly in order to find food and evade predators. It's also thought that they may even have a basic understanding of physics.

As for the sensible saying, 'Don't count your chickens before they're hatched', it isn't clear if adult chickens can actually count their own eggs.

Hens can identify an object when it's partially hidden. It was previously thought only humans could do this.

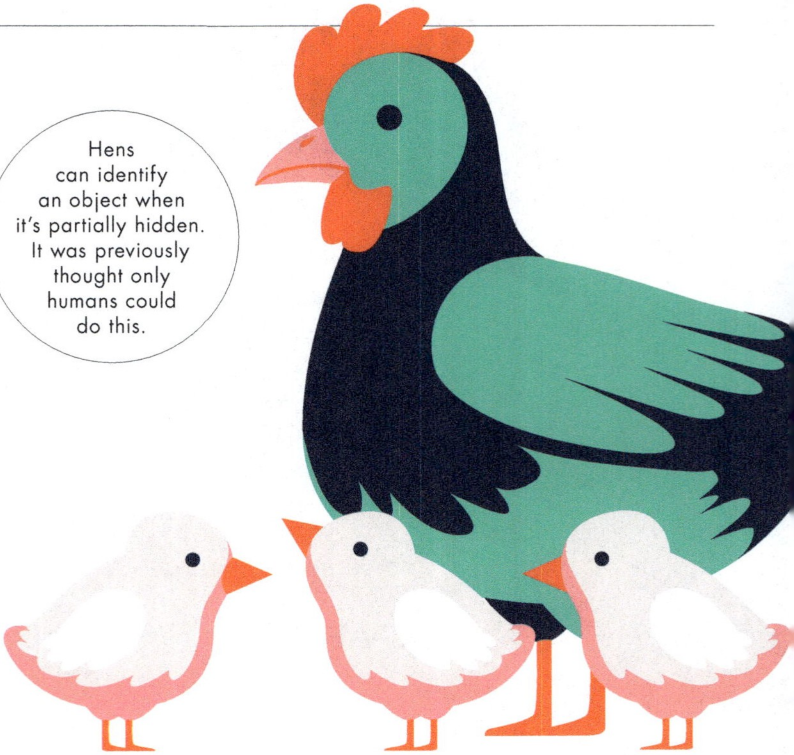

IMAGE SOURCE Getty Images

Robins tally up their food stores

Stealing food from the biggest hoard can be vital for survival

Male New Zealand robins are usually very devoted to their mates and will often go out of their way to cater to their partner's dietary preferences. When the females are sitting on eggs, males will happily bring them food several times an hour. However, in the harsh winter months food becomes very scarce, and even the most dedicated partners often hide food from each other.

Researchers have found that female robins watch their partners hiding food in tree stumps. They count which cache has the highest number of prey items and raid that particular one when the male's away. In return, the males are able to calculate which of their stores contains the most food and spend a disproportionate amount of time trying to defend these from other robins (including their mates). Tests found that the robins could easily identify between stores of similar sizes, such as one containing four grubs and one with seven.

When researchers showed robins a pair of mealworms and then hid them below a layer that only showed one worm, the birds dug furiously in search of the missing pair.

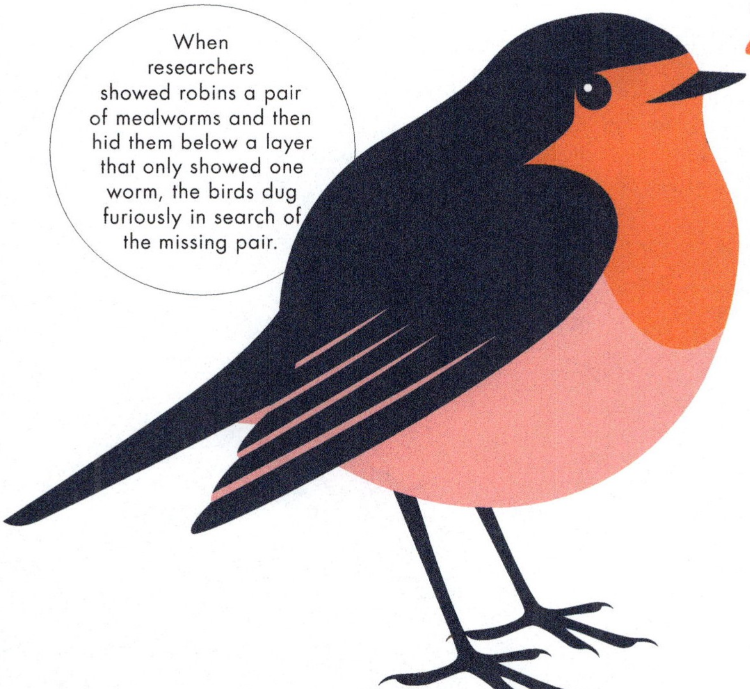

African grey parrots are thought to possess the mental and emotional skills of a five-year-old human.

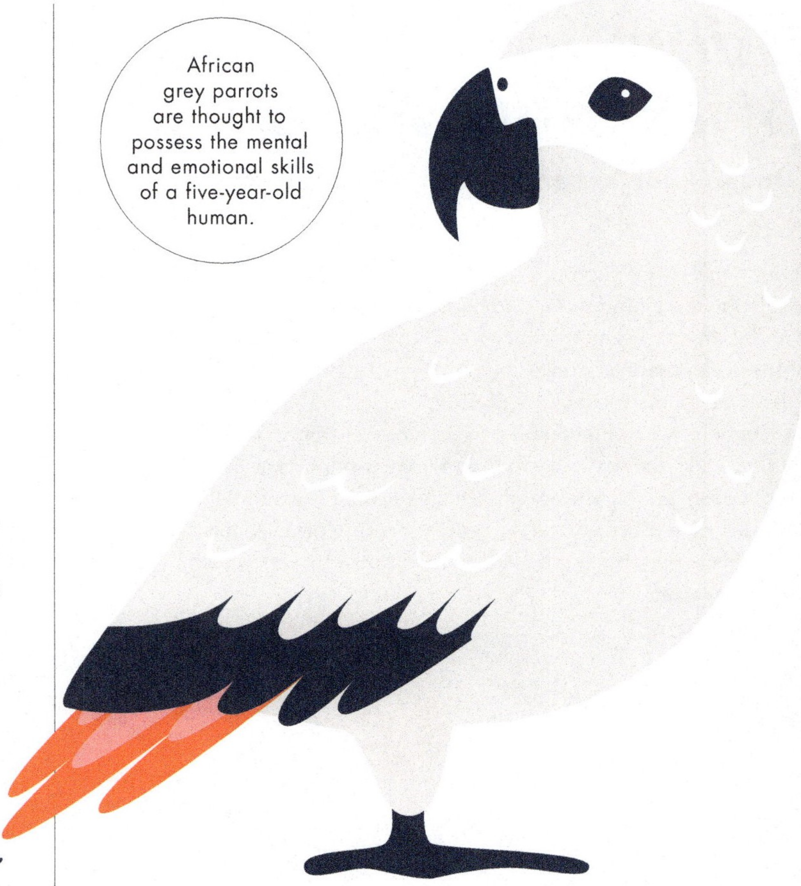

Grey parrots can do simple sums

These clever birds are capable of some impressive avian arithmetic

Grey parrots are known to be particularly intelligent, and they can perform as well as a four-year-old child in some tests. Despite not having true vocal cords they are able to produce sounds that mimic human speech. This means that they can learn how to say numbers, which makes it easier to test their ability to count.

A grey parrot called Alex was taught to recognise numbers up to eight and learnt to add up sets of objects to reach this number. Sadly he died at a young age, and the researchers working with him felt they had only touched the surface of his mathematical potential.

> FEMALE ROBINS COUNT WHICH CACHE CONTAINS THE MOST AND THEN RAID IT

Guppies prefer to stick together

Being part of a larger group can help guppies stay safe

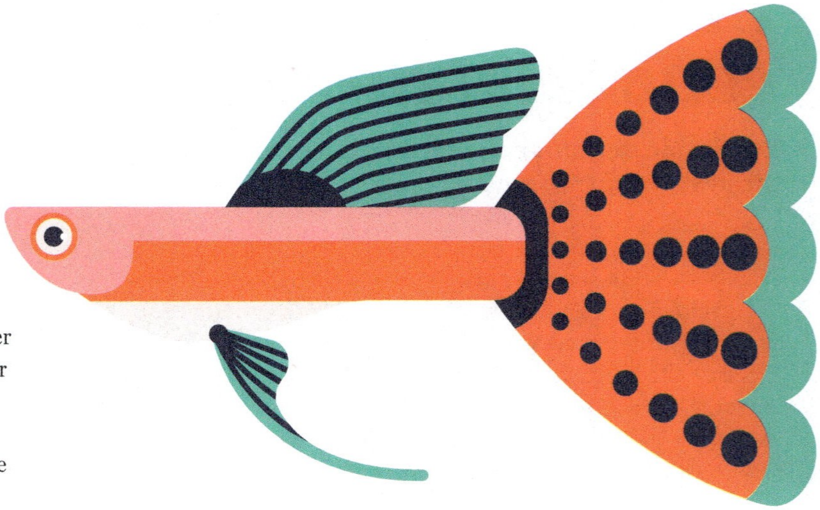

Guppies are small tropical fish, generally only a few centimetres long. Due to their size they make ideal prey for a huge range of birds and larger fish, so it is an advantage for them to try and stick together in groups to confuse predators and provide safety in numbers. Larger groups can also help the guppies look for food more successfully.

Guppies are able to estimate the number of fish in a group and actively choose to join the biggest one. Newborn guppies are also able to count up to four and correctly choose between food piles of different sizes.

> A LARGER HERD IS MORE LIKELY TO CONTAIN WEAK, OLD OR YOUNG ANIMALS, SO BEING ABLE TO JUDGE THE SIZE OF A HERD IS VERY BENEFICIAL

Studies have shown that wolves understand cause and effect. Domesticated dogs don't.

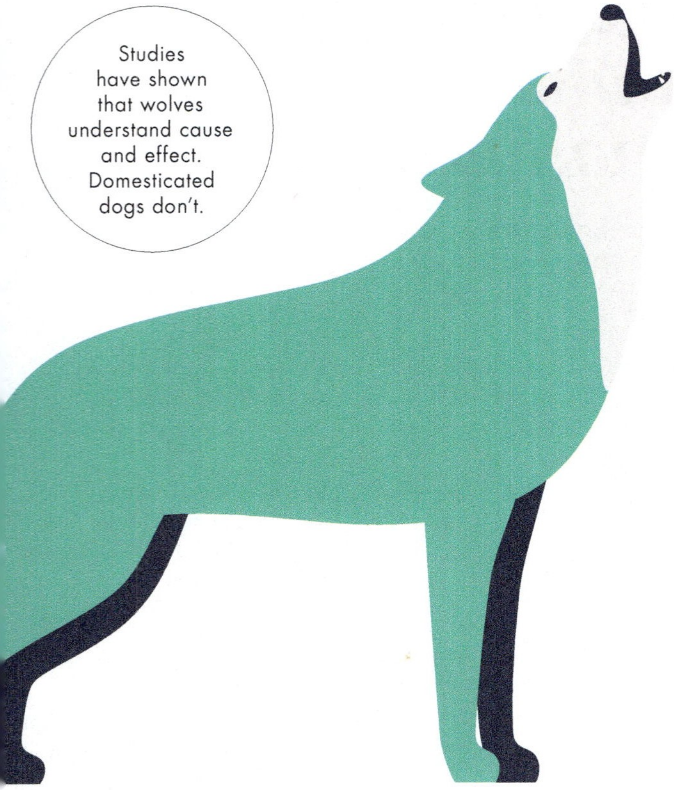

Wolves can count better than dogs

Unlike their domestic cousins, wolves can count their prey

Wolves hunt in packs and can take hours to chase down prey such as deer and bison. As hunting requires such a huge investment in both time and energy, it is important that they can quickly assess if it's worthwhile chasing any particular herd of prey. A larger herd is more likely to contain weak, old or young animals, so being able to judge the size of a herd is very beneficial.

Researchers have found that wolves are able to distinguish between different numbers of food items, even when the total was hidden from view. This shows that they were counting the individual items, not just judging which pile looked bigger. The ability to count is thought to help them decide where to hunt based upon the number of prey animals present in any particular area.

Strangely enough, when the same experiment was carried out with domestic dogs, they were unable to perform better than if they were just picking at random. Hundreds of years of domestication have made our canine companions totally reliant on us for food. There's no need for dogs to count when dinner is provided regularly by humans.

IMAGE SOURCE Getty Images

Chimpanzees can count and do sums

Being able to count helps chimpanzees choose the best groups to join and places to eat

Chimpanzees are one of our closest relatives (only the bonobo is thought to share slightly more DNA with us), so it's not too surprising that they are very intelligent. Among other skills, chimps can use tools, be taught to recognise human words and use sign language, are able to follow complex instructions and can learn new skills from each other. In fact, they are thought to show roughly the same level of understanding as a three- to five-year-old child. Chimpanzees also have a phenomenal ability to memorise sequences, with a recent study showing that they can often do this faster than humans.

When it comes to counting, it has been found that chimpanzees can distinguish between small and large numbers. Some captive chimpanzees have also been taught to recognise Arabic numbers and to use these to add and subtract small amounts when trained using a reward-based system.

It is thought that chimpanzees use their counting skills in a wide variety of ways in the wild. They spend their time in small parties of five to ten individuals as part of larger communities of up to a couple of hundred. Meat is an important part of their diet, and hunting success increases with the number of male chimpanzees in a party, so being able to count is useful in determining which party to join. Counting might also help chimpanzees decide which areas and trees to forage in by focusing on places with the highest amounts of food.

Harvard scientists were able to teach Rhesus monkeys to associate ten Arabic numbers and 15 letters with values ranging from zero to 25.

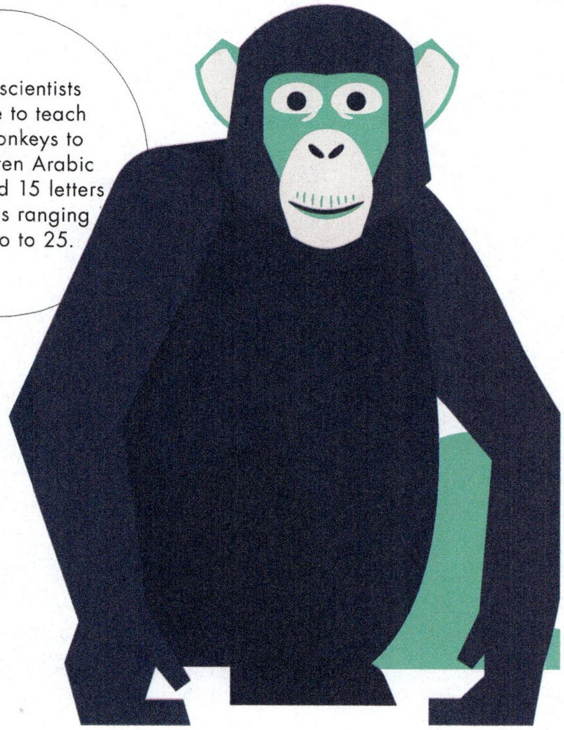

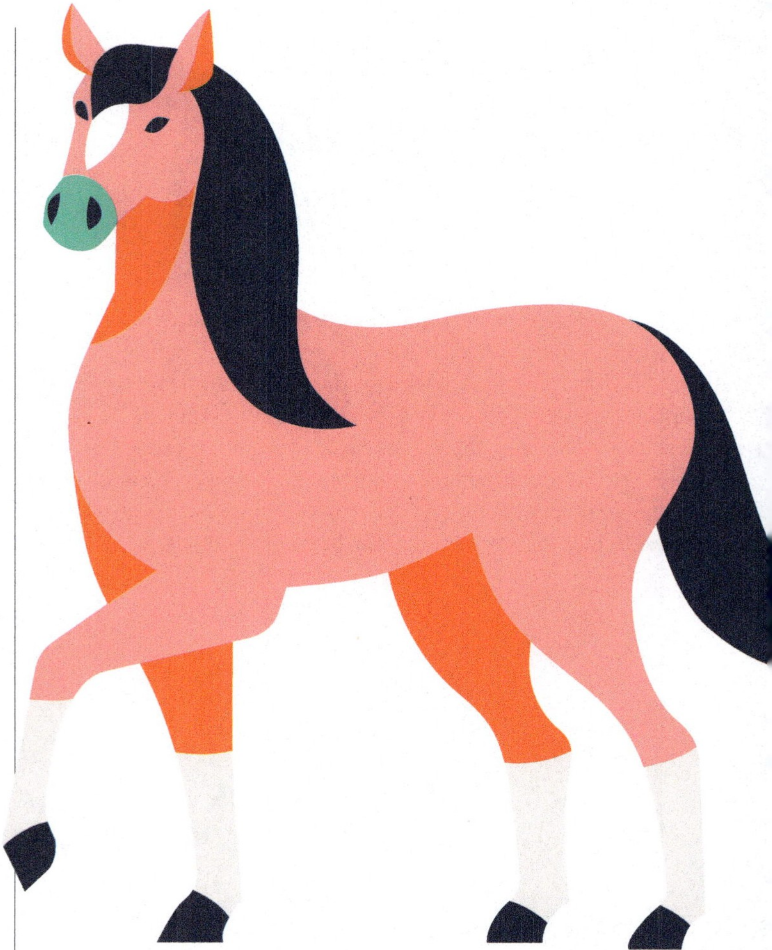

The horse that couldn't really count after all

Despite being the most famous counting animal, Clever Hans was actually a con

In the 1890s, a horse known as Clever Hans was supposedly taught to count by his owner Wilhelm von Osten. Wilhelm, a retired teacher, taught Hans to add, subtract, use fractions and even tell the time.

Hans' skills were so impressive that he was taken on a tour of Germany, thrilling audiences with his counting abilities. When Wilhelm asked him a question, Hans would tap his hoof repeatedly to count out his answer.

However, all wasn't as it seemed. Hans was in fact responding to visual cues from his owner that were imperceptible to humans. Even so, he continued to be a public sensation for a long time.

So can horses really count? Research suggests they can count small numbers. In one study, horses always picked the bucket with the most apples.

> FEMALE COOTS ARE ABLE TO KEEP TRACK OF HOW MANY EGGS THEY HAVE IN THEIR NEST IN TOTAL AND REJECT ONES THAT AREN'T THEIRS

Coots count their eggs

Knowing when a clutch is big enough is a helpful skill

American coots often live in quite high densities and have large clutches of up to ten eggs. This means that there is a lot of competition for food, and the youngest birds in any one clutch often starve. To try and mitigate this, females will often lay their last few eggs in other coot nests. Some birds will even bypass creating their own nest at all and lay all their eggs in host nests.

Researchers found that the females seem to be able to keep track of how many eggs they have in their nest in total and often reject ones that aren't theirs. If the parasitic eggs look different from their own they push them to the edge of the nest so they are less likely to stay warm and hatch. They then carry on laying more eggs of their own. But if they can't tell the difference between the imposter eggs and their own ones they stop laying eggs as soon as they have a big enough clutch in total.

This difference in behaviour implies they can count how many eggs they have in their nest and lay more or stop laying accordingly.

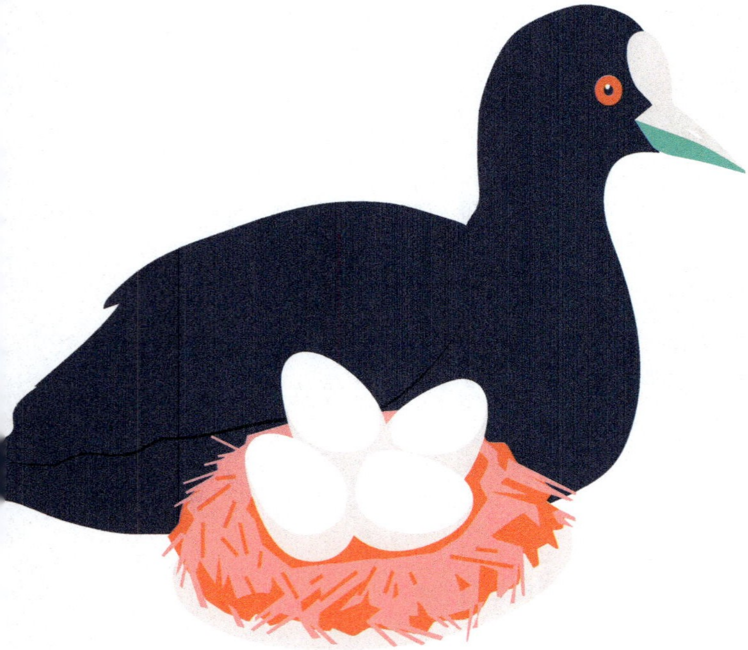

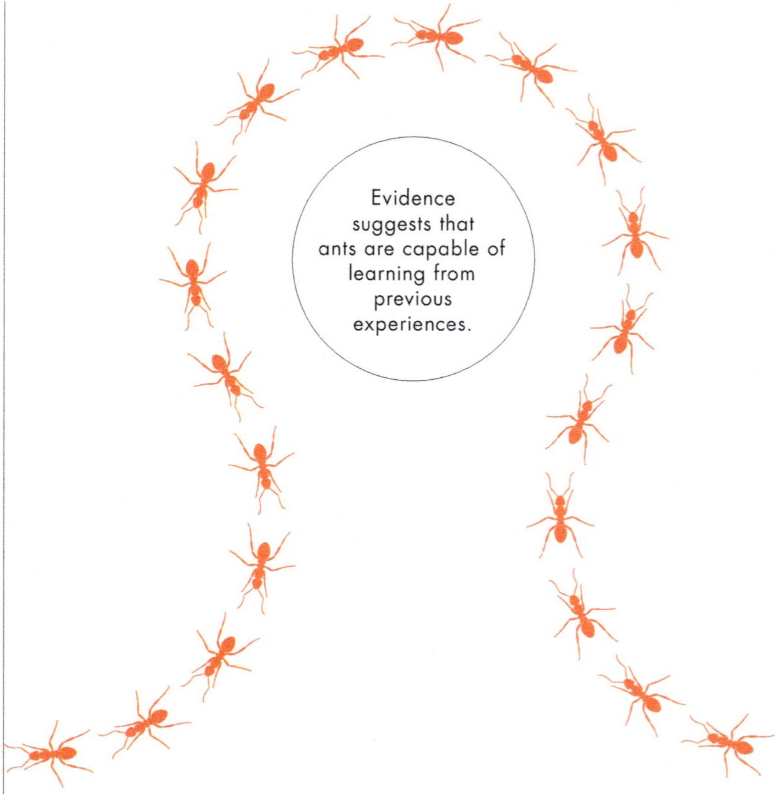

Ants count steps

Desert ants count steps like a pedometer

Desert ants live in very barren landscapes, so navigation can be rather challenging. Despite this they seem to have an uncanny knack of being able to always take the most direct route home. This is very important, as temperatures can get so high that the ants are only able to survive for a few minutes outside their nests.

It was once assumed that they used the position of the Sun or stars to work out how to return to their nests, but researchers discovered they were also able to do this even without these cues. After many experiments it turned out that the ants are actually able to count the number of steps that they have taken in any particular direction. They then use trigonometry to work out which angle they need to walk home in, using polarised light to ensure they keep their bearing right.

IMAGE SOURCE Getty Images

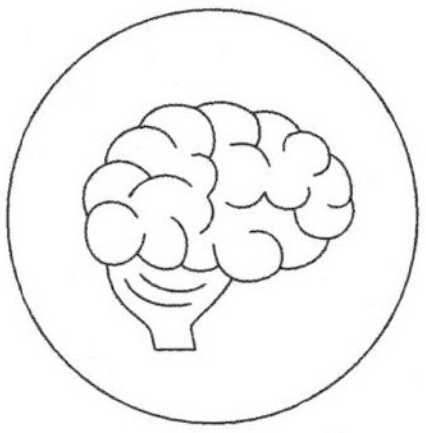

Animal sleeping habits

We set aside time for our beds, but these animals have had to find novel ways to fit in their 40 winks while travelling and avoiding being eaten

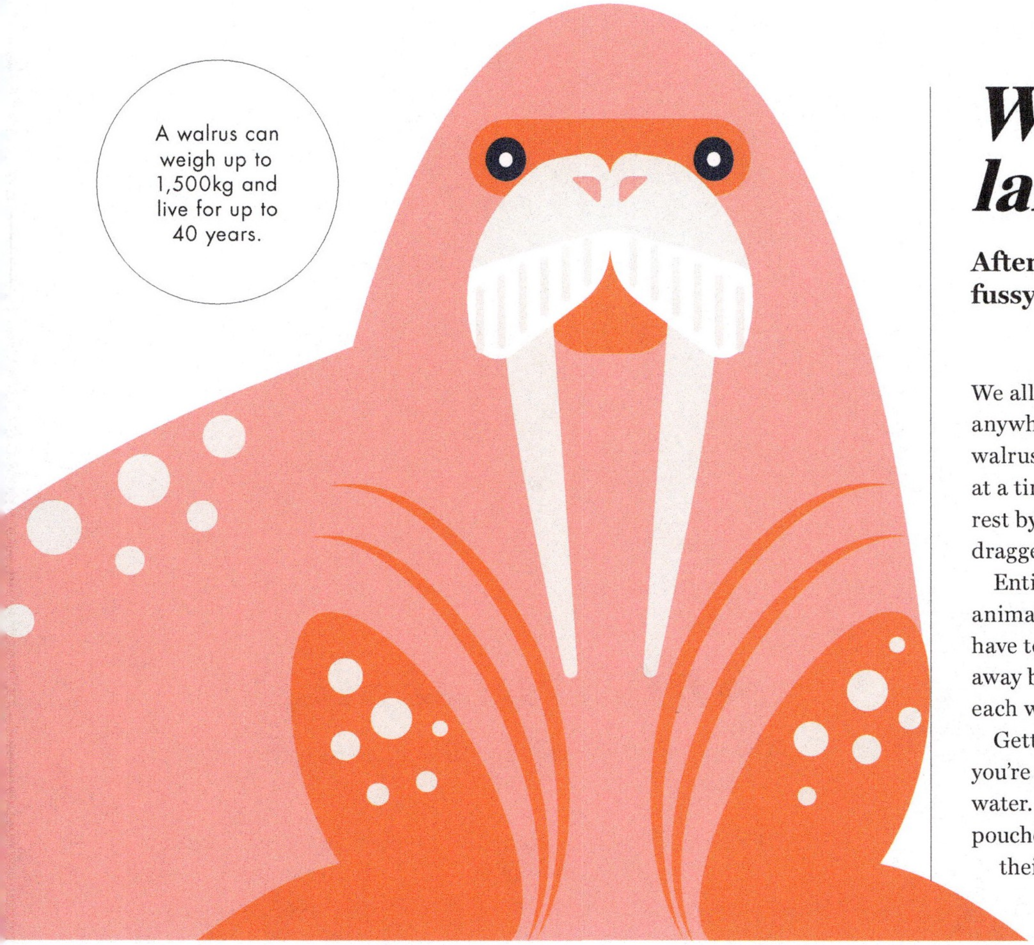

A walrus can weigh up to 1,500kg and live for up to 40 years.

Walruses nap on land and in water

After staying awake for days, walruses aren't fussy about where they sleep

We all know a person who can fall asleep just about anywhere, but even they'd be put to shame by a sleepy walrus. Walruses can stay awake and active for 84 hours at a time, but they make up for such a long time without rest by sleeping for up to 19 hours once they've eventually dragged themselves back onto land.

Entire shorelines can be covered in these snoozing animals as they rest against rocks and each other – some have to disentangle themselves from the pile and creep away because there's a huge variation in how much sleep each walrus needs.

Getting tired while swimming isn't a problem when you're a walrus; they've evolved the ability to nap in the water. By filling pockets in their necks called pharyngeal pouches with up to 50 litres of air, they can nod off with their heads bobbing above the surface. They can even anchor themselves to sea ice with their tusks so that they don't drift away.

"WALRUSES CAN STAY AWAKE AND ACTIVE FOR 84 HOURS AT A TIME, BUT THEY MAKE UP FOR IT BY SLEEPING FOR AROUND 19 HOURS"

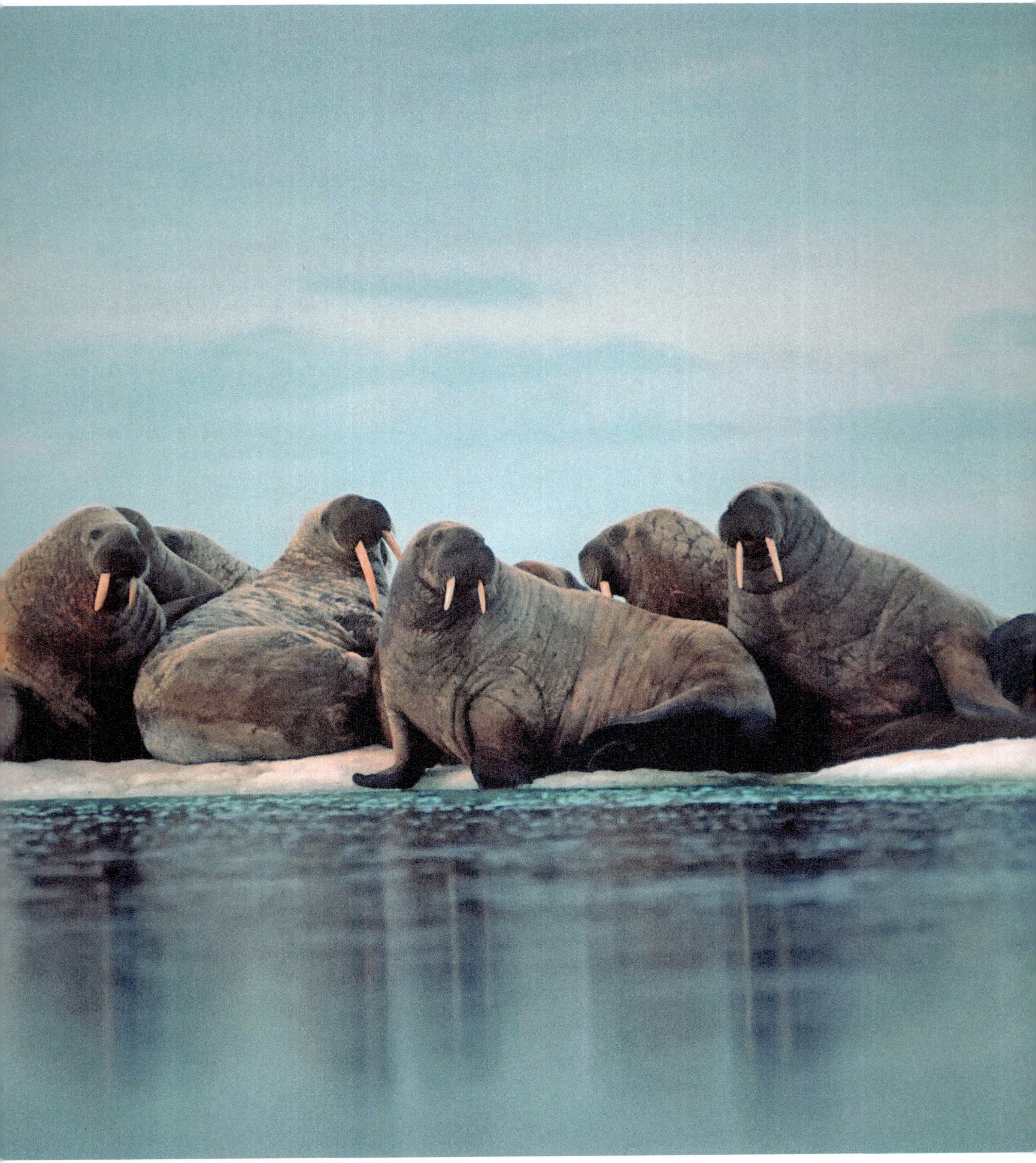

IMAGE SOURCE Getty Images

Parrotfish like to tuck themselves in at night

It might not look very appealing, but a parrotfish's cocoon is absolutely vital for its survival

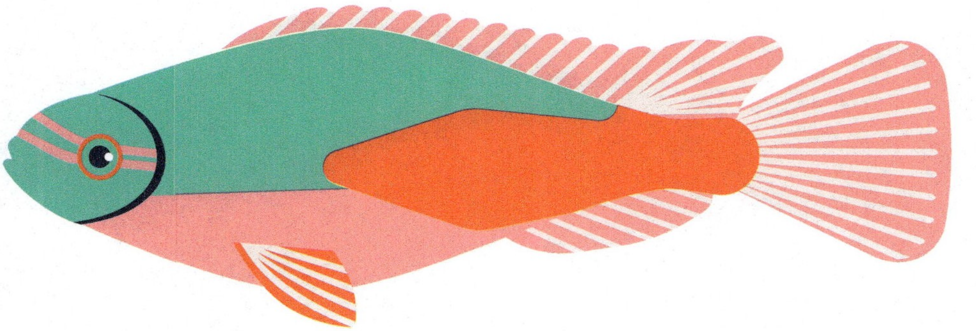

THE COCOON KEEPS AWAY PARASITES ROAMING THE NIGHT IN SEARCH OF BLOOD

Campers and holidaymakers will be familiar with the idea of wiggling into a sleeping bag as the day draws to a close, but it's unlikely that they made it themselves.

Before going to sleep each night, members of several parrotfish species enclose themselves in a case constructed using their own mucous secretions. While this may sound like a disgusting way to sleep, the cocoon acts like a mosquito net to keep away parasites roaming the night in search of blood, as the structure allows water in but is too fine for unwanted visitors to fit through.

The mucous probably also masks the fish's scent so that predators don't discover them, and it could act as a warning system, as the fish will notice any disturbance to their slippery sleeping bag before the danger gets too close.

Common swifts have to sleep on the wing

Until recently these birds baffled scientists with their record-breaking flights

Many migratory birds spend huge stretches of time on the wing without landing, but the common swift takes it to the extreme.

These little birds, which grow to around 16 centimetres, fly between their African wintering grounds and their breeding grounds further north, spending up to ten months in the air without landing. Warm air during the day helps them to travel with less effort, and their aerodynamic wings are highly efficient, but this incredible feat still raises a question: when do they sleep?

Researchers fitted trackers to swifts to monitor their movements and found that they climbed high in the air at dawn and dusk. After gaining several kilometres, the birds began a slow glide down again. The descent lasted about half an hour, and the scientists think this could give them enough time for a power-nap before they regain consciousness and continue their journey.

THESE LITTLE BIRDS SPEND UP TO TEN MONTHS IN THE AIR WITHOUT LANDING

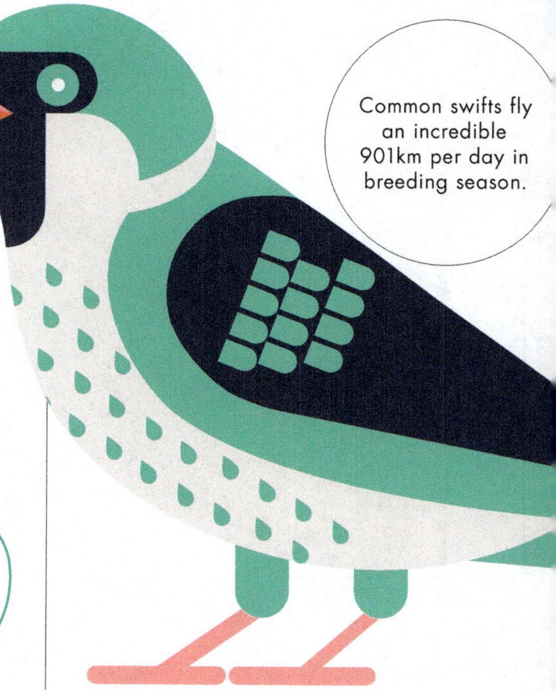

Common swifts fly an incredible 901km per day in breeding season.

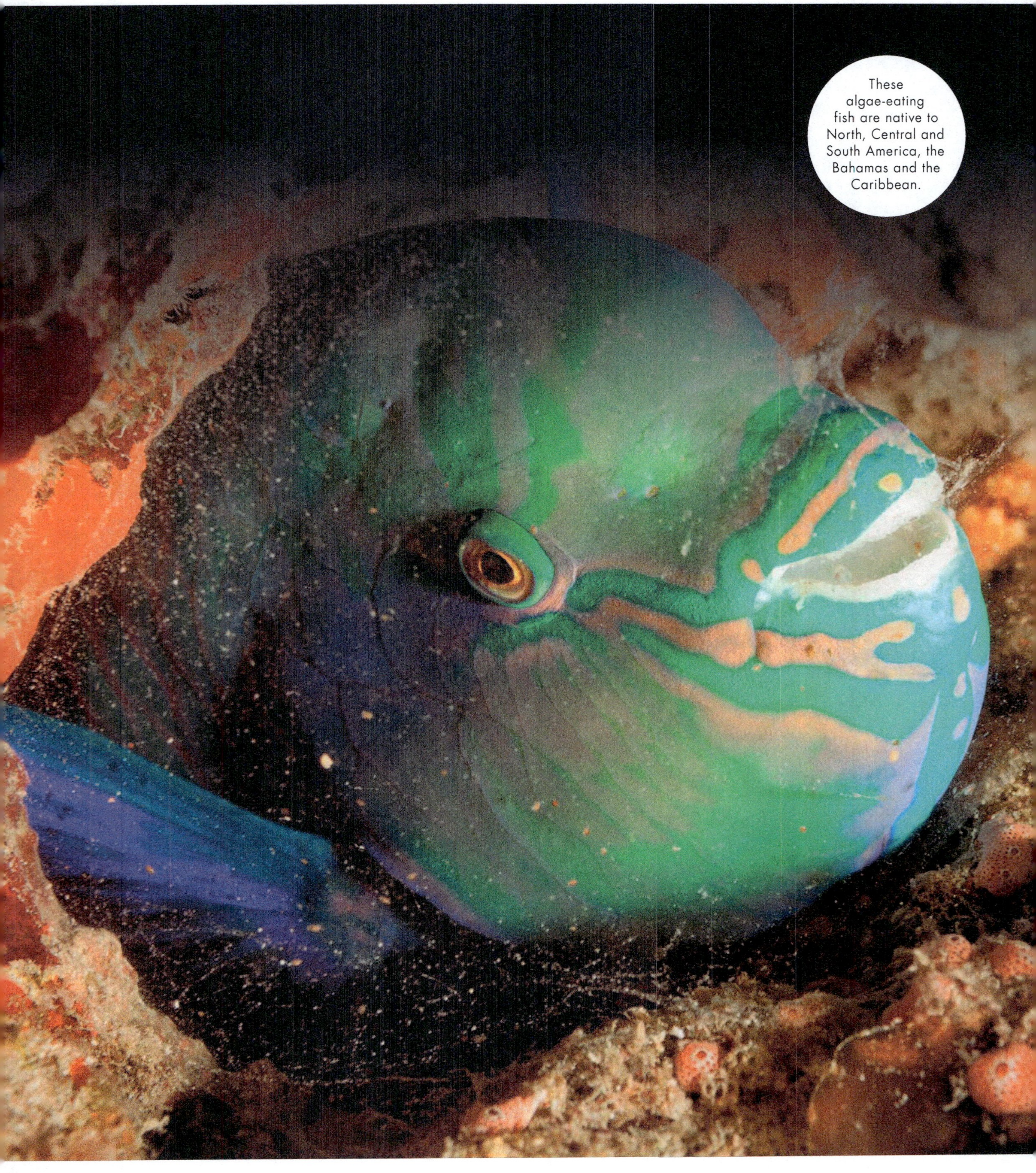

These algae-eating fish are native to North, Central and South America, the Bahamas and the Caribbean.

IMAGE SOURCE Getty Images

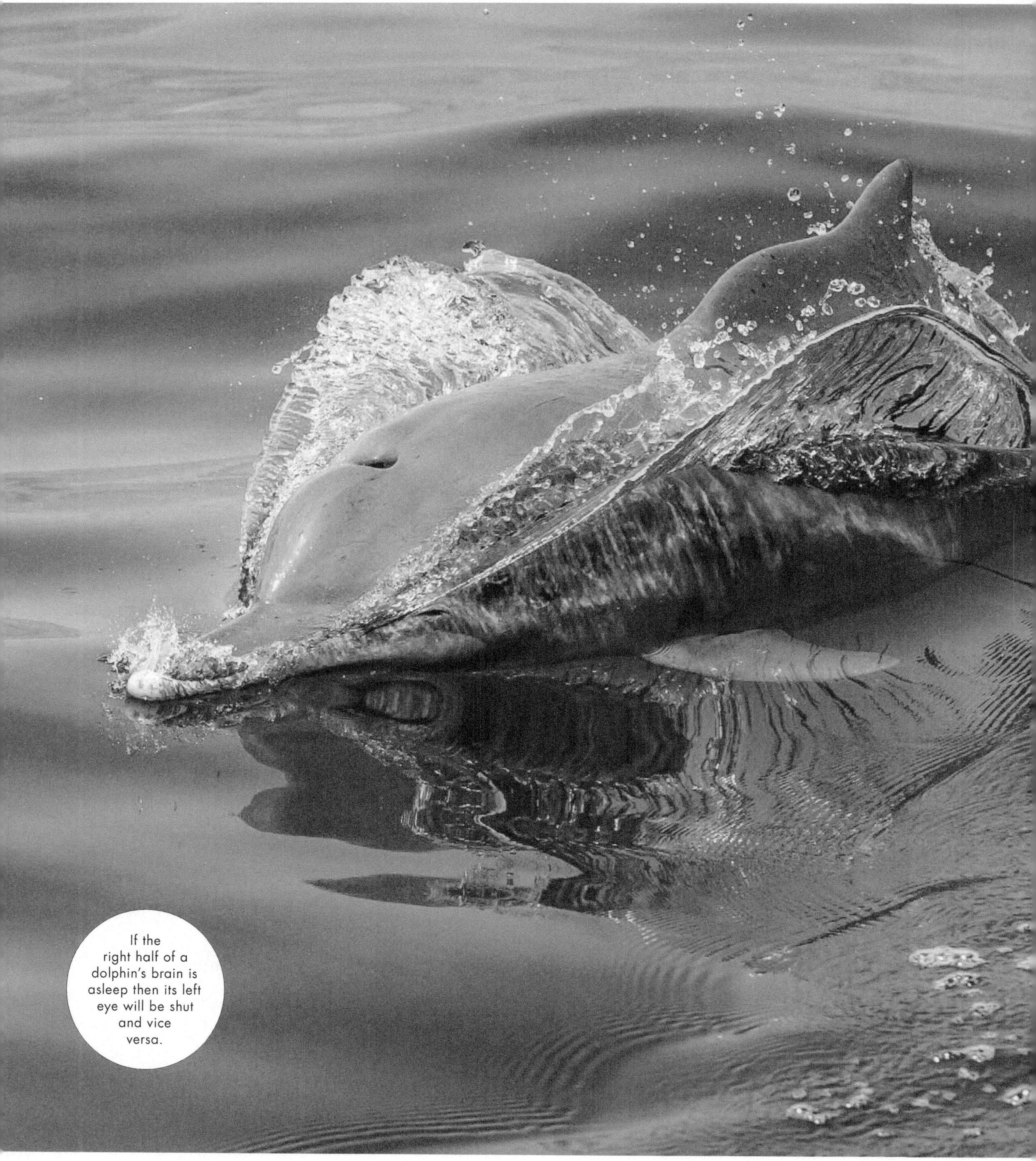

If the right half of a dolphin's brain is asleep then its left eye will be shut and vice versa.

Zebras can't risk a lie-down

With predators all around, zebras need to be prepared for a quick getaway

For prey animals, lying down to sleep is risky as getting up could cost crucial seconds should a predator approach. To make sure they're always ready to run, horses and zebras often get their shut-eye while standing up.

A series of muscles, tendons and ligaments collectively known as the 'stay apparatus' work together to allow animals like cows to stay standing with little effort, but in the case of equids (horses, zebras and asses) it also gives them the ability to lock their limbs while resting. Zebras can't go into a deep sleep while standing, but they can take a nap without their legs collapsing.

When they really need to restore their energy, zebras lie down to sleep, often taking turns with others so there's always a watchful eye looking out for danger, which often comes in the form of prowling lionesses.

> ZEBRAS HAVE THE ABILITY TO LOCK THEIR LIMBS WHILE RESTING

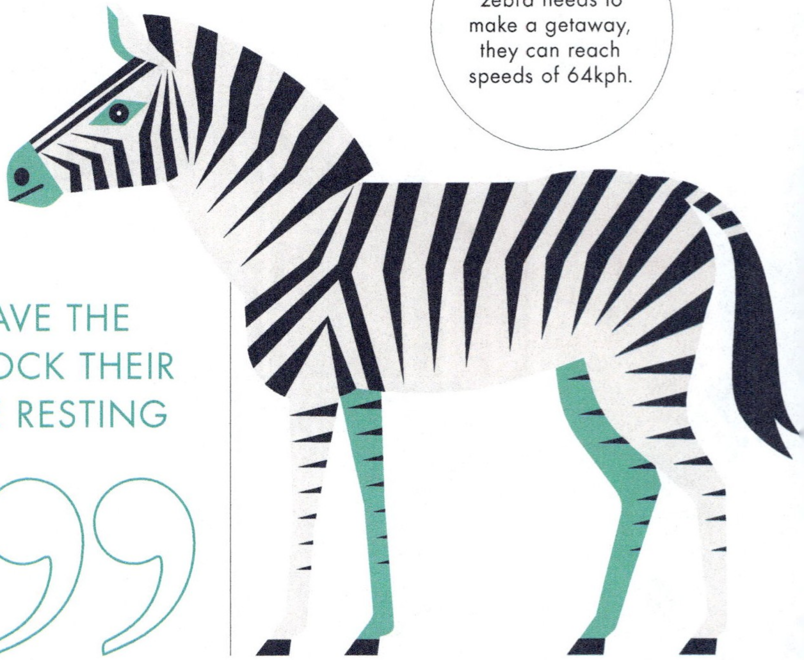

In the event a zebra needs to make a getaway, they can reach speeds of 64kph.

Dolphins sleep with one eye open

These aquatic mammals have found a way to nap without drowning

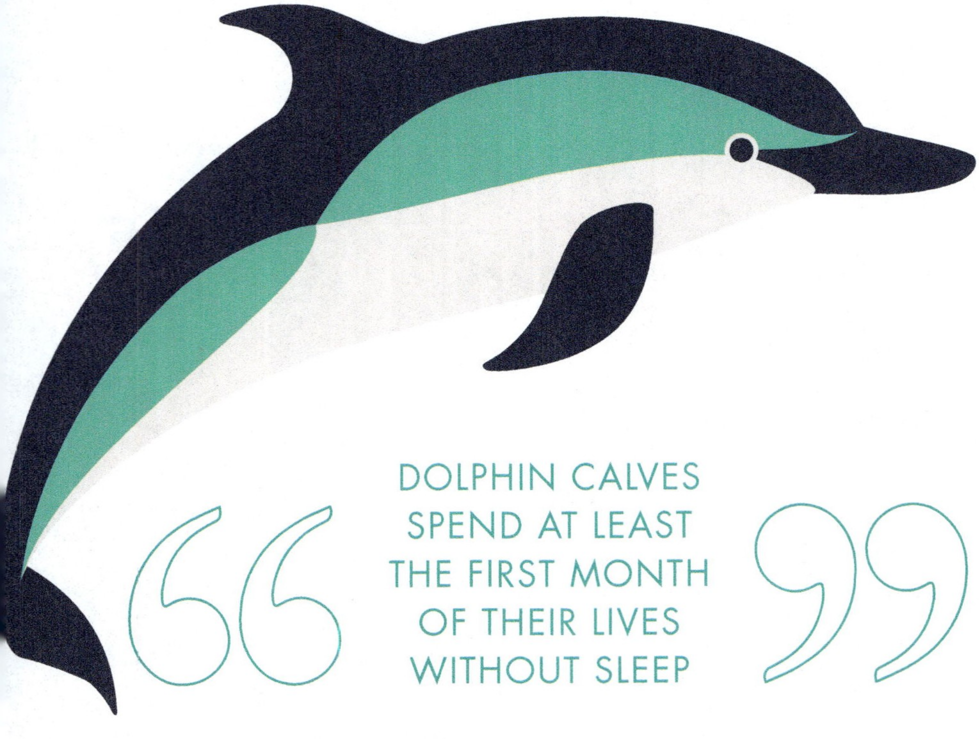

> DOLPHIN CALVES SPEND AT LEAST THE FIRST MONTH OF THEIR LIVES WITHOUT SLEEP

Some animals never leave the water and have no choice but to sleep while they swim. Dolphins (as well as ducks, iguanas and some whale species) rejuvenate using unihemispheric sleep, where one half of their brain shuts down and rests while the other stays awake and alert.

Always having at least half a brain taking in the surroundings keeps pods of dolphins out of trouble and means they can still swim and surface when they need oxygen. Sometimes they enter a deep sleep and stay at the surface, something referred to as 'logging' because of the way the pods float.

Most young animals rest more than adults, but calves spend at least the first month of their lives without sleep. Constantly swimming puts calves in a better position should they need to escape, and the movement maintains their body temperature until they've built up enough blubber.

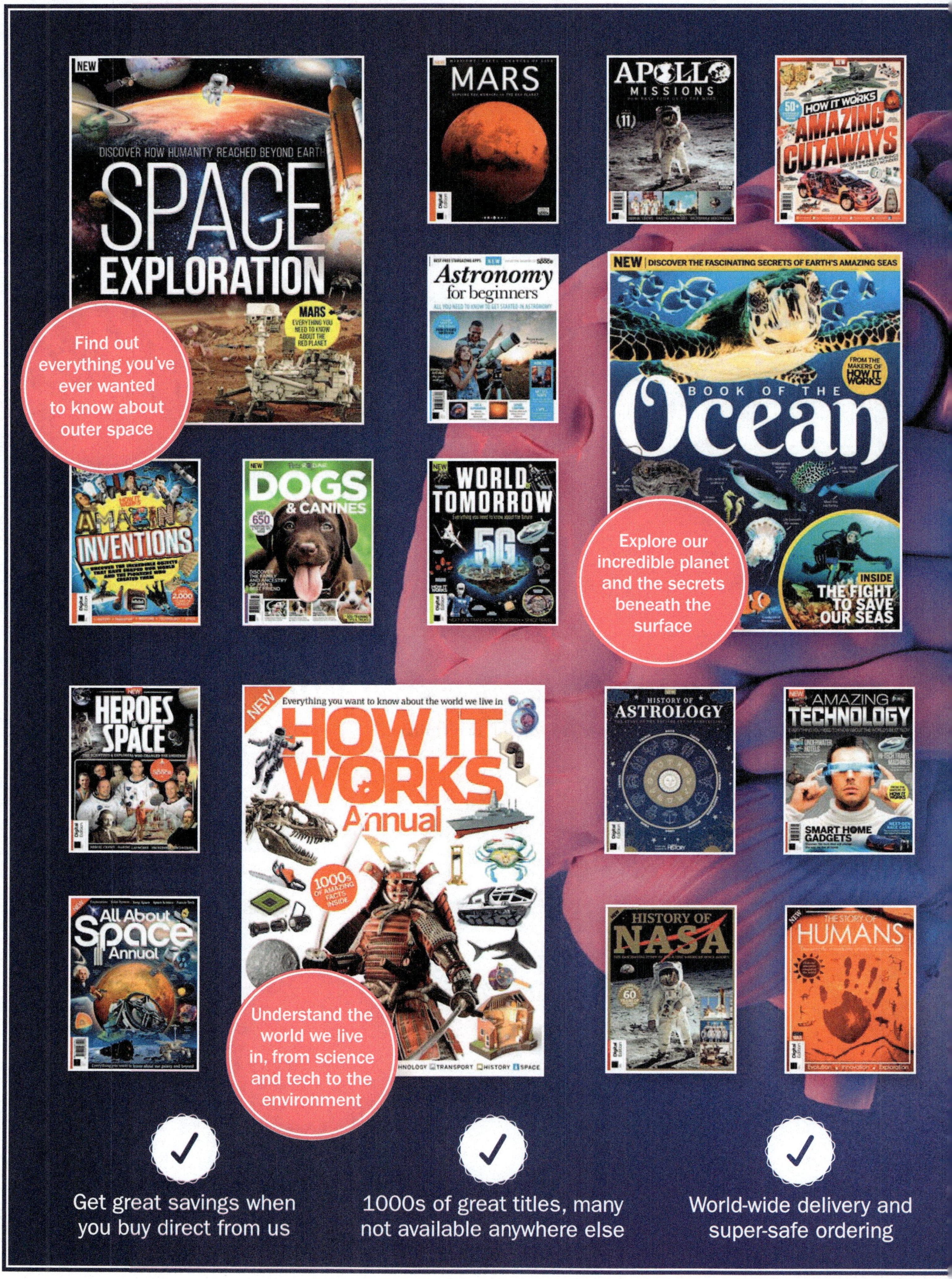

NEW
DISCOVER HOW HUMANITY REACHED BEYOND EARTH
SPACE EXPLORATION
MARS
Find out everything you've ever wanted to know about outer space
MARS
APOLLO MISSIONS
HOW IT WORKS AMAZING CUTAWAYS
Astronomy for beginners
NEW DISCOVER THE FASCINATING SECRETS OF EARTH'S AMAZING SEAS
FROM THE MAKERS OF HOW IT WORKS
BOOK OF THE Ocean
INSIDE THE FIGHT TO SAVE OUR SEAS
Explore our incredible planet and the secrets beneath the surface
AMAZING INVENTIONS
DOGS & CANINES
WORLD OF TOMORROW
5G
HEROES OF SPACE
NEW
Everything you want to know about the world we live in
HOW IT WORKS Annual
1000s OF AMAZING FACTS INSIDE
Understand the world we live in, from science and tech to the environment
HISTORY OF ASTROLOGY
AMAZING TECHNOLOGY
SMART HOME GADGETS
All About Space Annual
HISTORY OF NASA
THE STORY OF HUMANS
Get great savings when you buy direct from us
1000s of great titles, many not available anywhere else
World-wide delivery and super-safe ordering

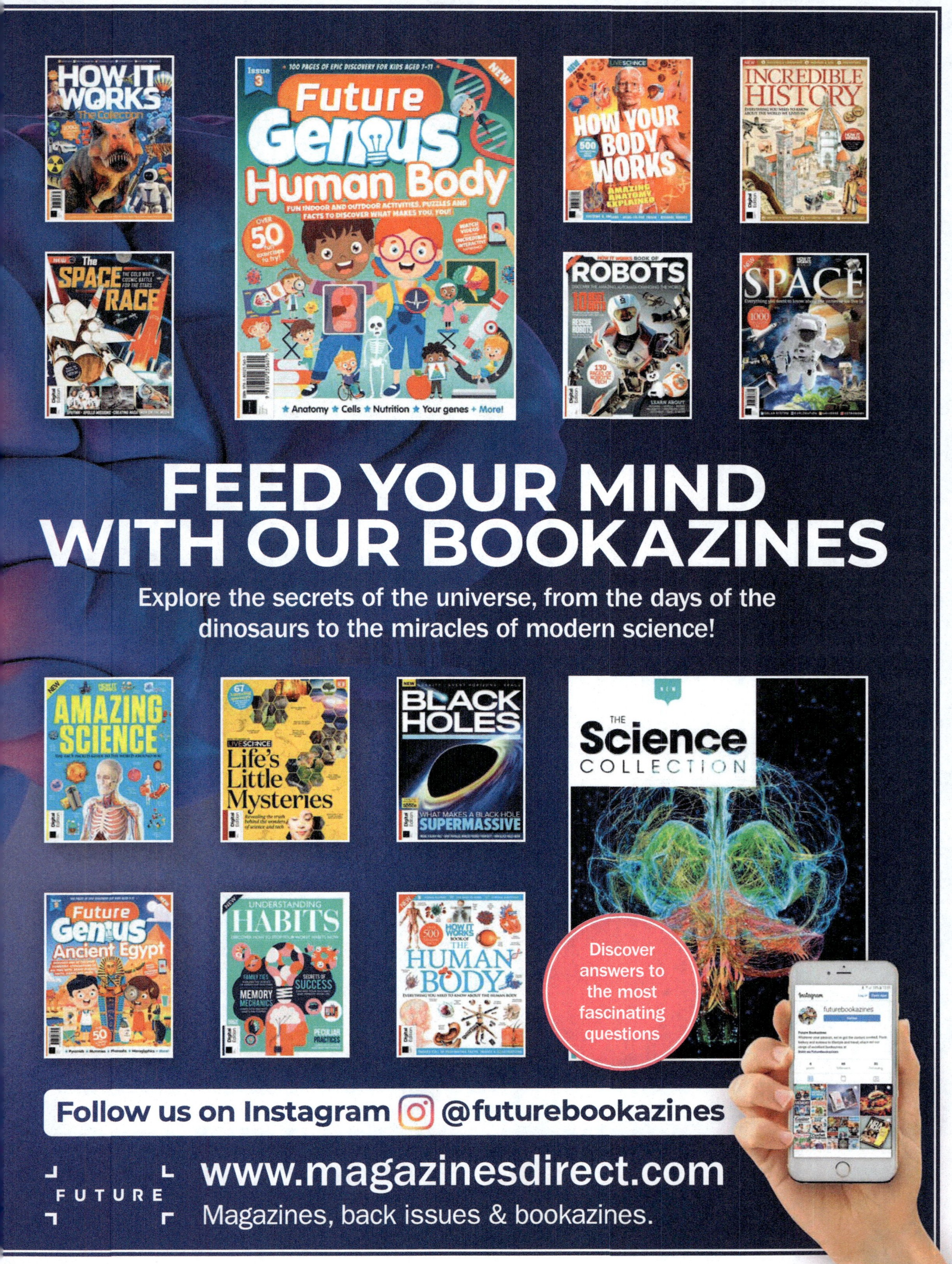
FEED YOUR MIND
WITH OUR BOOKAZINES
Explore the secrets of the universe, from the days of the dinosaurs to the miracles of modern science!
Discover answers to the most fascinating questions
Follow us on Instagram @futurebookazines
FUTURE
www.magazinesdirect.com
Magazines, back issues & bookazines.

Printed in Dunstable, United Kingdom

91218507R00078